OSCE for
Emergency Medicine Practical Exam

OSCE for
Emergency Medicine Practical Exam
Including Short Cases & Multiple Choice Questions

Editor

Devendra Richhariya
MBBS MD MBA (Hospital Administration)
Fellowship Intensive Care Medicine
PG Diploma in Medical Toxicology
Senior Emergency Physician
Gurugram, Haryana, India

Forewords

TV Ramakrishnan
Nadeem Qureshi

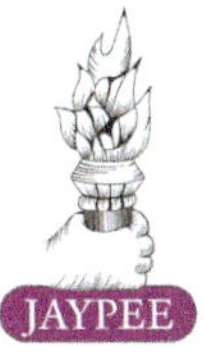

JAYPEE BROTHERS MEDICAL PUBLISHERS
The Health Sciences Publisher
New Delhi | London

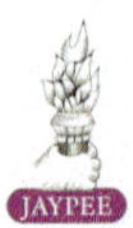

Jaypee Brothers Medical Publishers (P) Ltd

Headquarters
EMCA House
23/23-B, Ansari Road, Daryaganj
New Delhi 110 002, India
Landline: +91-11-23272143, +91-11-23272703
+91-11-23282021, +91-11-23245672
E-mail: jaypee@jaypeebrothers.com

Corporate Office
4838/24, Ansari Road, Daryaganj
New Delhi 110 002, India
Phone: +91-11-43574357
Fax: +91-11-43574314
E-mail: jaypee@jaypeebrothers.com

Overseas Office
J.P. Medical Ltd.
83, Victoria Street, London
SW1H 0HW (UK)
Phone: +44 20 3170 8910
E-mail: info@jpmedpub.com

EU GPSR Authorised Representative
Logos Europe, 9 rue Nicolas Poussin
17000, La Rochelle, France
Phone: +33 (0) 6 67 93 73 78
E-mail: contact@logoseurope.eu

Website: www.jaypeebrothers.com
Website: www.jaypeedigital.com

Inquiries for bulk sales may be solicited at: jaypee@jaypeebrothers.com

OSCE for Emergency Medicine Practical Exam Including Short Cases & Multiple Choice Questions

First Edition: 2024
Reprint: **2025**

ISBN: 978-93-5696-622-2

Printed in India

Dedicated to

My parents

Contributors

Amritesh Ranjan MBBS MD (Pediatrics)
Associate Professor
Department of Pediatrics
Muzaffarnagar Medical College
Muzaffarnagar, Uttar Pradesh, India

AN Venkatesh
MBBS MRCEM (UK) FEM (RCGP-UK) PGCGM (XLRI)
Senior Consultant and Regional Director (Karnataka Region)
Department of Emergency Medicine
Apollo Hospitals
Bengaluru, Karnataka, India

Atur Mahant MBBS MRCEM (UK)
Attending Consultant
Department of Emergency Medicine
Fortis Hospital
Mumbai, Maharashtra, India

Awaneesh Katiyar
MBBS MS MCh PGDDM
Assistant Professor
Department of Trauma Surgery and Critical Care
Muzaffarnagar Medical College
Muzaffarnagar, Uttar Pradesh, India

Bhawana Sharma MBBS DNB IDCCM
Consultant
Department of Critical Care
Medanta—The Medicity
Gurugram, Haryana, India

Devendra Richhariya
MBBS MD MBA (Hospital Administration)
Fellowship Intensive Care Medicine
PG Diploma in Medical Toxicology
Senior Emergency Physician
Gurugram, Haryana, India

Gouri Ranade
MBBS DNB (Anes) FRCA EDIC
Consultant
Department of Emergency Medicine and Critical Care
Deenanath Mangeshkar Hospital
Pune, Maharashtra, India

J Joshua Vijay
MBBS MEM MRCEM MBA (HHSM)
Consultant
Department of Emergency Medicine and Critical Care
Apollo KH Hospital
Melvisharam, Tamil Nadu, India

Khusrav Bajan
MD EDIC
Head
Department of Emergency Medicine
Consultant (Critical Care)
PD Hinduja Hospital and Medical Research Centre
Mumbai, Maharashtra, India

M Rajadurai
MD (Anes) FEM (RCGP-UK) FCCC FLM
Senior Consultant and Head
Department of Emergency Medicine and Critical Care
Apollo KH Hospital
Melvisharam, Tamil Nadu, India

M Sai Surendar
MD DEM FICM Dip (Diab) MACEP
National Joint Secretary
Society for Emergency Medicine, India (SEMI)
Chennai, Tamil Nadu, India

Mahesh Vyankatrao Salunke
MBBS MD IDCCM
Associate Consultant
Critical Care Medicine
PD Hinduja Hospital and Medical Research Centre
Mumbai, Maharashtra, India

Maitha Almazrouei MBBS
Chief Resident
Department of Emergency Medicine
Cleveland Clinic
Abu Dhabi, UAE

Manish Agrawal MBBS MD (Pediatrics)
Professor and Head
Department of Pediatrics
Muzaffarnagar Medical College
Muzaffarnagar, Uttar Pradesh, India

Mona Lisa Janarthanan
MBBS DNB (Emergency Medicine)
Assistant Professor
Department of Emergency Medicine
Sri Ramachandra Institute of Higher Education and Research
Chennai, Tamil Nadu, India

Nadeem Qureshi MD FAAP FCCM
Professor of Pediatrics
School of Medicine, St Louis University
Cardinal Glennon Children's Hospital
St Louis, Missouri, USA

Nilanka Mudithakumara
MBBS DSp Med PG Dip Med Phys
Registrar
Department of Emergency Medicine
National Hospital
Colombo, Sri Lanka

Nishi Trivedi MBBS MD DVL
Consultant Dermatologist
Aadya Hospital Vedanta Complex
Ahmedabad, Gujarat, India

Olita Shilpakar
MD DM (Emergency Medicine) FRCP (Edin)
Assistant Professor
Department of Emergency Medicine
Institute of Medicine
Tribhuvan University Teaching Hospital
Kathmandu, Nepal

Omar Ghazanfar
MBBS MSc DM EBCEMMBA
Assistant Professor
Department of Emergency Medicine
Cleveland Clinic Lerner College of Medicine
Abu Dhabu, UAE

Patibandla Sree Sowjanya
MBBS MD MBA PhD
Chief Emergency Physician
Department of Emergency Medicine
Yashoda Hospitals
Hyderabad, Telangana, India

Preeti Dwivedi
MBBS DNB (Pediatrics)
Assistant Professor
Department of Pediatrics
Muzaffarnagar Medical College
Muzaffarnagar, Uttar Pradesh, India

S Senthilkumaran
MD FCCM FRCP (Edin & Lond) PhD
Medical Director
Department of Emergency and Critical Care
Manian Medical Centre
Erode, Tamil Nadu, India

Sakthi Muthalraju
MBBS DNB (EM) MRCEM
Consultant
Department of Emergency Medicine
Deenanath Mangeshkar Hospital
Pune, Maharashtra, India

Sandeep Gore
MBBS MRCEM (UK) EBCEM (Europe) FAEM (CMC, Vellore) MBA (BITS Pilani) E-EAC (ELSO)
Director
Department of Emergency Medicine
Fortis Hospital
Mumbai, Maharashtra, India

Sanjay Shah
MS DNB FNB (Trauma) EPHM (IIM-C)
Senior Consultant and Trauma Surgeon
Head
Department of Emergency Medicine
Apollo Hospital International Limited
Ahmedabad, Gujarat, India

Sharath TR MBBS MD EDAIC
Clinical Assistant
Department of Critical Care Medicine
PD Hinduja Hospital and Medical Research Centre
Mumbai, Maharashtra, India

Shweta Ashok
MBBS MEM FICM MBA (HHSM)
Consultant and In-charge
Matsaya Clinics
Chennai, Tamil Nadu, India

Tejas D Patel MBBS MD (Dermatology)
Consultant Dermatologist
Aroma Skin and Laser Clinic
Aravalli, Gujarat, India

TV Ramakrishnan
MBBS MD (Anesthesiology)
Head
Department of Emergency Medicine
Sri Ramachandra Institute of Higher Education and Research
Chennai, Tamil Nadu, India

Venugopalan PP
MBBS DA DNB MNAMS MEM (GWU)
Director and Lead Consultant
Department of Emergency Medicine
Aster MIMS, Aster DM Healthcare
Kozhikode, Kerala, India

Foreword

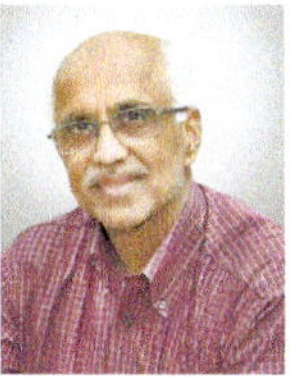

An Objective Structured Clinical Examination (OSCE) is a performance-based test which allows for the standardized assessment of clinical skills. The OSCE format was first described by Harden in 1975 and has been extensively studied and widely adopted by educational institutions for high-stake examinations.

Considering that the development and administration of an OSCE is a laborious and resource-intensive endeavor, its use should be reserved for skills that cannot readily be assessed in a valid and reliable way using other examination formats. Candidates/trainees are assessed on skills like completing a physical examination, obtaining a history, interpreting data, or managing an emergent medical issue. It is ideally suited for assessing skills in trainees in emergency medicine as these cannot be assessed in acutely ill patients!

While OSCE is a reliable and valid method of assessment of skills, MCQs can reliably assess the breadth of knowledge in any subject. Case-based or scenario-based MCQs are useful in assessing knowledge about diagnosis and management of emergent conditions in medicine.

I have had the good fortune to know Dr Devendra Richhariya for almost a decade now and have found him to be an astute clinician as well as a very dedicated and passionate teacher of emergency medicine. Development of valid and reliable OSCE is a significant undertaking with several steps involved. Creating MCQs, especially case-based ones, is a demanding task. Therefore, one should appreciate Dr Devendra Richhariya for having successfully undertaken this arduous task of publishing an entire book of OSCEs and MCQs!!

A well-written repository on OSCE and MCQs, like this book, is a treasure for every faculty involved in the training and assessment of emergency medicine residents.

TV Ramakrishnan
MBBS MD (Anesthesiology)
Head
Department of Emergency Medicine
Sri Ramachandra Institute of Higher Education and Research
Chennai, Tamil Nadu, India

Foreword

Dear Readers,

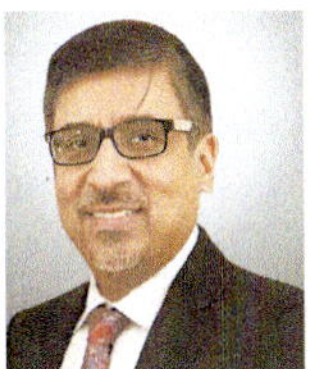

It is with immense enthusiasm that I introduce you to, *OSCE for Emergency Medicine Practical Exam Including Short Cases and Multiple Choice Questions,* an indispensable resource meticulously curated to empower medical professionals in navigating the intricacies of Emergency Medicine. Within the confines of this book, you will unearth a wealth of knowledge, thoughtfully organized to bolster your comprehension and mastery of vital concepts through Objective Structured Clinical Examination (OSCE) scenarios and Multiple Choice Questions (MCQs).

In Section I, we embark on a transformative journey into the practical application of Emergency Medicine knowledge through immersive OSCE scenarios. From mastering the nuances of Arterial Blood Gas (ABG) Analysis to refining your proficiency in Point-of-Care Ultrasound, each chapter presents authentic scenarios mirroring the intensity and complexity of real-life emergencies. With comprehensive explanations and meticulous guidance, you will cultivate the confidence to navigate, assess, diagnose, and manage a diverse array of emergencies with precision and efficacy.

Chapter 4 of the Part I serves as a gateway to a comprehensive exploration of essential drugs and instruments, equipping you with the requisite tools to administer timely and effective interventions in emergency settings. Meanwhile Chapter 5 onward delve into OSCE specific to various emergent conditions. Each chapter is meticulously crafted to offer tailored OSCE scenarios pertinent to the respective specialty, fostering a profound understanding of management strategies and protocols essential for clinical practice.

Furthermore, Chapter 15 delves into the intricate realm of Pediatric Emergencies, acknowledging the unique challenges and considerations inherent in caring for pediatric patients in emergency situations. By spotlighting pediatric-specific scenarios, this section delivers invaluable insights into the assessment and management of pediatric emergencies, empowering practitioners to deliver optimal care to the most vulnerable members of our society.

At the helm of this seminal work is Dr Devendra Richhariya, a distinguished figure in Emergency Medicine renowned for his groundbreaking contributions. As a leading authority in the field, Devendra has authored numerous acclaimed books, cementing his status as a trailblazer in medical education and clinical practice.

As you embark on your journey through the pages of *OSCE for Emergency Medicine Practical Exam Including Short Cases and Multiple Choice Questions*, I implore you to approach each scenario with an open mind and an unwavering commitment to continuous learning. Whether you are a seasoned emergency medicine physician, a resident in training, or a medical student preparing for licensure examinations, this book stands as an indispensable tool for refining your clinical acumen and elevating patient care to unprecedented heights.

My deepest gratitude extends to the esteemed contributors and editors who have poured their expertise and passion into the creation of this seminal resource. May *OSCE for Emergency Medicine Practical Exam Including Short Cases and Multiple Choice Questions* serve as a beacon of enlightenment and guidance in your pursuit of excellence in Emergency Medicine.

Wishing you boundless success and fulfillment in your medical odyssey.

Nadeem Qureshi
MD FAAP FCCM
Professor (Pediatrics)
School of Medicine, St Louis University
Cardinal Glennon Children's Hospital
St Louis, Missouri, USA
nqureshi25@hotmail.com

Preface

"An Examination should be viewed as an opportunity not a life-changing event."

–Narendra Modi

Medical education generally has four phases: Premedical, undergraduate, postgraduate, and continuing medical education (CME). The main aim of medical education is to help medical students acquire ethical and professional skills aptitude. The medical education system helps in developing strong clinical skills, effective communication, and the ability to perform under pressure. The medical education system adopts various methods of assessment for evaluation of their students like theoretical and Objective Structured Clinical Examination (OSCE). OSCEs are a highly effective tool in medical education evaluation because they allow a student to practice and demonstrate clinical skills in a standardized medical scenario. An OSCE is a framework consisting of multiple stations, an approach to the assessment of clinical competence, assessed in a planned or structured way. Medical students need to develop strong clinical skills, effective communication, and the ability to perform under pressure for clearing the OSCE examinations. Few important tips need to be followed by the medical students to clear the OSCE, such as get your basic right, stay focused, know your weakness and strength, achieve confidence and perfection with practice...practice...and practice.

I am confident that this book will help the medical students in achieving strong clinical skills.

Devendra Richhariya

Acknowledgments

I would like to thank all the authors for providing manuscripts in spite of their busy schedules.

Special thanks go to publisher, Shri Jitendar P Vij (Group Chairman), Mr Ankit Vij (Managing Director), and all members of M/s Jaypee Brothers Medical Publishers (P) Ltd, New Delhi, India, for invaluable contribution. I acknowledge the technical support given by Ms Avighna Richhariya.

Contents

SECTION I OSCE in Emergency Medicine

SECTION 2 MCQs in Emergency Medicine

SECTION 1 OSCE in Emergency Medicine

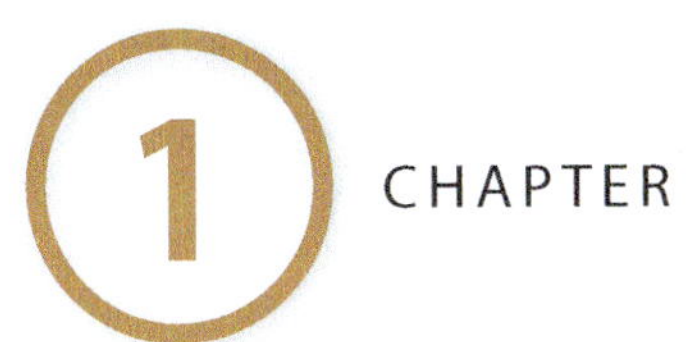

Arterial Blood Gas Analysis OSCE

Khusrav Bajan, Sharath TR, Mahesh Vyankatrao Salunke

QUESTIONS

Q1. **A 45-year-old male admitted with history of acute abdominal pain, profuse vomiting for 4 days duration followed by obstipation for a day. Later he became drowsy, responding only to painful stimuli. Arterial blood gas (ABG) and X-ray abdomen provided to emergency physician.**

pH—7.48, $PaCO_2$—52 mm Hg, PaO_2—83 mm Hg, HCO_3—32 mEq/L, Lactate—0.6 mmol/L, Na^+—131 mEq/L, K^+—2.8 mEq/L, and Cl^-—91 mEq/L.

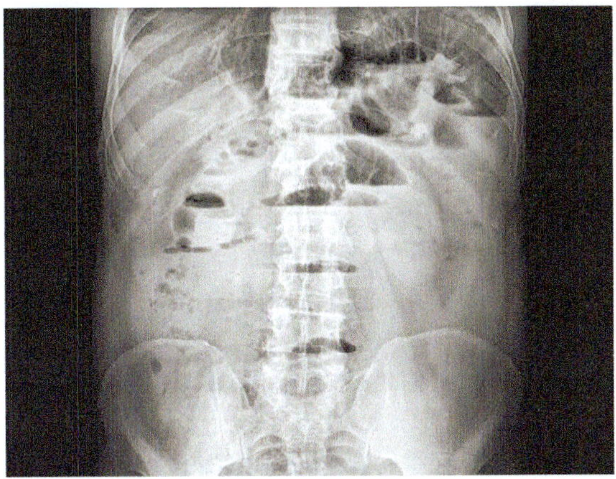

a. What is the clinical diagnosis?
b. What is the acid-base disorder?
c. Enumerate investigations and treatment.

Q2. **A 75-year-old man, a known case of (k/c/o) heart failure with reduced ejection fraction (HFrEF) (EF-30%) with congestive hepatomegaly on thiazide diuretics, was brought to emergency room (ER) with history of vomiting and disorientation since morning, associated with reduced urine output. Renal function tests were suggestive of increased serum creatinine to 2.8 mg/dL and blood urea nitrogen (BUN) 85 mg/dL (previous serum**

creatinine—1.2 mg/dL and BUN—25 mg/dL). ABG and electrolytes are provided to emergency physician.

pH—7.55, $PaCO_2$—46 mm Hg, PaO_2—75 mm Hg, HCO_3—36 mmol/L, Na—121 mEq/L, K—3 mEq/L, and Cl—99 mEq/L

a. Interpret the acid-base disorder.
b. What are the other causes of this acid-base disorder?
c. What are the causes of disorientation in this patient?

Q3. **A 30-year-old male presented to ER with fracture of femur following a road traffic accident (RTA), no other major injuries were evident in the primary survey. He was disoriented and irritable with SpO_2 of 82% on room air with respiratory rate of 38 breaths/min.**

pH—7.523, $PaCO_2$—30 mm Hg, PaO_2—75 mm Hg, and HCO_3—23 mmol/L

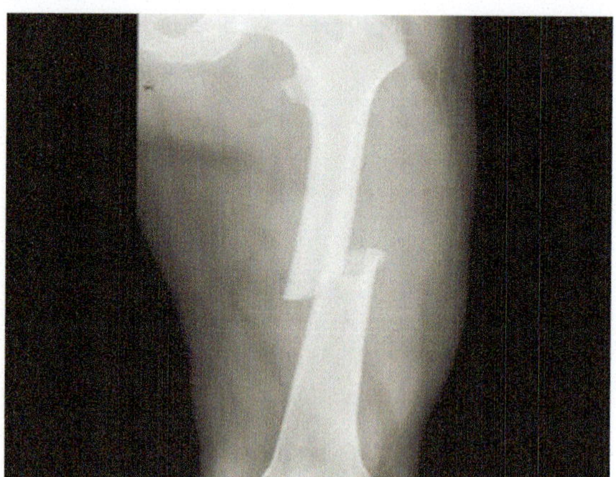

a. What are the abnormalities in this ABG?
b. What are the causes for tachypnea and hypoxia?
c. What are systemic manifestations observed in this case and treatment?

Q4. **A 42-year-old type 1 diabetic lady, who has been on insulin since the age of 13 years, presents with a 4-day history of dysuria which has progressed to severe right flank pain. She has a temperature of 38.8°C, a WBC of 14,000, her breath has fruity smell, and she is disoriented. Hemo glucose test (HGT)—500 mg/dL. Urine ketones and serum β-hydroxybutyrate are positive.**

pH—7.23, Na—127 mEq/L, $PaCO_2$—25 mm Hg, K—3.1 mEq/L, PaO_2—118 mm Hg, HCO_3—12 mmol/L, and Cl—91 mEq/L

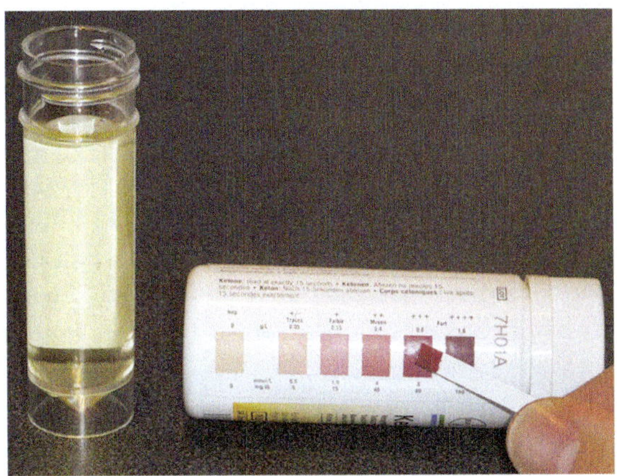

a. Explain the ABG disorder including Gap analysis.
b. Why the sodium is low in this case?
c. What are the other causes of ketosis?
d. What are the other causes of this ABG disorder?

Q5. **A 45-year-old male was undergoing posterior fossa craniectomy under general anesthesia for cerebellar meningioma excision in sitting position. While surgeon was opening dura mater, anesthesiologist noticed sudden hypotension, bradycardia, and drop in end-tidal carbon dioxide ($ETCO_2$) tracing.**
pH—7.22, $PaCO_2$—70 mm Hg, PaO_2—40 mm Hg, and HCO_3—27 mmol/L

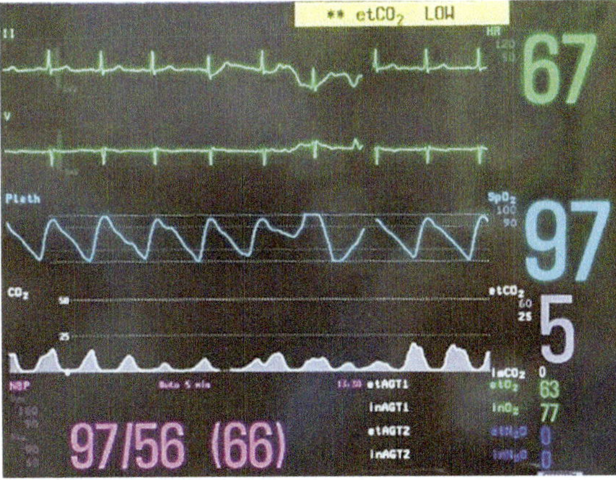

a. Interpret the given ABG.
b. What is the diagnosis?
c. Explain the relation between $PaCO_2$-$ETCO_2$ and other causes of high $PaCO_2$ with low $ETCO_2$.

Q6. A 55-year-old patient presented with history of fever, cough with greenish expectoration for 7 days. His chest X-ray (CXR) is shown below. His laboratory tests show a white blood cell (WBC) of 18,000/mm^3. On examination, he is hemodynamically unstable with heart rate (HR) of 120 beats/min and blood pressure (BP) of 80/50 mm Hg. The patient was intubated in ER, central venous catheter (CVC) line secured, and vasopressors and IV fluids started. Nasogastric tube is inserted due to abdominal gaseous distension. He had a high nasogastric aspirate of 1,000 mL in the first 2 hours. Interpret the following ABG.

pH—7.44, $PaCO_2$—12 mm Hg, PaO_2—55 mm Hg, HCO_3—10 mEq/L, Na—130 mEq/L, K—2.9 mEq/L, and Cl—80 mEq/L

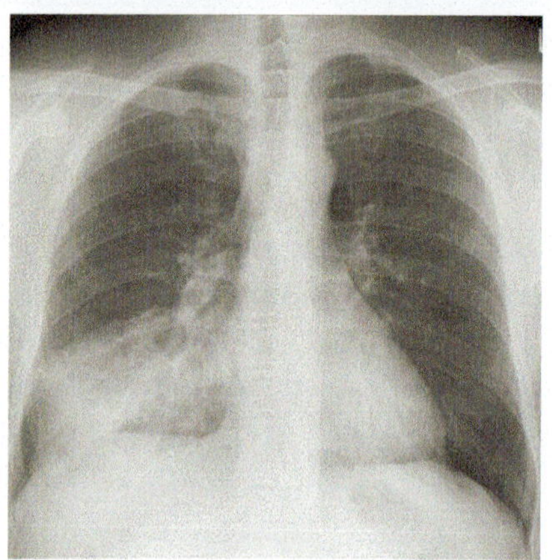

a. Interpret the ABG in detail.
b. What is the clinical diagnosis?

Q7. A 27-year-old girl presents to ER complaining of a tightness in the chest, shortness of breath as well as irritability with some tingling in the fingers and mouth. She has no significant past medical history and not on any regular medication. She had just given a job interview 2 hours ago. CXR is normal and ABG is performed on the patient while she was breathing room air and ABG results are available to the emergency physician:

pH—7.58, $PaCO_2$—20 mm Hg, PaO_2—95 mm Hg, and HCO_3—22

a. Interpret the ABG.
b. Enumerate the other causes of this ABG disorder.
c. How do you treat this case in ER?

Q8. A 74-year-old man, k/c/o chronic obstructive pulmonary disease (COPD) on home bilevel positive airway pressure (BiPAP) usage

for 2 years, is now admitted to the ER with chest pain and sudden onset of breathlessness. He gives history of recent travel to the USA. On examination, his BP is 90/50 mm Hg and SpO_2 of 72%. He is put on nonrebreathe mask (NRBM) at 15 L/min and IV fluids started. As the nurses are getting him attached to the ECG, he has a cardiac arrest. CPR was commenced and the patient is intubated immediately and after 6 minutes he achieved return of spontaneous circulation (ROSC). Following ROSC, he is hypotensive, drowsy, and tachycardic. Immediately, the patient is shifted to intensive care unit (ICU). The ECG did not show any ST/T changes. Beck's triad is negative. Screening 2D-ECHO revealed dilated right atrial/right ventricular (RA/RV) with severe pulmonary arterial hypertension (PAH) and D-shaped interventricular septum.

An ABG performed on NRBM at 15 L/min reveals the following:
pH—7.14, $PaCO_2$—63.1 mm Hg, PaO_2—50.1 mm Hg, HCO_3—14.9 mEq/L, and BE—9.7 (-2 to +2)

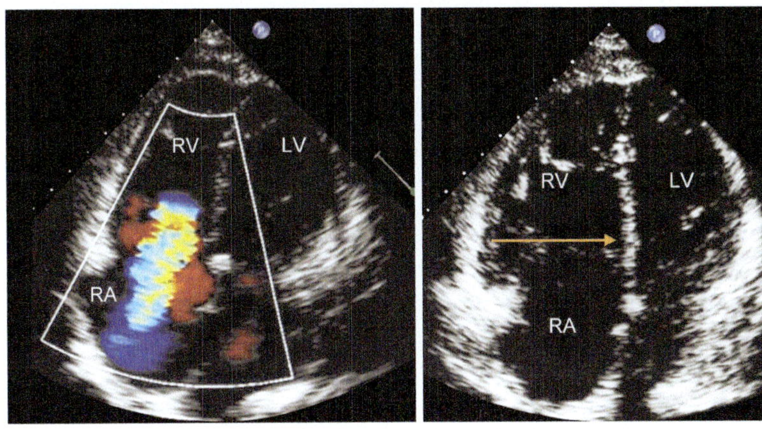

a. Interpret the ABG.
b. Discuss the probable cause of cardiac arrest in this case and how do you manage the patient?

Q9. **A 14-year-old boy is rescued from a house fire and was brought to the ER. The fire fighters estimate he is likely to have been trapped in a smoke-filled room for up to 20 minutes before rescue. The boy is heavily contaminated with soot and smells strongly of smoke. On preliminary examination, he has not sustained any thermal injuries. He appears to be confused. He was observed in the ER with close monitoring. He is mildly tachypneic with dusky extremities and lips. His vitals are stable with SpO_2 of 99% on the face mask at 10 L/min.**

Arterial blood gas is done 10 hours later, interpret the ABG given below:

pH—7.36, $PaCO_2$—34 mm Hg, PaO_2—150 mm Hg, HCO_3—18 mEq/L, Na—146 mEq/L, Cl—94 mEq/L, and lactate—3 mmol/L (0.5–1.5)

a. Describe given ABG.
b. What is the most likely diagnosis and which additional test would you need to make a definitive diagnosis?
c. Which of the provided value is falsely high—SpO_2 or PaO_2 and how do you treat?

Q10. **A 38-year-old male went on a mountain trek along with his friends. At around 7,500 feet height, he started complaining of headache, nausea, vomiting, dyspnea, tachypnea, and irritability. He was admitted to hospital with SpO_2 of 84% and on oxygen at 6 L/min. He was hemodynamically stable. His ABG and CXR show:**

pH—7.52, $PaCO_2$—26 mm Hg, PaO_2—56 mm Hg, HCO_3—22 mEq/L, Na—135, K—3.5, and Cl—112

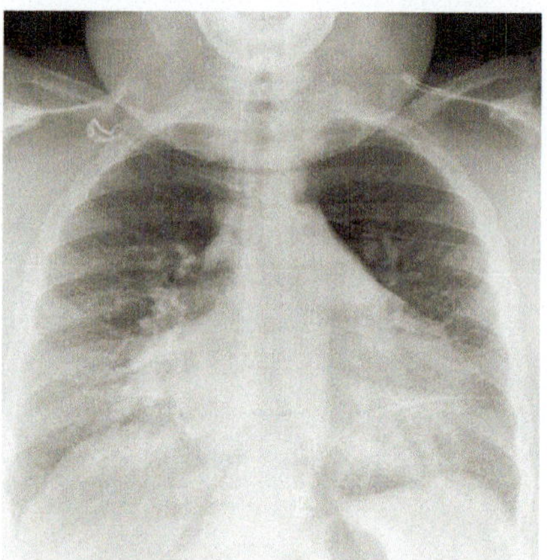

a. How would you describe the acid-base disorders?
b. Calculate PAO_2-PaO_2 gradient.
c. What are the high-altitude conditions?
d. How to treat the high-altitude pulmonary edema (HAPE)?

Q11. **A 58-year-old, 70 kg male patient with k/c/o hypertension (HTN) and diabetes mellitus (DM) on treatment, was brought to the ER with case of altered sensorium since 1 day with breathlessness and fever since 3 days. On receiving the patient, his vitals are HR of 130 beats/min, BP of 90/50 mm Hg, and SpO_2 of 70% on room air. On local examination, he has right leg cellulitis. Initially, he was**

kept on noninvasive ventilation (NIV) but in view of worsening respiratory distress he was intubated and kept on ventilator on volume control (VC) mode with tidal volume (TV) 300 mL, RR 30 breaths/min, positive end-expiratory pressure (PEEP) of 8 cmH_2O, inspiratory to expiratory (I:E) ratio of 1:2, and FiO_2 of 100%. CVC inserted and vasopressors started. After 1 hour of intubation, ABG was done which shows:

pH—7.148, glucose—279.6 mg/dL, $PaCO_2$—72 mm Hg, Lactate—5.84 mmol/L, HCO_3—18 mEq/L, PaO_2—52 mm Hg, and serum creatinine 2.0 mg/dL

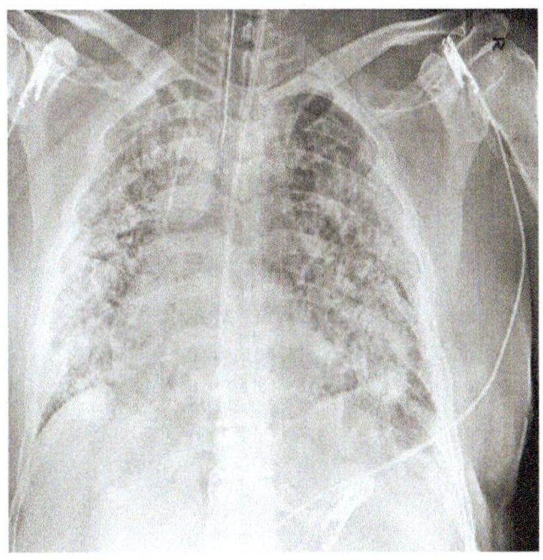

a. How would you interpret the ABG?
b. What are the ventilatory management goals in acute respiratory distress syndrome (ARDS) to treat hypoxemia?
c. What are the other causes of type I respiratory failure?

Q12. **A 50-year-old male was brought to emergency department (ED) with history of irrelevant talk and irritability. Initial assessment shows SpO_2 of 100% (10 L oxygen via a NRBM) and RR of 34 breaths/min. Chest clears on auscultation, HR—90 beats/min, BP—120/70 mm Hg, and capillary refill time 2 seconds centrally. GCS score 13/15 (E3, V4, and M5) and temperature 37.0°C. Clothes were stained with vomit but there were no signs of external injury. Later patient remains aggressive and irritable. ABG analysis is available. Other investigations are computed tomography (CT) brain: mild right subdural hematoma (SDH). Paracetamol/ salicylates: not detected. Blood methyl alcohol 35 mg/dL**

pH 7—0.28, blood glucose 74 mg/dL, pCO_2—28 mm Hg, lactate—10 mmol/L, PO_2—150 mm Hg, Na^+—140 mmol/L, HCO_3—10 mEq/L, K^+—5 mmol/L, Cl—100 mmol/L, and measured osmolality 330 mOsm/kg

a. Interpret ABG results and also calculate the osmolar gap.
b. What are the other causes for an elevated osmolar gap?
c. What are the clinical features of methanol poisoning?
d. How to treat methanol intoxicated patient?

Q13. A 17-year-old girl came to the ED after an argument with her boyfriend the previous night. He says that she took two strips (total 30 tablets) of tablets Dolo (paracetamol 650 mg/tablet). She complained of abdominal pain and nausea with two episodes of vomiting. Vitally she is stable. Her ABG on day 3 is given below.

pH—7.15 (7.35-7.45), Na^+—130 mmol/L, PO_2—82 (80-100), K^+—3.7 mmol/L, pCO_2—23 (35-45), Cl^-—109 mmol/L, HCO_3—9 (22-26), and BE—18 (-2 to +2)

Her other laboratory tests on admission are serum bilirubin 1.0, serum glutamic-oxaloacetic transaminase (SGOT) of 45 IU/L, serum glutamic-pyruvic transaminase (SGPT) of 55 IU/L, alanine aminotransferase (ALT) of 25 IU/L, prothrombin time/international normalized ratio (PT/INR) of 15/1.25. On third day, the laboratory test changed to serum bilirubin 3.0, SGOT of 1,200 IU/L, SGPT of 1,450 IU/L, ALT of 3,500 IU/L, and PT/INR of 45/3.5.

a. Interpret the ABG.
b. How do you manage the patient?

Q14. A 68-year-old male patient, operated case of duodenal perforation (resection anastomosis) with gastrointestinal septic shock and profuse diarrhea, is on ventilator with inotropic supports. Despite treating with adequate fluids, antibiotics, and high vasopressors, his BP remains low (90/40 mm Hg). We did ABG on ventilatory setting as VC with TV of 360/RR of 32 breaths/min/FiO_2 of 100%/PEEP of 14. The reports are as follows:

pH—7.10, blood glucose—279.6 mg/dL, PCO_2—52 mm Hg, lactate—5.84 mmol/L, PO_2—72 mm Hg, Na^+—136 mmol/L, HCO_3—10 mEq/L, K^+—5.00 mmol/L, and Cl^-—100 mmol/L

a. Interpret the ABG.
b. How do you manage the patient?

Q15. A 28-year-old male patient presented with history of fever, abdominal pain, and vomiting. Resident in the ER resuscitated the patient with IV fluids and started vasopressors in view of hypotension. Later the resident draws blood sample for ABG analysis and gets confused as to whether the sample is of arterial or venous origin and draws repeat sample to confirm the same. Given below are the results of both the samples.

Sample 1: pH—7.35, $PaCO_2$—30 mm Hg, PaO_2—62 mm Hg, and HCO_3—15 mEq/L

Sample 2: pH—7.27, $PaCO_2$—48 mm Hg, PaO_2—45 mm Hg, and HCO_3—17 mEq/L

a. How does one differentiate between ABG and venous blood gas (VBG) samples?
b. What is the role of A-V CO_2 gap in sepsis resuscitation?

ANSWERS

Ans. 1

a. It is a case of acute abdomen—bowel obstruction
b. Interpretation of ABG:
   - *pH of 7.48 is alkalosis:* Primary respiratory or metabolic
   - Metabolic (pH and HCO_3 in the same direction)
   - Compensated? In metabolic alkalosis for every one change in HCO_3, $PaCO_2$ should change by 0.7 in the same direction. Expected $PaCO_2$ = 0.7 [(HCO_3) + 20]. After applying formula, 0.7 (32) + 20 = 42 (actual $PaCO_2$ = 52 mm Hg). Overcompensation cannot happen, hence, there is coexisting respiratory acidosis as well.
   - *Diagnosis:* Mixed disorder—metabolic alkalosis with coexisting respiratory acidosis
c. Investigations and management—Nasogastric tube insertion, contrast-enhanced computed tomography (CECT) (Abdomen + Pelvis), IV fluids, and potassium correction. Antibiotics if sepsis is suspected—surgery reference

Ans. 2

a. Interpretation of ABG
   - pH of 7.55 is alkalosis
   - Primary respiratory or metabolic—metabolic (pH and HCO_3 in the same direction)
   - Compensated? In metabolic alkalosis for every one change in HCO_3, $PaCO_2$ should change by 0.7 times.
   - Expected $PaCO_2$ = 0.7 [(HCO_3) + 20] = 46.2 (actual $PaCO_2$ = 46 mm Hg), so respiratory compensation adequate
   - Diagnosis: Metabolic alkalosis
b. Metabolic alkalosis is of two types:
   i. *Chloride responsive (urinary Cl < 10 mEq/L):* Vomiting, dehydration, naso-jejunal (NJ) aspiration, diuretics, hypokalemia, and hyperaldosteronism
   ii. *Chloride resistant (urinary Cl > 10 mEq/L):* Steroids, Bartter syndrome, Gitelman syndrome, and Liddle's syndrome
c. Causes of altered sensorium in this patient—hyponatremia, uremia, and acute metabolic alkalosis

Ans. 3

a. Interpretation of ABG:
    - pH of 7.523 is alkalosis
    - pCO_2—30.1 (pH and $PaCO_2$ in the opposite direction)
    - *Respiratory alkalosis:* Acute or chronic? Look for renal compensation
    - For every 10 decreases in $PaCO_2$, HCO_3 should decrease by 2 and 5 in acute and chronic respiratory alkalosis respectively. Here, $PaCO_2$ has decreased by 10 (Expected $HCO_3 = 23$, observed = 23)
    - Hence, acute respiratory alkalosis

b. Causes for tachypnea and hypoxia are:
    - Acute respiratory alkalosis secondary to hyperventilation due to pain/contused lung/fat embolism.
    - Hypoxemia (normal PaO_2: 60–100 mm Hg) secondary to fat embolism from long bone fracture causing V/Q mismatch due to pulmonary vascular endothelial injury from free fatty acids.
    - Possibility of direct chest injury should be ruled out clinically and radiologically.

c. *Systemic manifestations of fat embolism:* Gurd and Wilson criteria can be used to diagnose fat embolism. Fever, petechial rash, retinal/urinal fat globules respiratory, neurological, renal

   Treatment: Largely supportive and symptomatic, support airway, breathing, and circulation, treat the underlying cause—fixation of fracture, IV steroids (controversial), mechanical ventilation—noninvasive ventilation (NIV)/high-flow nasal oxygen (HFNO)/mechanical ventilation

Ans. 4

a. Interpretation of ABG:
    - pH of 7.23 is acidosis
    - Primary respiratory or metabolic? Metabolic (pH and HCO_3 in the same direction)
    - Compensated? In metabolic acidosis for every one change in HCO_3, $PaCO_2$ should change by 1.5 times
    - Expected $PaCO_2 = 1.5\ [(HCO_3) + 8] = 26$ (actual $PaCO_2 = 25$ mm Hg)
    - So, adequate respiratory compensation
    - Anion gap (AG) (normal = 12); $AG = Na - (HCO_3 + Cl) = 127 - (12 + 91) = 24$
    - High anion gap metabolic acidosis (HAGMA)
    - Is there any additional acid-base disorder? Use delta ratio to find out coexisting disorders, if any
    - Delta ratio = $(AG - 12)/(24 - HCO_3)$ = (delta AG/delta bicarbonate) $=(24 - 12)/(24 - 12) = 1$
    - Delta ratio HAGMA and metabolic alkalosis >1, HAGMA =1, HAGMA + non-anion gap metabolic acidosis (NAGMA) <1
    - Diagnosis: HAGMA due to diabetic ketoacidosis (DKA)

b. *Pseudohyponatremia*—very common in diabetic ketoacidosis/ hyperosmolar hyperglycemic state (DKA/HHS) due to hyperosmolarity leading to shift of water from the intracellular to extracellular compartments.

Na* (adjusted) = Na* (measured) + 2.4 × [(Glucose – 100)/100]. Roughly for every 100 raises in sugars from 100 mg/dL, add 2 mEq (1.6 - 2.6 mEq) of Na to get the adjusted Na

However, patients with DKA can have normal or high Na depending on the patient's hydration status

c. *Causes of ketosis:* Diabetic ketosis, starvation, high fat, and low carbohydrate (ketogenic) diet, and alcohol

d. *Causes of HAGMA. MUDPILES (CAT):* M—*M*ethanol; U—*U*remia; D—DKA; P—*P*araldehyde; I—*I*ron, *I*soniazid; L—*L*actic acidosis; E—*E*thanol, *E*thylene glycol; S—*S*alicylate/aspirin; C—*C*arbon monoxide; A—*A*minoglycosides; T—*T*heophylline

(HAGMA: high anion gap metabolic acidosis; NAGMA: normal anion gap metabolic acidosis)

Ans. 5

a. Interpretation of ABG:
   - *pH of 7.22 is acidosis:* Primary respiratory or metabolic
   - Respiratory (pH and $PaCO_2$ in the opposite direction)
   - Compensated? HCO_3 compensation (baseline 24 mmol/L)

Every 10 mm Hg change in $PaCO_2$ from 40 mm Hg (HCO_3 compensation—baseline 24 mmol/L)		
	Acute	**Chronic**
Respiratory acidosis	1	4
Respiratory alkalosis	2	5

   - $PaCO_2$ has increased by 30, as per the table HCO_3 should increase to 28 (25 + 3) for acute and (25 + 12) 37 for chronic respiratory acidosis, actual HCO_3 = 27
   - Diagnosis: *Acute respiratory acidosis with hypoxemia*

b. It is a case of massive venous air embolism from dural venous system, mostly seen in sitting position surgeries. There is a sudden drop in $ETCO_2$ tracing, hypotension, and bradycardia which are unexplained by other causes. Fatal dose—quantity 3-5 mL/kg (200-300 mL of air for an adult) and as well as rate of air embolism (rapid infusion even in small quantity of air is more fatal). However, ABG shows hypoxia, hypercapnia, and respiratory acidosis. Normally, $PaCO_2$ is higher than $ETCO_2$ by 2-5 mm Hg. It is considered significant when the difference is more than 10-15 mm Hg.

c. Isolated drop in $ETCO_2$ tracing with high $PaCO_2$ is noted in V/Q mismatch (air/fat/thromboembolism) Cardiac arrest, breathing circuit obstruction/ disconnection, mucus plug/lung collapse

Ans. 6

a. Interpretation of ABG:
   - pH—7.44
   - Normal primary respiratory or metabolic, pH normal and $PaCO_2$ abnormal, probably mixed disorder
   - Compensated? Let us presume for a *metabolic acidosis* HCO_3 drop is 15 (25–10)
   - $PaCO_2$ compensation should be between 44 and 22 as per the standard calculations (for one HCO_3 drop, expect 1.5 times drop in $PaCO_2$).
   - But actual $PaCO_2$ is 10 (over compensation cannot occur). Hence, there is also a coexisting *respiratory alkalosis.*
   - AG = 130 – (10 + 80) = 40 (High) High AG metabolic acidosis
   - *Delta ratio:* To rule out coexisting metabolic disorders, *Delta AG/ Delta* HCO_3 = *(AG – 12)/(24 –* HCO_3*)* = (40 – 12/24 – 10) = 28/14 = 2. The ratio is >1, hence, there is a coexisting metabolic alkalosis as well due to hypokalemia.
   - *Diagnosis:* HAGMA with coexisting metabolic alkalosis and coexisting *respiratory alkalosis. (Triple ABG disorder)*

b. It is a case of pneumonia with septic shock with hypokalemia

Ans. 7

a. Interpretation of ABG:
   - pH of 7.58 is alkalosis
   - Primary respiratory or metabolic respiratory (pH and $PaCO_2$ in the opposite direction)
   - Acute or chronic? Expected HCO_3 = Two drops in HCO_3 for 10 drops in $PaCO_2$ in acute (actual HCO_3 = 22)
     - Adequate metabolic compensation
     - *Diagnosis:* Acute respiratory alkalosis

b. Respiratory alkalosis causes:
   - *Physiological:* Pregnancy, anxiety, pain, high altitude
   - *Pathological:* Fever, hysterical hyperventilation syndrome, sympathomimetic overdose (amphetamine and ketamine), hypoxemia (pneumonia/pulmonary embolism/sepsis), aspirin overdose, and hyperthyroidism

c. Treatment:
   - CXR and PaO_2 are essentially normal. Ask relevant history to rule out possible differentials.
   - *Any overdose:* Sympathomimetics? *Prolonged travel/oral contraceptive (OC) pills* usage—deep vein thrombosis (DVT) causing pulmonary embolism? Domestic *fights/performance anxiety—hysterical hyperventilation syndrome?*

- This patient is probably having hysterical hyperventilation syndrome.
- An untreated condition can lead to convulsion and muscle spasms.
- Intervention—use paper bag to facilitate rebreathing of CO_2, reassurance, and use of mild sedatives is sufficient enough to treat the case.

Ans. 8

a. Interpretation of ABG:
  - pH of 7.14 is acidosis
  - Primary respiratory or metabolic? Respiratory (pH and $PaCO_2$ in the opposite direction)
  - Compensated? Expected HCO_3 = For 20 increases in $PaCO_2$ (63.1–40), HCO_3 should have been 26 (24 + 2) if acute or 32 (24 + 8) if chronic respiratory acidosis. Actual HCO_3 = 14.9 with base excess of -9, 7 (low)
  - Also HCO_3 and $PaCO_2$ move in the opposite direction, which they should not. Hence, coexisting metabolic acidosis as well
  - Diagnosis: *Respiratory acidosis and metabolic acidosis*

b. A 74-year-old male known COPD and has a recent travel history with sudden onset of breathlessness and chest pain leading to cardiac arrest should warrant evaluation of massive pulmonary thromboembolism (PTE), cardiac tamponade, or acute myocardial infarction (MI) as immediate differentials. ECG is normal and Beck's triad is negative for tamponade.
  - As the patient has severe hypotension, tachycardia along with hypercapnia plus hypoxemia on ABG and POCUS findings showing RA/RV dilatation with MR secondary to acute pulmonary HTN favors the diagnosis of acute PTE.
  - Supportive measures and mechanical ventilation to be continued.
  - Depending on the clinical profile, patient should be taken up for immediate thrombolysis.

Ans. 9

a. Interpretation of ABG:
  - pH of 7.36 is acidosis
  - Primary respiratory or metabolic? Metabolic (pH and HCO_3 in the same direction with high lactate)
  - Compensated? In metabolic acidosis for every one change in HCO_3, $PaCO_2$ should change by 1.5 in the same direction
  - Expected $PaCO_2 = 1.5\,[(HCO_3) + 8] = 35$ (Actual $PaCO_2$ = 34 mm Hg)
  - $AG = Na - (Cl + HCO_3) = 146 - (94 + 18) = 34$ (High)
  - Respiratory compensation adequate (Normal = 12)
  - *Diagnosis:* HAGMA due to high lactates

b. It is a case of CO poisoning which commonly presents with nausea, vomiting, headache, and confusion. Carboxyhemoglobin (COHb) saturation correlate poorly with symptoms but levels above 50% may cause cardiac arrest and seizures. High index of clinical suspicion is key to early diagnosis.
c. CO binds to Hb with 200 times the affinity of O_2 and, therefore, is carried on the Hb molecule (COHb) in preference to O_2.
   - Therefore, the percentage of Hb saturated with O_2 is markedly reduced in CO poisoning, even when the PaO_2 is falsely normal. O_2 delivery to tissues is inadequate (tissue hypoxia), leading to cellular hypoxia and cytochrome oxidase inhibition causing lactic acidosis—metabolic acidosis. Most pulse oximeters are unable to distinguish COHb from oxyhemoglobin, therefore, fail to reflect the true SpO_2 in CO poisoning.
   - *Hence, SpO_2 is spuriously high in this patient.*
   - *Treatment:* 100% oxygen, hyperbaric oxygen therapy (HBOT)—it is 200 times more effective than normobaric O_2 delivery in reversing the symptoms.

Ans. 10

a. Interpretation of ABG:
   - pH of 7.52 is alkalosis
   - pCO_2 of 26 is low (decrease by 40 – 26 = 14). Hence, pH and pCO_2 moving in the opposite direction.
   - Compensation for respiratory acid-base disorders
   - For acute respiratory alkalosis, for every 10 decreases in pCO_2 decrease in HCO_3 is 2.
   - Here decrease in pCO_2 is (40 – 26= 14), expect decrease in HCO_3 to 21.
   - PO_2 is low 56 mm Hg on 6 L/min oxygen—symptomatic of (s/o) hypoxia.
   - Diagnosis is acute respiratory alkalosis with hypoxia.
b. (PAO_2-PaO_2) gradient
   - *P Alveolar O_2 = FiO_2 × (Atomic pressure – H_2O vapor pressure) - [pCO_2/respiratory quotient(RQ)]*
   - Normal atmospheric pressure at sea level is 760 mm Hg, H_2O pressure 47 mm Hg, and RQ is 0.8.
   - Normal PAO_2 – PaO_2 gradient is 5-15 mm Hg.
   - Atmospheric pressure drops by 26 mm Hg for every 1,000 feet above sea level.
   - At 7,500 feet P_{atm} is 565 mm Hg (760 – 195)
   - $PAO_2 = FiO_2 \times (P_{atm} - PH_2O) - PaCO_2/RQ$

$$= 0.45 \times (565 - 47) - 26/0.8$$
$$= 0.45 \times (518) - 32.5$$
$$= 233.1 - 32.5$$
$$= 200.6$$

- $PAO_2 - PaO_2 = 200.6 - 56 = 144.6$
- Classification of hypoxia based on A-a gradient
    - *Normal A-a gradient:* Alveolar hypoventilation (elevated $PaCO_2$), low PiO_2 ($FiO_2 < 0.21$ or barometric pressure < 760 mm Hg) at high altitude.
    - *Raised A-a gradient:* V/Q mismatch, diffusion defect, right-to-left shunt (intrapulmonary or cardiac), and increased O_2 extraction

c. *High-altitude conditions:* High-altitude pulmonary edema (HAPE), high-altitude cerebral edema (HACE), high-altitude bronchitis/pharyngitis, chronic mountain polycythemia, UV keratitis (snow blindness), peripheral edema, acute exacerbation of COPD/CAD, high-altitude retinopathy, and hypothermia

d. *Management of high altitute pulmonary embolism (HAPE):* Oxygen support, acetazolamide, immediate evacuation to lower altitudes or simulated descent in hyperbaric chamber, β-agonist inhalers and nebulization, and tablet nifedipine 10 mg stat, then 20–30 mg TID, consider steroids, HFNC, NIV, or ET intubation for airway protection

Ans. 11

a. Interpretation of ABG:
    - pH of 7.148 is acidosis
    - High pCO_2 is 72, it is increased by (72 – 40) = 32
    - *Compensation:* For acute respiratory acidosis, for every 10 increase in $PaCO_2$ rise in HCO_3 is 1, that is rise in pCO_2 here is 32 (72 – 40) expected rise in HCO_3 is 28.
    - But actual HCO_3 is 18. When $PaCO_2$ and HCO_3 are moving in the opposite direction, the ABG disorder is mixed, i.e., coexisting metabolic acidosis as well in this case.
    - A PO_2 of 52 is low with 100% FiO_2. PF ratio is 52 s/o severe hypoxia.
    - *Diagnosis:* Mixed disorder, acute respiratory acidosis with metabolic acidosis with hypoxia (PF ratio <100).
    - Acute respiratory acidosis probably due to low tidal volume, inadequate minute ventilation, decreased lung compliance secondary to ARDS

b. *Ventilatory management in ARDS* such as lung protective ventilation, i.e.,
    - Start mechanical ventilation with assist-control (AC) mode with following initial parameter: TV—6 mL/kg of predicted body weight, PEEP—5-10 cmH_2O, and RR ≤ 35 breaths/min
    - Mechanical ventilation goals: PaO_2—55-80 mm Hg or $SaO_2 \geq 88\%$, plateau pressure ≤ 30 cmH_2O, driving pressure (plateau pressure—PEEP) < 15, pH goal 7.3-7.35, mechanical power < 7
    - Other rescue therapies used are recruitment maneuvers, prone ventilation, high-frequency oscillation (HFO) (not proven),

extracorporeal carbon dioxide removal (not proven), and rescue ventilation with extracorporeal membrane oxygenation (ECMO).

c. *Other causes of type I respiratory failure (hypoxia):* Pneumonia, pulmonary embolism, pulmonary edema, pneumothorax, low FiO_2 (high altitude), V/Q mismatch (low V/Q), and intrapulmonary shunt

Ans. 12

a. Interpretation of ABG:
   - PH of 7.28 is acidosis
   - HCO_3 is 10, it is decreased by (24 – 10) = 14, (pH and HCO_3 are in the same direction), so it is a metabolic acidosis.
   - *Compensation:* Expected change in $pCO_2 = [(1.5 \times HCO_3) + 8] = (1.5 \times 10) + 8 = 23$
   - Expected $PaCO_2 = 23$; Actual $PaCO_2 = 28$ (compensation ongoing)
   - *Anion gap = $([Na^+] + [K^+] - ([Cl^-] + [HCO_3])$*
   - Anion gap = (140 + 5) – (100 + 10) = 35 mmol/L (normal anion gap is 10–12)
   - *Osmolar gap = osmolality (measured) – osmolarity (calculated)*
   - Calculated osmolarity = $2[Na^+] + [glucose]/18 + [BUN]/2.8$
     $= (2 \times 140) + 74/18 + 50/2.8 = 301$
   - Osmolar gap = 330 – 301 = 29 (normal osmolal gap < 10 mOsm/kg)
   - *Diagnosis:* HAGMA with high osmolar gap due to methanol poisoning.

b. *Other causes of an elevated osmolar gap*: Mannitol, ethanol, glycine (transurethral resection of prostate syndrome—caused by excessive absorption of electrolyte-free irrigation fluid), hypertriglyceridemia, and hypergammaglobulinemia

c. *Effect of blood methanol level:* Blood level g/dL and clinical effects
   - *0.02 g/dL:* Decrease inhibition and slight feeling of intoxication
   - *0.08 g/dL:* Decrease in cognitive and motor function
   - *0.2 g/dL:* Slurred speech, motor in coordination, irritability, and poor judgment
   - *0.3 g/dL:* Light coma and depressed vitals
   - *0.4 g/dl:* Death

d. *Treatment of methanol poisoning:*
   - Maintain the patients airway, breathing, and circulation
   - *Bicarbonate to reduce acidemia:* 1–2 mEq/kg HCO_3
   - Alcohol dehydrogenase (ADH) inhibition by:
     - *Fomepizole:* 15 mg/kg intravenously followed by 100 mg/kg every 12 hours till the acidosis get corrected.
     - *Ethanol:* 10 mL/kg of 10% ethanol infused over 60 minutes followed by maintenance infusion of 10% ethanol solution at 1 mL/kg/hours
   - Extracorporeal removal by hemodialysis

- *Cofactor therapy:* Folic acid, thiamine, and pyridoxine help to optimize metabolic pathway.
- Obtaining confirmatory alcohol concentration
- *Gastrointestinal decontamination:* Limited role

Ans. 13

a. Interpretation of ABG:
   - PH of 7.23 is acidosis
   - HCO_3 is 9, it is decreased by (24 – 9) =15. So, it is metabolic acidosis.
   - *Compensation:* Change in $pCO_2 = [(1.5 \times HCO_3) + 8] = (1.5 \times 9) + 8 = 21.5$
   - Expected $PaCO_2$ =21.5; Actual $PaCO_2$ = 23 (compensated)
   - *Anion gap =* $([Na^+] - ([Cl] + [HCO_3])$
   - Anion gap = (130) – (109 + 9) = 12 mmol/L (normal)
   - *Diagnosis:* Metabolic acidosis due to paracetamol overdose

b. Management of acetaminophen overdose:
   - Manage ABC and supportive care
   - Gastric lavage within 1 hour of ingestion (although no evidence for mortality reduction) and activated charcoal
   - *N-acetyl cysteine (NAC)* promotes conjugation of circulating paracetamol
   - Greatest effect if given <12 hours after ingestion
     - *Intravenous 20 hours regimen*—150 mg/kg in 200 mL D5 over 15 minutes, then 50 mg/kg in 500 mL D5 over 4 hours, then 100 mg/kg in 1 L of D5 over 16 hours.
     - *Oral 72 hours regimen*—140 mg/kg PO once, then 70 mg/kg PO every 4 hours × 17 doses.
     - Repeat ALT and paracetamol levels 2 hours before completion of NAC
   - *Management if < 8 hours after ingestion:* Give acetyl cysteine if >12 g or >150 mg/kg has been ingested, regardless of current plasma level (do not wait for blood result). Use activated charcoal and acetyl cysteine
     - Intravenous 20 hours regimen—150 mg/kg in 200 mL D5 over 15 minutes, then 50 mg/kg in 500 mL D5 over 4 hours, then 100 mg/kg in 1 L of D5 over 16 hours.
     - *Oral 72 hours regimen*—140 mg/kg PO once, then 70 mg/kg PO every 4 hours × 17 doses.
     - Repeat ALT and paracetamol levels 2 hours before completion of NAC
   - *Management if >8 hours after ingestion*: Only give acetyl cysteine if >12 g or >150 mg/kg has been ingested, regardless of current plasma level. Do not use after activated charcoal. Other treatment modalities are therapeutic plasma exchange and liver transplant.

Ans. 14

a. Interpretation of ABG:
   - PH of 7.10 is acidosis
   - HCO_3 is 10, it is decreased by (24 – 10) =14. So, it is metabolic acidosis.
   - *Compensation:* Change in $pCO_2 = [(1.5 \times HCO_3) + 8] = (1.5 \times 10) + 8 = 23$
   - Expected $PaCO_2 = 23$; Actual $PaCO_2 = 52$ (noncompensated), both in fact HCO_3 and pCO_2 are moving in the opposite directions, which they should not, hence, it is mixed disorders.
   - *Anion gap = ([Na⁺] – ([Cl] + [HCO₃]))*
     Anion gap = (136) – (100 + 15) = 21 mmol/L (increased)
     Delta AG = AG – 12 = 21 – 12 = 9
     Delta $HCO_3 = 24 - HCO_3 = 24 - 10 = 14$
     Delta ratio = Delta AG/Delta HCO_3 = 9/14 = <1
   - *Diagnosis:* HAGMA with NAGMA and coexisting respiratory acidosis.

b. Management:
   - ABG is suggestive of severe hypoxia with PF ratio <100, and acute respiratory acidosis probably due to lung protective ventilatory strategy (very low TV used). There is associated hyperlactatemia and hyperglycemia. This patient also requires urgent attention to improve ventilation and oxygenation with rescue therapies such as recruitment maneuvers, prone ventilation, $ECCO_2R$, and/or ECMO. To correct severe metabolic acidosis by giving bicarbonate correction as per formula
   - *Amount of $NAHCO_3$ in mEq = 0.5 × weight in kg × (Bicarbonate deficit)*
     = 0.5 × weight in kg × (Desired bicarbonate – actual bicarbonate)
     = 0.5 × weight in kg × (24 – actual bicarbonate)
     Half of total dose should be given in 4–8 hours and remaining half should be given within total 24 hours. Simultaneously, steps should be taken to control hyperglycemia after ruling out DKA.

Ans. 15

a. VBG sample will always have $PaCO_2$ value above 42. Hence, sample 1 is of ABG and sample 2 is probably of VBG.

Differentiating features of arterial and venous blood gases in normal individuals		
	Arterial	***Peripheral venous***
pH	7.36–7.44	7.32–7.38
Partial pressure of O_2 (PaO_2) in mm Hg	95–100	40
Partial pressure of CO_2 ($PaCO_2$) in mm Hg	36–44	42–50
Saturation SO_2 in %	>95%	65–75%
HCO_3 in mEq/L	22–26	23–27

b. A venous saturation < 70% and A-V-CO_2 gap >6 mm Hg has been found to have significant lower cardiac output. Normalization of increased CO_2 gap has been shown to correlate with improvement in tissue perfusion. Hence, CO_2 gap of ≥6 mm Hg is an addition marker to identify inadequate resuscitation after achieving target $ScvO_2$ of 70%.
   - A delta $PaCO_2$/(A-V) CO_2 ratio of 1.4 predicts the presence of anaerobic metabolism and global tissue hypoxia.

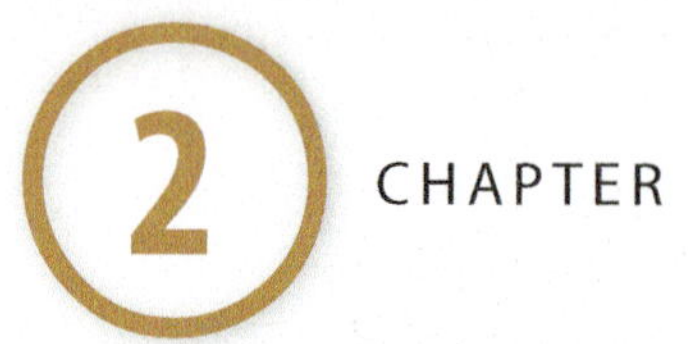

CHAPTER 2 Point-of-Care Ultrasound (POCUS) in Emergency OSCE

Sandeep Gore, Atur Mahant

QUESTIONS

Q1. **A 46-year-old diabetic and hypertensive male had a recent travel to the United States for a vacation. During his stay, he had contact with a friend who was noted to be coronavirus disease (COVID) positive. Today, the patient sought consult with complaints of chest discomfort, breathing difficulty, and uneasiness for 2 days. Upon assessment, his vital signs are blood pressure (BP): 90/60 mm Hg, heart rate (HR): 115 bpm, SpO_2: 85% in room air (RA), temperature: 36.9°C, and a respiratory (RR) of 30 breaths/min. You performed a bedside ultrasound which showed the following image:**

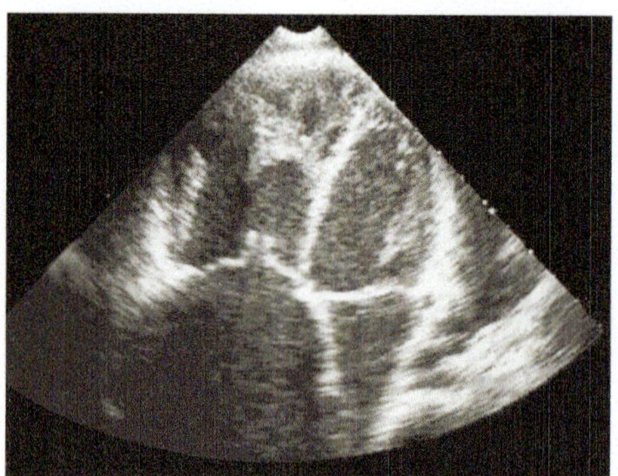

a. What is the most probable diagnosis?
b. Describe the image and two signs on ultrasound which supports the diagnosis?
c. State the gold standard imaging modality for this condition. What are its limitations?
d. What is the gold standard treatment for the above case?

Q2. **A 25-year-old female presents to the emergency department with complaints of breathlessness, pricking chest pain, and fever. Upon examination, patient is hemodynamically unstable. Physical examination revealed engorged neck veins and muffled heart sounds. Bedside ultrasound reveals the following:**

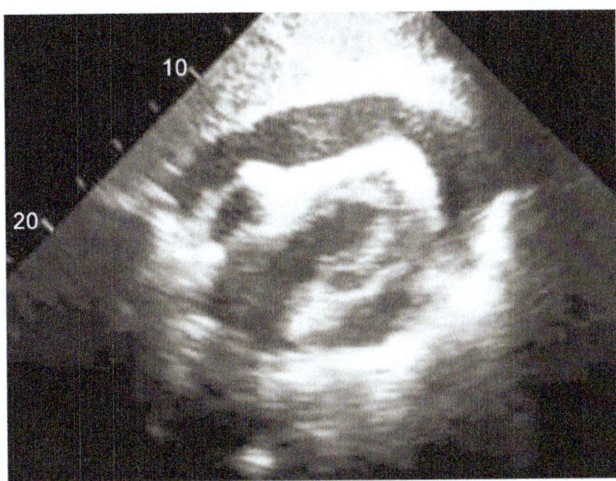

a. What are the causes of the condition above?
b. Identify the type of shock and its pathophysiology.
c. What are the resuscitation measures and definitive treatment required for the condition?

Q3. **A 75-year-old male presented to the emergency department with complaints of chest pain radiating to the back, breathing difficulty, and blackouts for 2 hours. He has no significant past medical history. Vital signs are BP: 60 mm Hg systolic, HR: 105 bpm, SpO_2: 90% RA, temperature: 37°C, and a respiratory rate (RR) of 19 breaths/min. Pulses are not elicited well. ECG shows sinus tachycardia with early repolarization. The provisional chest X-ray report is unremarkable. A bedside ultrasonography was performed.**

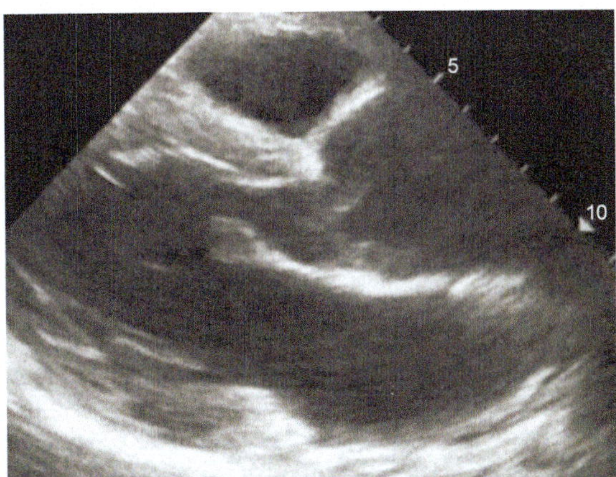

a. Name two findings which should be seen on the X-ray which would raise the suspicion of the diagnosis.

b. State the physical examination findings of patients with this condition.
c. State two classifications used to stage and manage the diagnosis.
d. Name the definitive investigation and its emergency management.

Q4. A 20-year-old basketball player had sudden onset of chest pain, breathing difficulty, and sweating while he was walking home from the championship final. He was unable to walk further due to the pain. He called his friend who brought him into the emergency. Upon arrival, you note him to be in distress with the following vital signs: BP: 90/60 mm Hg, HR: 105 bpm, SpO_2: 90% RA, temperature: 36.9°C, and a RR of 25 breaths/min. After starting oxygen, you order for an ECG which was normal. Cardiac marker results are awaited. However, the patient is in severe discomfort and demands urgent resolution. You investigate him with an ultrasound shown in below image.

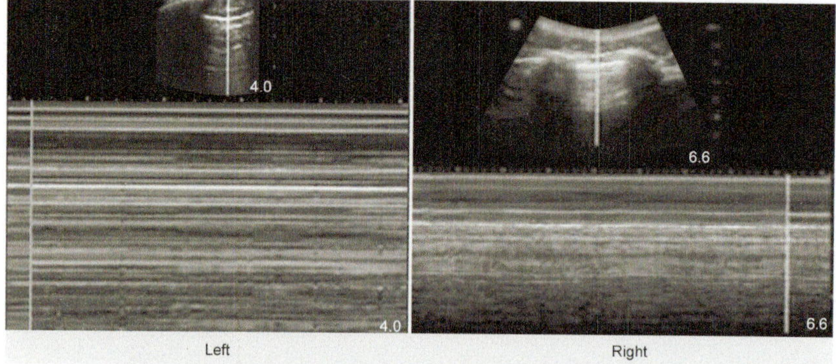

a. State the bedside lung ultrasonography in emergency (BLUE) protocol algorithm.
b. What is the diagnosis and which point of care ultrasound (POCUS) feature is required to confirm the diagnosis?
c. State the British Thoracic Society (BTS) guidelines for the management.
d. Identify the landmarks of the procedure if a chest drain is required.

Q5. An 83-year-old male was brought to the emergency department with complaints of fever in the last 1 week associated with cough. He noted the cough to be productive. He had associated breathlessness since a few days which was exacerbated on exertion. Today, he is worried that he has chest pain. Upon primary survey, patient is hypoxic, tachypneic and has a blood pressure of 80 mm Hg systolic. His arterial blood gas shows early

signs of acute respiratory distress syndrome (ARDS) with a lactate of 5.6. Upon examination, you notice that his cardiovascular and respiratory symptoms are clear. You opt for a bedside ultrasound which revealed this abnormality.

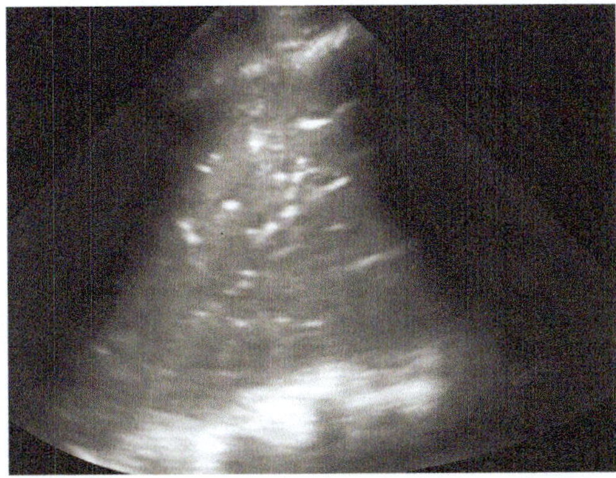

a. Which areas would have been screened if you are conducting the above protocol? Describe their anatomical positions.
b. Differentiate the BLUE and rapid ultrasound in shock (RUSH) protocol.
c. What finding is demonstrated above and what is the most probable diagnosis?
d. Which protocol is used to guide fluid management in the case above?

Q6. A 42-year-old female underwent a hysterectomy for abnormal uterine bleeding. She was advised bed rest for 3 weeks. 3 days prior to consult, patient noted to have pain over her left leg with swelling. The emergency medicine consultant has asked you to perform a bedside ultrasound.

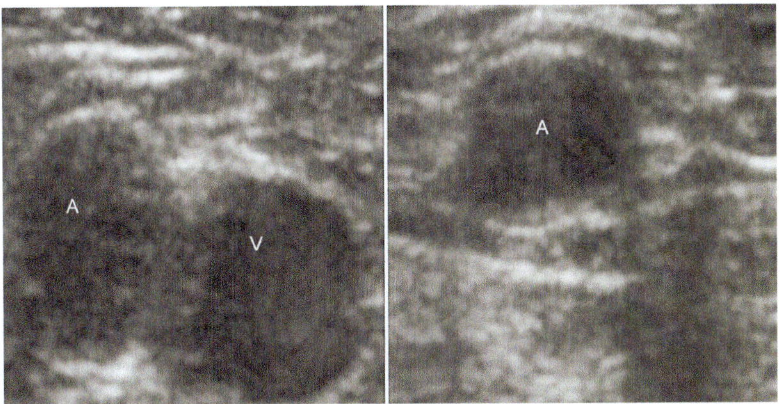

a. Name the POCUS imaging which is used to screen for the diagnosis and how does it aid in the diagnosis?
b. State the score and its components to diagnose the condition.
c. Does the patient require other imaging? What is the treatment?

Q7. **A 47-year-old woman is brought in the resuscitation area by the ambulance. The paramedics say she was extricated from her car. Unfortunately, her copassenger died on the scene. She is conscious but confused, complaining of pain in her "tummy". Primary survey has been addressed but you notice she complains of persistent tummy pain.**

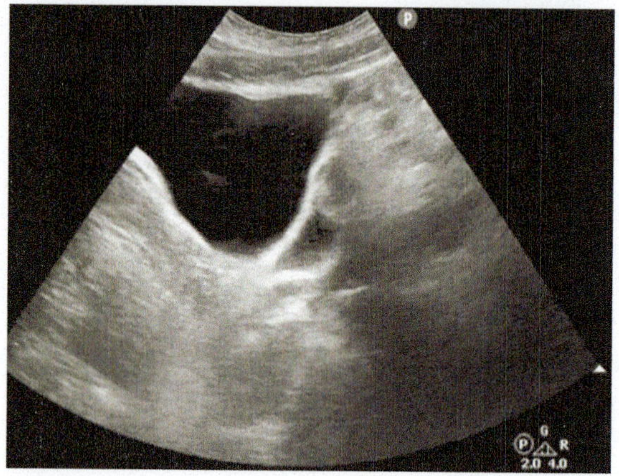

a. Describe the image above. You noticed that the patient is hypotensive and has the above findings. What should be your immediate disposition?
b. What are the four areas which should be visualized using bedside ultrasound?
c. Which site accumulates the fluid first and why? How does it differ from the pediatric age group?

Q8. **A 26-year-old female had onset of right shoulder pain and abdominal pain with vomiting for 3 days. She attributed this to a urinary tract infection for which she self-medicated with unrecalled antibiotics. Today she had onset of vaginal bleeding which alarmed her. She is anxious and presented to the emergency with her friend. Upon assessment, her vital signs are BP: 80 mm Hg systolic, HR: 120 bpm, SpO_2: 99% RA, temperature: 36.9°C, and a RR of 25 breaths/min. You notice her abdomen to be severely tender. You have started IV fluids and pain medications to provide relief. To investigate further, you apply the bedside ultrasound on the abdomen which revealed the following:**

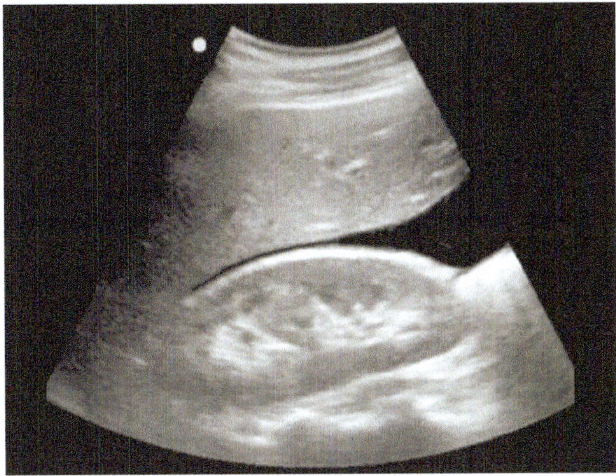

a. What is the most probable diagnosis considering the clinical presentation?
b. What is shown in the image above and which conditions can produce such findings?
c. What is the initial and definitive management?

Q9. **A 56-year-old male came with complaints of abdominal pain, vomiting, and abdominal distension in the last 2 days. The patient's abdomen is diffusely tender and you notice hyperactive bowel sounds. You suspect intestinal obstruction.**

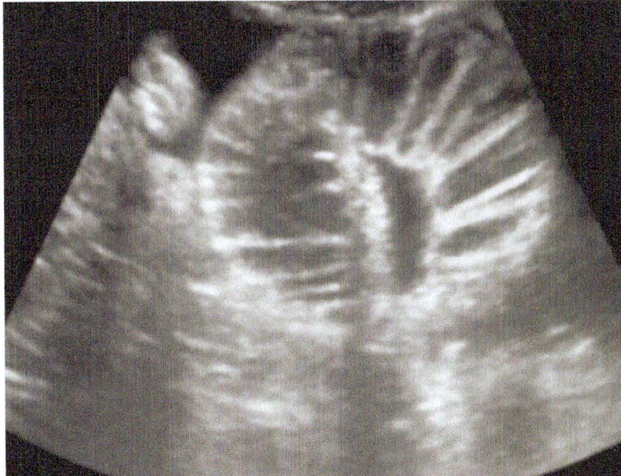

a. What finding will you illicit on a bedside ultrasound?
b. What is the most common cause of the finding?
c. What complications are possible if the diagnosis is not treated promptly?

d. Which imaging is essential to confirm the diagnosis and plan the management for the patient?

Q10. **A 51-year-old hypertensive and diabetic male presents to the emergency department with left facial swelling in the last 2 days. He is also complaining of pain and feverish feeling. His vitals include BP of 140/80 mm Hg, HR of 103 bpm, temperature of 100.80°C, RR of 20 breaths/min, SpO_2 of 97% on RA. Examination reveals the patient to be unwell with a focal area of swelling anteriorly to his left ear that is warm and tender to palpation. You notice his dentition to be poor. You notice few areas of swelling on the left side which are tender. You suspect a diagnosis of parotitis. You see the following image on the USG screen:**

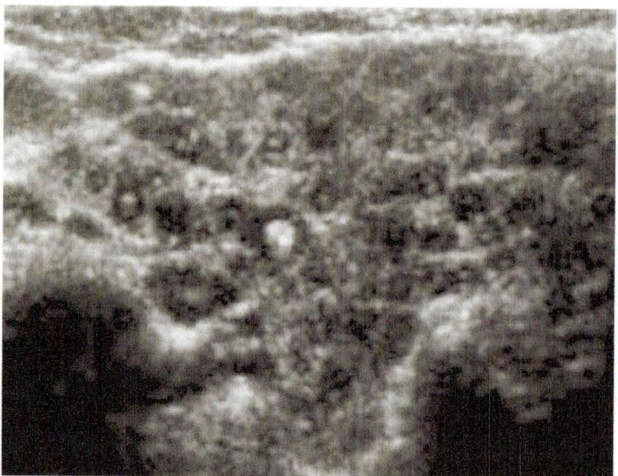

a. Identify the sign in the above image.
b. Is this condition more common in elderly or children? What are the most common etiologies in the respective age groups?
c. What are the indications to refer the patient to an ENT?

Q11. **A 52-year-old female patient presented at the emergency department with a 3-week history of facial swelling, significant hearing loss, cough, nasal congestion, hoarseness, and swelling of the arms, chest, and upper back. Upon examination, vital signs are within normal range. Physical examination shows swollen face that included swelling of the tongue and lips, right arm swelling >left arm, and decreased hearing. Blood workup, ECG, and chest X-ray are unremarkable. Upon bedside ultrasound, you notice the following:**

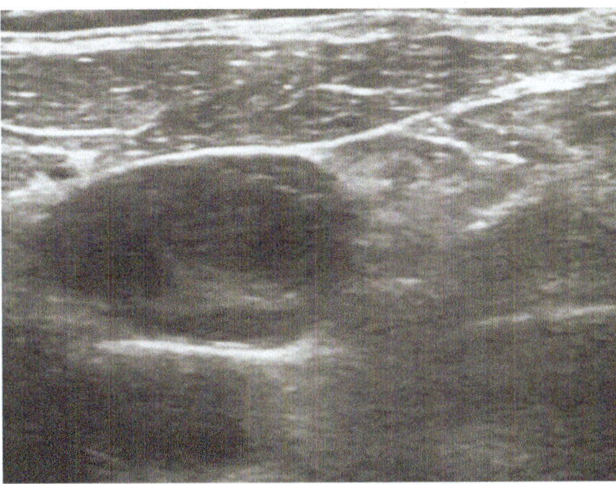

a. What is the diagnosis?
b. Which sign can be appreciated on physical examination?
c. What is the imaging modality of choice and its management?

Q12. A 16-year-old female presented to the emergency department with complaints of chest pain, fever, and cough and colds for 1 week. She is in respiratory distress, febrile, and hypotensive on arrival. ECG shows nonspecific ST-T changes with sinus tachycardia. You interpret the cardiac function to be poor and see the following on the short axis

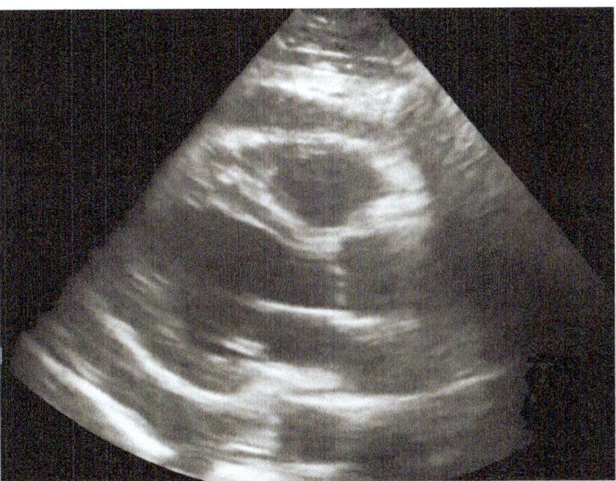

a. What is the most common cause for the above findings?
b. You have administered fluids and started inotropes but there is no improvement. Which treatment should be considered in this patient and explain its mechanism?
c. What complication could result from this condition and how will POCUS aid in its diagnosis?

Q13. An 18-year-old male presented with sudden onset of right-sided abdominal and scrotal pain since 1 hour. He was playing soccer when he had onset of the pain. He has no other complaints. He is hemodynamically stable. Physical examination reveals mild tenderness over the painful area with swelling of the scrotum.

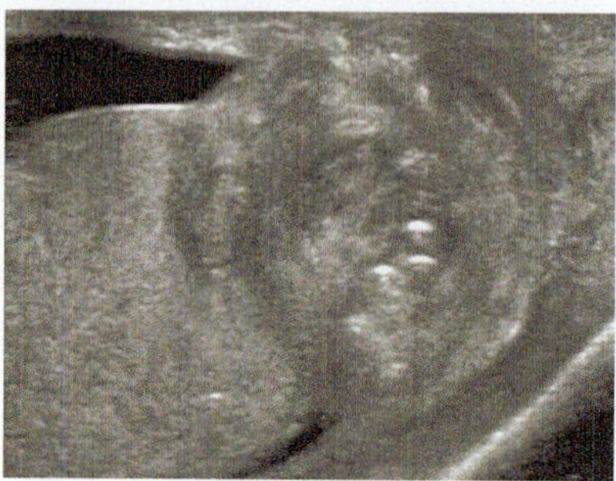

a. Identify the sign in the above image.
b. Describe the emergency department management and definitive management of the condition.
c. What are the time goals which should be met?

Q14. An 80-year-old hypertensive and diabetic male with a history of ischemic heart disease (IHD) presented to the emergency department with abdominal pain radiating to the groin area and back since a few days. He has an associated fever and burning sensation while passing urine. The patient is hemodynamically stable, and you suspect pyelonephritis. As a keen fellow in your emergency POCUS course, you want to screen the kidneys. Upon performing the POCUS, you notice the following:

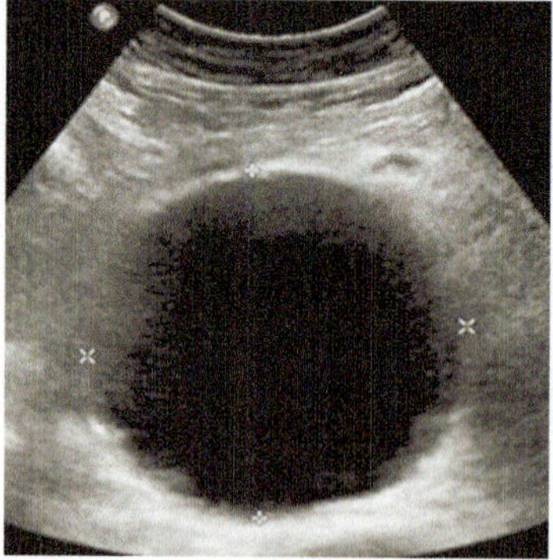

a. What are the risk factors for the condition above?
b. What is the risk of abdominal aortic aneurysm (AAA) rupture per year based on diameter?
c. What are the indications of AAA repair?

Q15. A 40-year-old diabetic patient was presented to the emergency department with complaints of swelling over the right leg, pain, fever, and difficulty in breathing. The patient had no previous hospitalizations and was previously healthy and compliant with her diabetic medications. Upon assessment, the patient is noted to be febrile with sugars of 360 and ketones of 0.2. Upon examination of the limb, you notice swelling, redness, and warmth upon palpation. The formulated differentials include a deep venous thrombosis, cellulitis, and abscess.

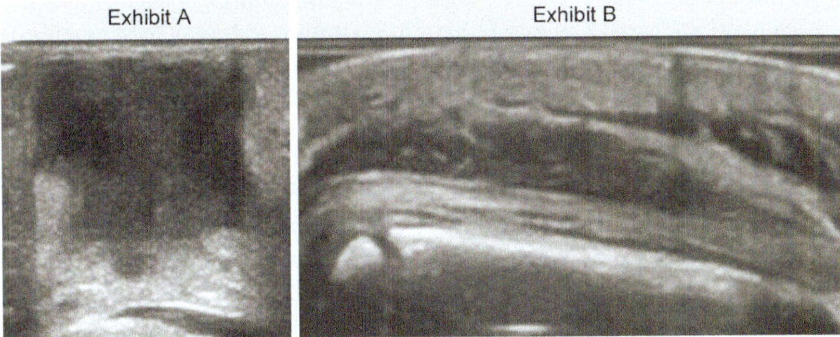

a. Identify the diagnosis seen in the two images above.
b. How does the management of both the conditions differ?
c. Which imaging modality should be used to rule out an underlying condition?

ANSWERS

Ans. 1

a. Pulmonary embolism—recent history of travel with chest pain. Hemodynamically unstable with hypoxia. Right atrial/right ventricular (RA/RV) dilatation on ultrasound.
b. The image shows RA/RV dilatation. Other signs consistent with pulmonary embolism are:
   - *McConnell sign:* RV free wall akinesis sparing the apex
   - *D sign:* A D-shaped left ventricle or flattening of the interventricular septum with a D-shaped configuration
c. Computed tomography (CT) pulmonary angiography. It utilizes a contrast agent; so, it is contraindicated in patients with allergies to the contrast and renal patients. Furthermore, pregnant females should not be exposed to a CT scan; hence, a VQ scan, chest X-ray, and ultrasound can aid in the diagnosis and the management.
d. Thrombolysis with injection alteplase 100 mg over 2 hours

Ans. 2

a. Aortic dissection (thoracic), end-stage lung cancer, acute myocardial infarction (MI), heart surgery or invasive procedures, bacterial or viral infections, trauma, Iatrogenic (central line), heart tumors and leukemia, kidney and heart failure, and radiation therapy to the chest connective tissue disorders [systemic lupus erythematosus (SLE)/dermatomyositis]
b. Obstructive shock. The fluid surrounding the heart impairs right ventricular filling resulting in the inability to produce adequate cardiac output. The cardiac function and blood volume is undisturbed.
c. Follow the ABCDE (Airway, Breathing, Circulation, Disability, and Exposure) approach. Avoid fluid administration as it may lead to volume overload and further deteriorate the condition. Pericardiocentesis is the definitive management.

Ans. 3

a. *Wide mediastinum:* It is >8.0–8.8 cm at the level of the aortic knob on portable anteroposterior chest radiographs, double or irregular aortic contour, inward displacement of atherosclerotic calcification (>1 cm from the aortic margin). Depending on etiology, there may be signs of periaortic or mediastinal hematoma which include obscuration of the aortic knob, opacification of the aortopulmonary (AP) window, and deviation of mediastinal structures.
   - Esophagus or nasogastric tube to the right
   - Trachea to the right
   - Left main bronchus inferiorly
b. *Signs of an aortic murmur* (new diastolic murmur in the lower left sternal border). Discrepancy in blood pressure across four limbs (>20 mm Hg systolic and >10 mm Hg diastolic), signs of pericardial tamponade (dilated neck veins, diminished heart sounds, and decreased pulse or pulse pressure), Ischemic stroke, spinal ischemia leading to temporary or permanent paralysis in 1–3% of patients, and ischemic peripheral neuropathy.
c. *Classification:*
   - *DeBakey classification:*
     - *Type 1:* Ascending aorta and extending distally beyond the innominate artery
     - *Type 2:* Arising in the ascending aorta with extension till the level of the innominate artery
     - *Type 3:* Arising at or distal to the left subclavian artery with extension distally
   - *Stanford classification:*
     - *Type A:* Dissection originating from origin of aorta and involving distal area
     - *Type B:* Limited to the descending aorta

d. *CT aortogram* is the definitive investigation.

Primary goal: To minimize dissection extension.

Target a HR of 60 bpm using esmolol (drug of choice), labetalol, and metoprolol.

Decreased cardiac contractility can also be achieved with diltiazem or verapamil if β-blockers are contraindicated. Hypotension should be addressed. Check for signs of pericardial tamponade or internal hemorrhage and treat the condition. Crystalloid infusion and vasopressors to provide a mean arterial pressure of 65 mm Hg. Norepinephrine or phenylephrine infusions are preferred to optimize blood pressure. Hypertension is commonly encountered in type B dissections; the target blood pressure is 100–120 mm Hg systolic. Nitroprusside can be used to lower the blood pressure only after starting antiadrenergic therapy. Pain relief with opioids is ideal. The cornerstone of type A dissection is surgery while for type B its blood pressure management. Surgical intervention should be advised in type B for life-threatening complications such as ischemia of both kidneys causing reversible renal failure, intestinal and limb ischemia, progressive aneurysm extension, impending or frank rupture, or intractable pain.

Ans. 4

a. The BLUE protocol

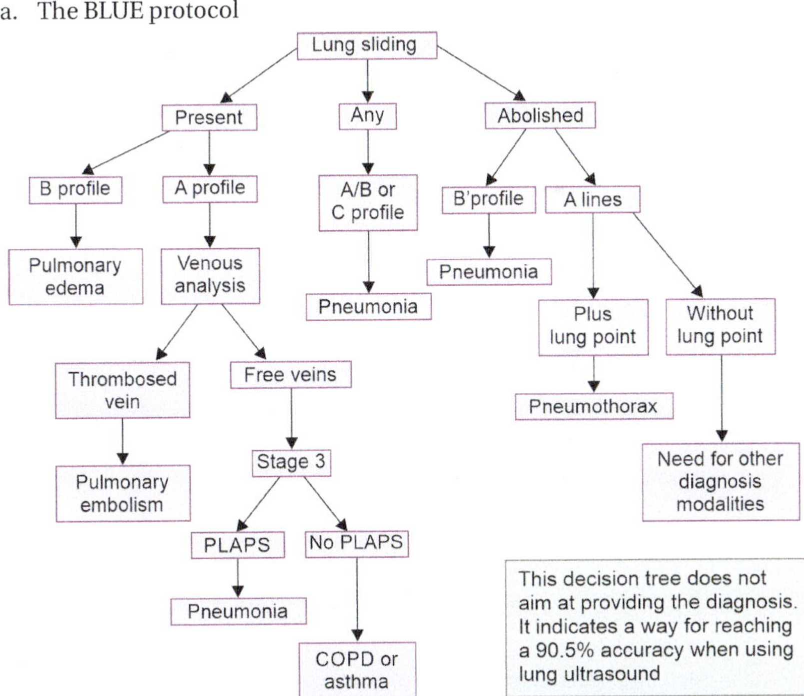

b. *Diagnosis:* Pneumothorax; Feature to confirm the diagnosis: Presence of a lung point.

c. BTS guidelines for management
d. The chest drain should be inserted in the "triangle of safety" which is bordered by anterior border of latissimus dorsi, lateral border of pectoralis major, apex of axilla, and level of nipple. The drain is usually inserted in the 5th intercostal space above the rib.

Management of spontaneous pneumothorax

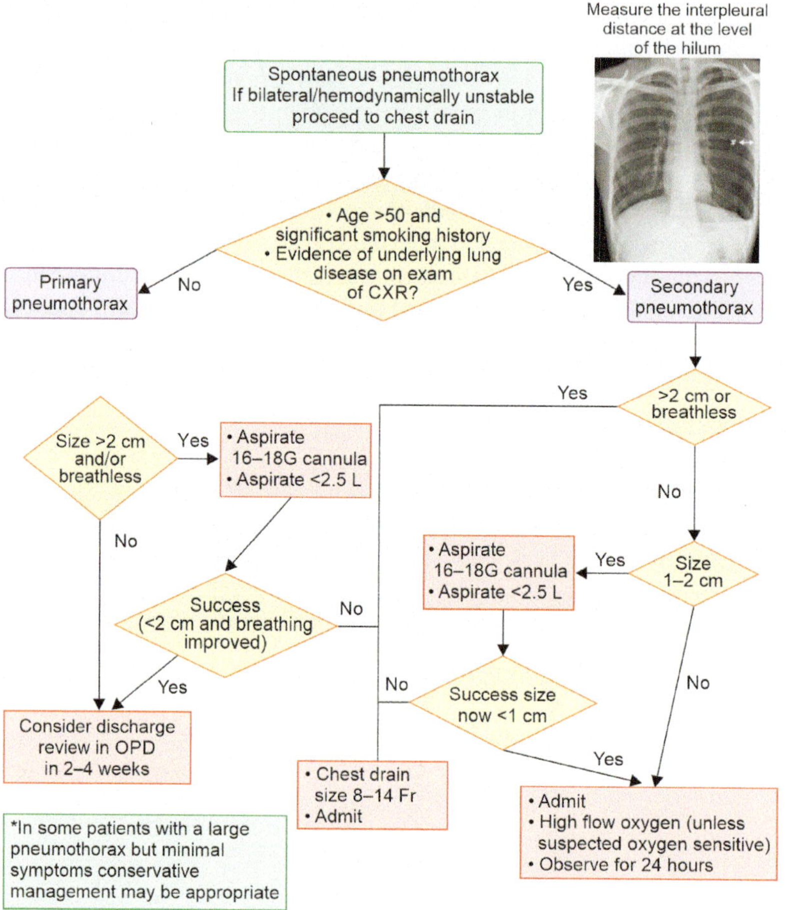

Guideline for management of pneumothorax

Ans. 5

a. Upper and lower lung points and posterior and/or lateral alveolar and/or pleural syndrome (PLAPS) view. Place four fingers of the hands below the clavicle and having the fingertips over the sternum, the upper point is located at the base of the second finger and third fingers. Place the other hand adjacent and below to the other, you will identify the lower point in the middle of the palm. The same is repeated on the other lung field. The PLAPS point, place the probe laterally till the posterior axillary line to identify the thoracic/abdominal border. It screens the posterolateral aspect of the lung.

b. BLUE protocol is to diagnose lung conditions while RUSH protocol is used to assess the cause of shock. The RUSH protocol assesses the pumps (heart), tank [inferior vena cava (IVC), lung, and abdomen], and pipes (aorta and veins).
c. Air bronchogram—suggestive of consolidation. Most likely to be lobar pneumonia.
d. FALLS protocol—fluid administration limited by lung sonography. It is a suggested approach for acute circulatory failure or undifferentiated shock. It uses the BLUE protocol to guide fluid therapy to guide the type of shock. It issued to assess for the development of new B lines and IVC volume to assess the amount of fluid to be administered.

Ans. 6

a. *Two-point compression test:* The noncompressibility of a vein signifies the presence of a deep vein thrombosis (DVT).
b. Wells score for DVT

Active cancer	1
Paralysis, paresis, or recent Plaster of Paris (POP) immobilization of a leg	1
Recently bedridden for >3 days or major surgery <12 weeks	1
Localized tenderness along the distribution of the deep venous system	1
Entire leg swelling	1
Calf swelling >3 cm, compared with asymptomatic leg	1
Pitting edema	1
Dilated superficial veins	1
Previous documented DVT	1
Another diagnosis more likely than DVT	–2
≤1 DVT unlikely ≥2 DVT is likely	

c. CT pulmonary angiography to visualize for pulmonary embolism. Injection enoxaparin 0.1 mg/kg

Ans. 7

a. The image shows the bladder with a hypoechoic region outside it. This is suggestive of free fluid in the abdomen in the case of trauma. The patient should be taken for exploratory laparotomy immediately.
b. Area needs to screened:
    - Hepatorenal space—free fluid between the liver and kidney

- Splenorenal space—free fluid between the spleen and kidney
- Suprapubic area—free fluid surrounding the bladder
- Subxiphoid area—free fluid around the heart

c. Hepatorenal space accumulates free fluid first as it is the most dependent area. The pediatric population accumulates fluid first around the bladder.

Ans. 8

a. *Ruptured ectopic pregnancy:* Patient is of reproductive age and has per vaginal (PV) bleeding. Additionally, she has signs of peritonitis by the presence of shoulder pain.
b. Free fluid is seen in the Morison's pouch—suggestive of free fluid in the abdomen. Other causes of free fluid are trauma, malignancy, organ rupture, chronic liver disease, right heart failure, pancreatitis, portal vein thrombosis, and hypoproteinemia.
c. *Management initial:* Airway, breathing, and circulation, maintenance, pain management, IV fluids, blood grouping and crossmatching, inotropes, and early involvement of gynecology team. Definitive management: Emergency laparotomy.

Ans. 9

a. *To-and-fro sign:* Movement of bowel contents back-and-forth due to increased peristalsis.
   Keyboard sign: The inner wall of the small intestine has plica circularis (or valves of Kerckring). These are especially prominent in the distal duodenum and jejunum. In small bowel obstruction, these become more prominent and look like a keyboard.
b. Intestinal obstruction
c. Bowel ischemia, perforation, infection, or aspiration pneumonia
d. CT abdomen with contrast to visualize the extend of obstruction and its cause. It will also identify signs of perforation and ischemia.
   The patient should be kept nil-per-os (NPO) with IV fluids, pain management, and broad-spectrum antibiotics. Nasogastric tube may be inserted if stomach decompression is required. Surgery team should be involved to plan for the surgical management.

Ans. 10

a. Pomegranate sign
b. Elderly (more common)—*Staphylococcus aureus*; Children—mumps
c. Facial nerve involvement, spread of infection into adjacent structures (deep fascial spaces and pharyngeal space), abscess formation, and no clinical improvement after 48–72 hours of antibiotics

Ans. 11

a. Superior vena cava (SVC) syndrome secondary to a thrombus
b. *Pemberton sign:* Bilateral arm elevation causes facial congestion

c. CT scan of the chest with contrast—complete occlusion of the SVC with thrombus extending into proximal portion of the brachiocephalic veins bilaterally
   Management—catheter-directed thrombolysis initiated with a 2 mg t-PA bolus followed by a 1 mg/hour t-PA infusion over 3 hours.

Ans. 12

a. Viral infection—coxsackie B virus
b. Extracorporeal membrane oxygenation (ECMO)—a venoarterial ECMO would allow venous blood to be filtered and returned to the arterial system which allows the cardiopulmonary system to recover. Intra-aortic balloon pump (IABP)—allows the heart to reperfuse its coronary arteries which can aid in the recovery. It is a short-term treatment modality.
c. *Dilated cardiomyopathy:* Severely enlarged and hypocontractile left ventricle. Decreased left ventricular ejection fraction. Global dilatation of the heart. Presence of valve dysfunction.

Ans. 13

a. Whirlpool sign—shown as a spiral twist along the course of the spermatic cord either in the external inguinal ring or in the scrotal sac.
b. Treat with IV pain management, keep nil orally. If delay in OT → manual detorsion to restore blood flow to the affected testicle. Definitive treatment—surgical detorsion and orchiopexy
c. Testis can become nonviable at 6 hours from onset of pain. Surgery should be performed within 6 hours of torsion or onset of symptoms.

Ans. 14

a. Advancing age, male gender, smoking, family history, atherosclerosis, hypertension, hypercholesterolemia, and other vascular aneurysm
b. Risk of abdominal aortic aneurysm rupture per year based of diameter of aneurysm.

AAA diameter (cm)	*Rupture risk (%/year)*
3–3.9	0%
4–4.9	1%
5–5.9	1–10%
6.0–6/9	10–22%
>7.0	30–50%

c. Indications of abdominal aortic aneurysm repair
   Male with AAA >5.5 cm
   Female with AAA >5 cm
   Rapid growth >1.0 cm/year
   Symptomatic AAA

Ans. 15

a. *Exhibit A—abscess:* Well-defined hypoechoic structure
Exhibit B—cellulitis: Subcutaneous hypoechoic regions
b. *Abscess:* Antibiotics with aspiration of abscess contents (send for culture and sensitivity)
Cellulitis: Antibiotics and probable surgical intervention for necrotizing infections
c. USG arterial and venous Doppler of lower extremities help to rule out any vascular insufficiency causing infections which are common in diabetic patients.

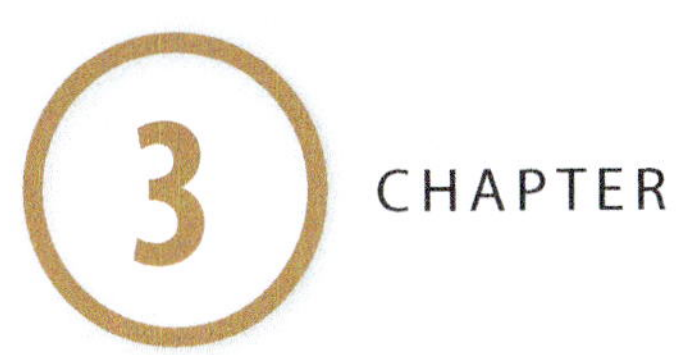

CHAPTER 3

HAZMAT PPE Infection Prevention Waste OSCE

TV Ramakrishnan, Mona Lisa Janarthanan

QUESTIONS

Q1. You are in a chemical spill field.

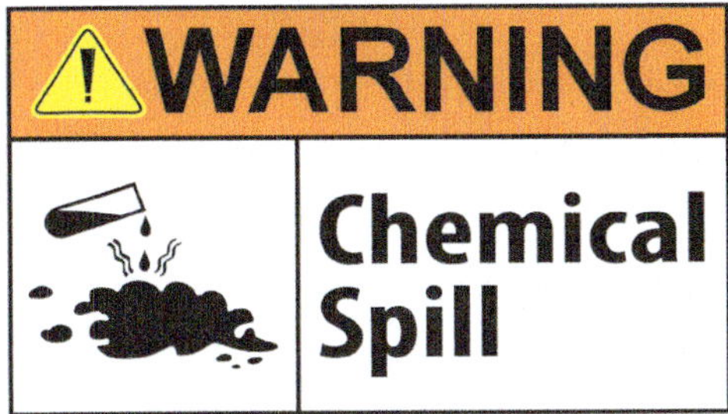

a. Define hazardous materials (HAZMAT)
b. How will you ensure the scene is safe?
c. What is the information you will provide after reaching the area to invite additional help?

Q2. You have received information regarding HAZMAT exposure and advised to go to field.

a. What are possible routes of exposure in affected individual?
b. What is primary contamination in the field?
c. What is secondary contamination?

Q3. In the scene, management of HAZMAT incident

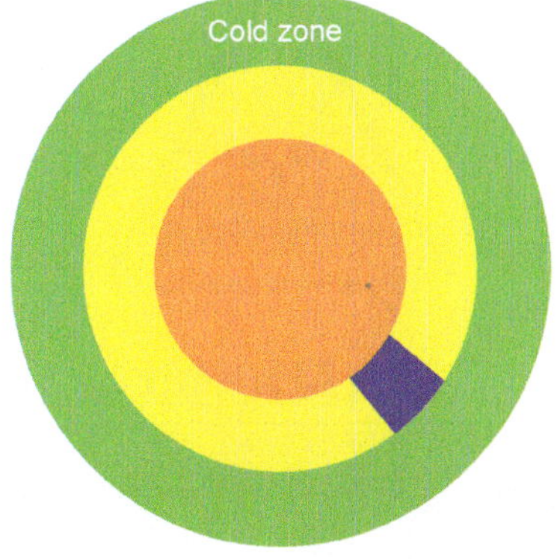

a. What are the different scene control zones?
b. Where does lifesaving procedures and decontamination happen?
c. Where does definitive patient care happen?
d. What are the types of decontamination?

Q4. As you prepare yourself in the HAZMAT scene with personal protective equipment (PPE).

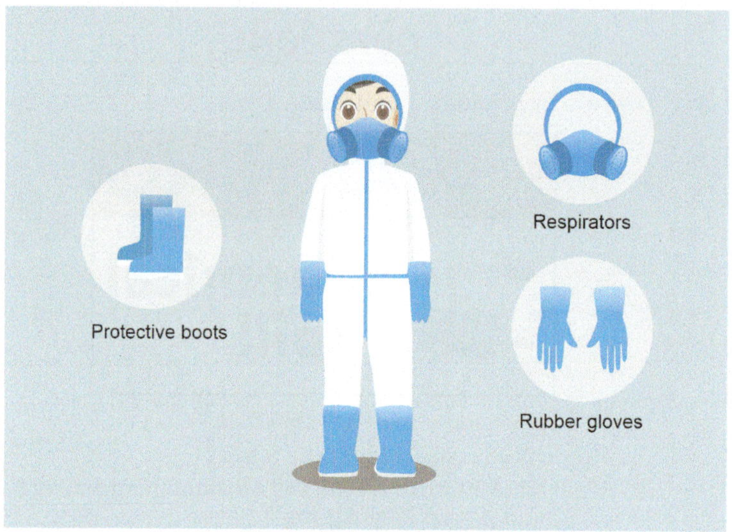

a. What are the levels of PPE in HAZMAT exposure?
b. Which level protects against gas and vapors?
c. What does level D protection mean?

Q5. Your team has been advised to arrive at a hazardous material exposure field of a fertilizer plant involving exposure to ammonia. Approximately 50 people are expected in the scene.

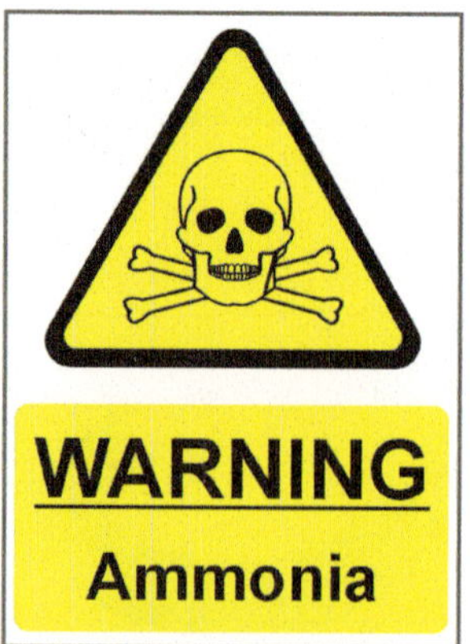

a. What types of exposures are expected and the symptoms?
b. What type of decontamination would be the best for them?
c. Which areas are difficult to decontaminate?
d. What is mass decontamination?

Q6. You are going into a hazardous exposure scene where people are exposed to a nerve gas agent suspected to be tabun.

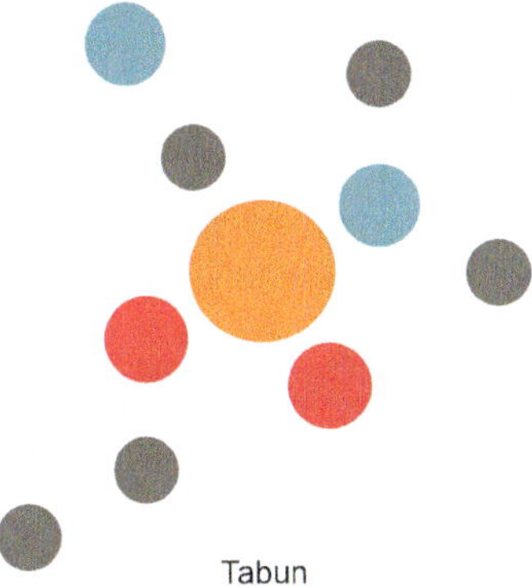

Tabun

a. What are the expected symptoms and time duration for it to develop?
b. Exposure has happened in open atmosphere, what precautions to be taken in scene safety?
c. Since the agent can vaporize, what important aspect should be taken care by emergency medical service (EMS) team while rescue?

Q7. *HAZMAT alert:* 20 people have been exposed to phosphorus in a fireworks factory.

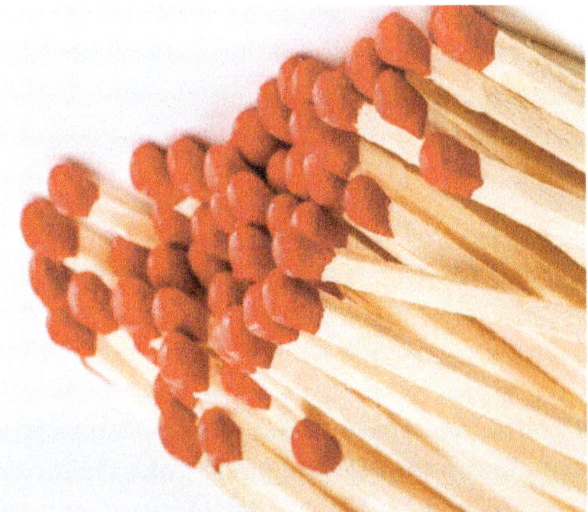

a. What are the routes of exposure?
b. Explain toxic manifestations.
c. Explain the decontamination of the patients.

Q8. You are called to attend an outbreak of hydrogen fluoride gas in a glass factory with EMS team.

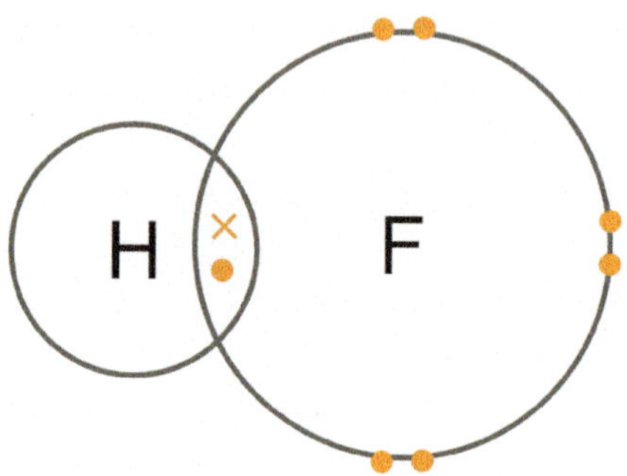

a. What are the toxic manifestations?
b. Explain the decontamination.
c. What is the specific skin care?
d. Name the antidote.

Q9. To limit the occurrence of HAZMAT exposure, there are various systems and responses which are formulated.

a. How can one identify the HAZMAT agent?
b. What is MSDS?
c. What are the warning properties of chemical exposure?

Q10. Healthcare-associated infections can be reduced by following infection prevention strategies by healthcare worker.

a. Is this statement true or false?
b. Who can act as source for the infection?
c. What can be the source of infection from a healthcare worker?

Q11. You have been asked to examine a patient with fever, cough, and rhinitis. Patient has history of recent travel.

a. What are the infection control precautions that need to be followed?
b. What are included in PPE?

Q12. A 30-year-old man presents with complaints of fever for 2 weeks. You have planned for taking blood cultures for the patient and have been advised to wash hands before the procedure.

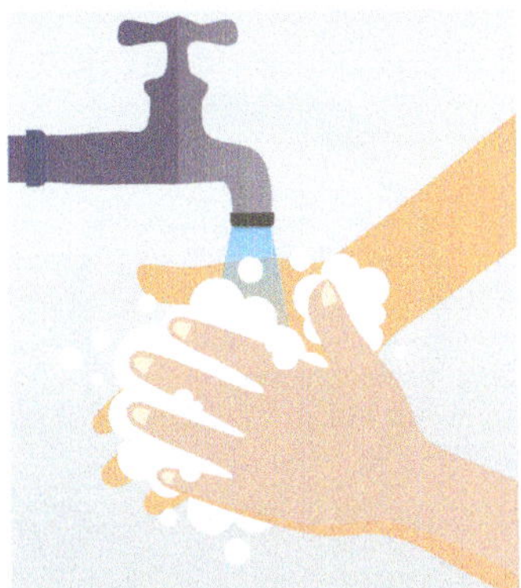

a. Explain five moments of hand wash advised by World Health Organization (WHO).
b. What are the steps of handwashing?
c. What is the WHO advised solution for handwashing?

Q13. A 30-year-old male diagnosed as COVID-19 with breathing difficulty. Patient is planned for intubation in view of respiratory failure.

a. What is the level of PPE recommended?
b. What are the different levels of PPE?
c. What are the other precautions for airborne transmission apart from PPE?

Q14. You are receiving a 40-year-old male with suspected influenza like respiratory infection in your emergency. Patient vitals are stable and needs admission for observation.

a. What level of PPE is used to examine the patient?
b. What are included in the specific PPE level?
c. What is the probable mode of transmission of the infection?
d. What are the other standard precautions to be taken in such infections?

Q15. You are preparing your emergency for sudden input of 15 patients with acute respiratory illness. You are preparing for all the needs to receive and treat them, checking on all the PPE needed by healthcare workers in this situation.

a. How will you manage on PPE in such crisis?
b. How do you decontaminate the PPE?

Q16. An infectious disease patient is admitted in the room where below mentions dial is observed by the resident doctors.

a. Identify the device.
b. Describe various type of isolation.

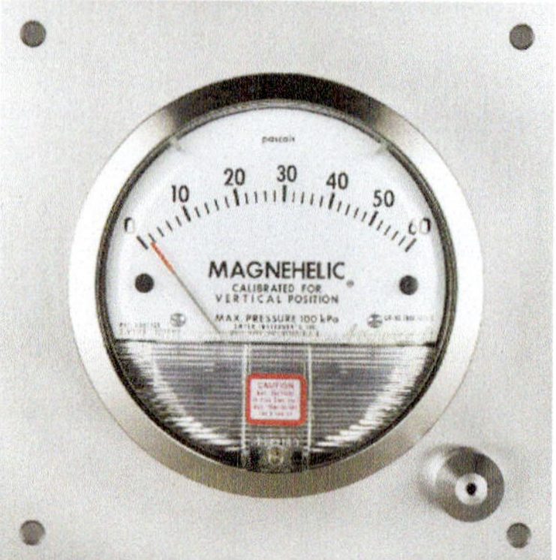

Q17. **Identify and mention the use of this product.**

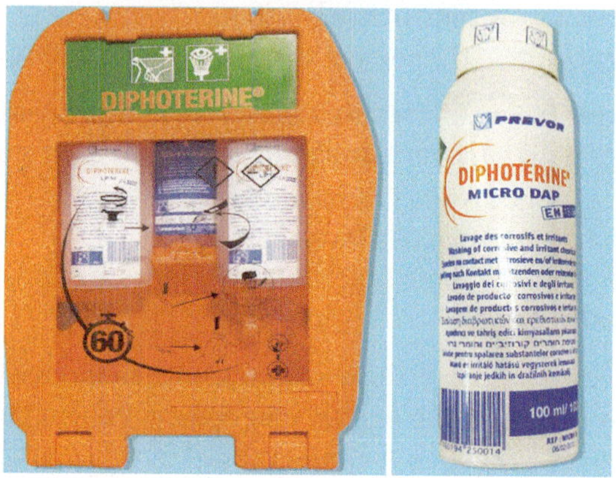

Q18. **Handwashing is an important precaution to prevent hospital acquired infections.**

What are the common antimicrobial agents used for hand-washing?

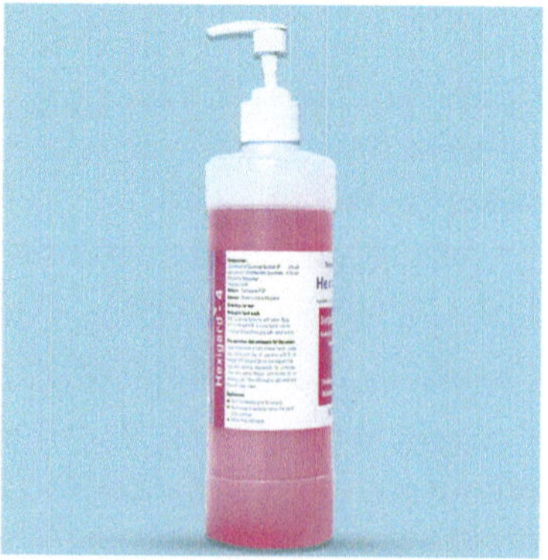

Q19. A housekeeping person is using below mentions solution for spill management of hazardous material in emergency room.

a. Write most common situation where sodium hypochlorite 1% solution is used.

b. After using this solution, how much time we should wait for next step?

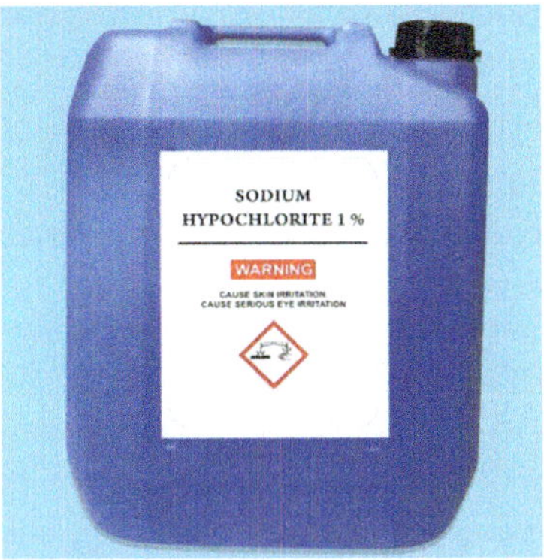

ANSWERS

Ans. 1

a. *Hazardous material* is defined as any substance or material that is capable of posing an unreasonable risk to human health, safety, or the environment when transported in commerce, used incorrectly, or not properly contained or stored.

b. Protect yourself first. Isolate the incident as much as possible to avoid further harm to other people. Identify the hazardous material. Notify to other EMS people, firefighters, law enforcement responders regarding the incident.

c. Your exact location, atmospheric conditions, exact name of the hazardous material—chemical ID number, number of victims including symptoms and signs, and type and number of additional resources needed. Location of incident command post and staging of resources.

Ans. 2

a. Inhalation, transdermal and transmucosal, ingestion injection (intravenous, intramuscular, and subcutaneous).

b. Primary contamination is decontamination of people or equipment due to direct contact with the initial hazardous material released (in hot zone).

c. Secondary contamination is contamination of healthcare professionals, other responders, and equipment's due to direct contact with a person or equipment covered with adherent solids/liquids that have been removed from the source of the hazardous material spill in the hot zone.

Ans. 3

a. There are three zones (1) hot zone (primary contamination), (2) warm zone, and (3) cold zone
b. Warm zone—access corridor
c. Cold zone
d. Dry decontamination—removal cloth and visible dust; Wet decontamination—with soap and water

Ans. 4

a. Four levels of PPE are:
   - *Level A:* Self-contained breathing apparatus, vapor protective suit, gloves, and boots
   - *Level B:* Supplied air respirator, full suit, gloves, and boots
   - *Level C:* Air purifying respirator, chemical resistant suit, gloves, and boots
   - *Level D:* Work overalls and no respiratory protection
b. Level A
c. *Level D:* It is used when there is no chemical hazard, common work wear overalls, no respiratory protection, gloves, goggles, and boots (optional)

Ans. 5

a. Exposure could be inhalation, skin absorption, mucus absorption, and ingestion
   Signs: Irritation of eyes, skin, throat, nose cough, breathing difficulty death due to respiratory failure
b. Decontamination with water or soap with water solution of skin
c. Axilla, groin, between buttocks, in-between fingers/toes—must be washed with brush and water thoroughly
d. When a large number of people are exposed to hazardous material—mass decontamination can be facilitated. Hose streams of water can be setup from two fire engines placed parallelly in warm zone, people are asked to disrobe themselves and runoff the water jet in-between engines.

Ans. 6

a. Symptoms tend to appear within seconds of exposure and lasts up to 18 hours. Symptoms—blurring vision, watering eyes, headache, drooling, excessive sweating, fasciculations, cardiac abnormalities, seizures, and cardiorespiratory arrest.
b. Open air exposure—patients should be moved uphill and upwind from the contamination site.
c. Vaporization can cause secondary contamination.

Ans. 7

a. Inhalation, skin and mucous membranes, and ingestion
b. Respiratory—irritation, cough, laryngospasm, breathing difficulty, and wheezing; Skin—chemical burns; Central nervous system (CNS)—anxiety,

confusion, seizures; Cardiovascular—arrhythmias, myocardial ischemia, and hypovolemia

c. Adequate oxygenation and ventilation; Thorough skin and eye decontamination—washing and eye irrigation

Ans. 8

a. Respiratory—irritation, cough, laryngospasm, breathing difficulty, wheezing; Skin—chemical burns causes severe pain, erode up to bones (hypocalcemia); CVS—hypocalcemia causes QT prolongation, ventricular tachyarrhythmias; Hyperkalemia causes tall T, bradycardia, and arrest
b. Needs "thorough decontamination"—minimum 15 minutes irrigation with water for one patient
c. Skin—topical calcium gluconate gel; Break the blisters to reduce absorption
d. IV calcium gluconate/calcium chloride

Ans. 9

a. One can identify the agent based on the chemical name and the specific classification provided—International Hazard Classification System (IHCS)
    - *Class 1:* Explosive substances and articles
    - *Class 2:* Gases
    - *Class 3:* Flammable liquids
    - *Class 4:* Flammable solids
    - *Class 5:* Oxidizing substances and organic peroxides
    - *Class 6:* Toxic and infectious substances
    - *Class 7:* Radioactive material
    - *Class 8:* Corrosive substances
    - *Class 9:* Miscellaneous dangerous substances and articles
b. MSDS—Material Safety Data Sheets—usually list one or more exposure limits for a substance, which can be used as benchmark to identify toxicity and select PPE.
c. Early warning properties—abnormal odor, irritation of eyes, and respiratory tract.

Ans. 10

a. True
b. Healthcare worker, patient contaminated surroundings, and hospital environment
c. Hands, body and skin, hair, and nose and mouth

Ans. 11

a. Precautions include hand hygiene, use of PPE, respiratory hygiene/cough etiquette by patients or healthcare worker, safe injection practices with proper disposal of sharps, device sterilization, environmental cleaning, and disinfection.

b. Gloves, masks, gowns, and protective eyewear

Ans. 12

a. Before direct contact or touching the patient, before performing clean/aseptic procedures on the patient, after contact with blood, body fluids, mucous membranes, nonintact skin, wound dressings, or visibly contaminated, after direct contact or touching the patient, and after touching the patient's surroundings or inanimate objects (including medical equipment) in the immediate vicinity

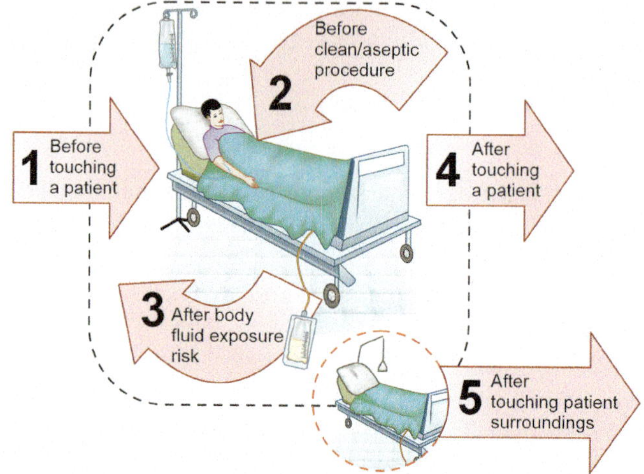

b. *Steps of handwashing* ***(Fig. 1)****:* Wet hands with water and liquid soap, rub palm to palm, dorsum of hands, between fingers, interlocking fingers, thumb, fingernails, and rinse and wipe dry

c. Water with liquid soap (or) alcohol-based hand rub

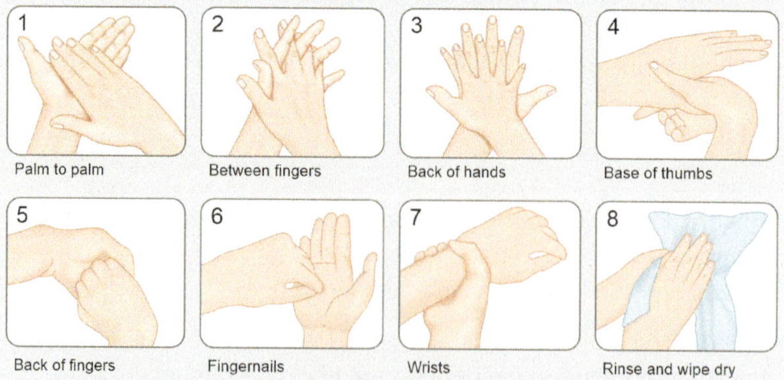

Fig. 1: Steps of handwashing.

Ans. 13

a. For all aerosol-generating procedures (AGPs), use level 3 PPE at any circumstances
b. Levels 1, 2, and 3
c. Place the patient in an airborne infection isolation room (AIIR)—monitored negative-pressure room with at least 6–12 air exchanges per hour. Room exhaust must be appropriately discharged outdoors or passed through a high-efficiency particulate air (HEPA) filter before recirculation within the hospital. A fit-tested certified N99/FFP3 respirator must be worn before entering the room; discard all PPEs except the respirator before exiting the room; transport of the patient should be minimized; the patient should wear a mask, if transport within the hospital is unavoidable; *Cough etiquette:* Patients and visitors should cover their nose or mouth when coughing, promptly dispose of used tissues, and practice hand hygiene after contact with respiratory secretions.

Ans. 14

a. Level 2 PPE
b. Disposable gloves, disposable apron, and disposable surgical mask with goggles or full-face visor. In case of high-risk direct physical contact, N95 respirator with goggles or full-face visor, disposable head cover/hood, and disposable shoe covers over closed shoes
c. Droplet transmission and later contact transmission
d. Place the patient in a single room, make sure eyes, nose, and mouth are fully covered before entering the room. Always wear a mask when within 1 m (3 feet) of the patient. Patients should wear a mask in the room and during transport in order to minimize the risk of environmental contamination. *Cough etiquette:* Patients and visitors should cover their nose or mouth when coughing, promptly dispose of used tissues, and practice hand hygiene after contact with respiratory secretions.

Ans. 15

a. Using appropriate PPE based on the suspected route of transmission. Prioritizing the use of specific PPE for only the highest risk of interventions on patient. Canceling nonemergency surgical procedures; proper reuse of PPE after decontamination; limiting staff usage as per need.
b. Most PPE are disposable or single use only. Decontamination with heat/ultraviolet reduces its efficacy against H1N1/SARS-CoV-2.

Ans. 16

a. Pressure meter to detect the pressure difference between negative or positive pressure rooms
b. Isolation rooms are broadly classified in four class **(Table 1)**

TABLE 1: Classification of isolation room.

	S—standard	*N—negative*	*P—positive*	*A—alternate*
Ventilation criteria	No pressure difference between room and adjacent corridor	Air pressure is less in room than adjacent corridor	Air pressure is more in room than adjacent corridor	Pressure can be adjusted either positive or negative
Indications	Contact or droplet	Airborne	Immunocompromised/ transplant patient, prevention of infection from outside environment	Not recommended
Examples	• Vancomycin-resistant *Enterococcus* • Gastroenteritis • Meningococcal disease • Hepatitis A • Cutaneous anthrax	• Measles • Chicken pox • Suspected or proven pulmonary/laryngeal tuberculosis	Prevention of infection in bone marrow transplant patient	Not recommended
Pressure	NA	• Room (negative) 30 Pa • Ensuite (negative) 30 Pa • Anteroom (negative) 15 Pa	• Room (positive) 30 Pa • Ensuite (positive) 30 Pa • Anteroom (positive) 15 Pa	NA

1. *Class-S—standard pressure rooms:* For patient with contact and droplet isolation. Normal air-condition room is appropriate.
2. *Class-N—negative pressure rooms:* It is used for airborne droplet nuclei isolation. Also known as "airborne infection isolation" or "infectious isolation unit". Negative pressure gradient is maintained from the room to the anteroom and the ambient air. Air change rate of 12 air changes per hour.
3. *Class-P—positive pressure rooms:* Rooms are positive pressure relative to ambient air used for immunocompromised and transplant patient.
4. *Class-A—alternating pressure (negative/positive):* Room with alternate negative and positive pressure, usually not recommended as there is difficulty in maintaining the appropriate airflow.

Ans. 17

Diphoterine is an emergency rinsing solution for eye and skin chemical splashes. It quickly eliminates the residual chemical product on the skin or on the eye when applied rapidly. Diphoterine has amphoteric chelating and hypertonic properties which minimize the severity of chemical burn.

Ans. 18

Common antimicrobial agents used for handwashing are:

- Water
- Plain soap (nonantimicrobial)
- Alcohol (ethanol, isopropanol, or combination of two)
- Chlorhexidine
- Chloroxylenol
- Hexachlorophene
- Quaternary ammonium compounds

Ans. 19

a. Sodium hypochlorite 1% is most common disinfectant solution to clean the spills of blood, body fluid, and other potentially infectious fluids.

b. Cover the area with absorbent like tissue paper, cover the spill with 1% sodium hypochlorite for 10–20 minutes contact time. Clean up spill and discard into infectious waste bin, and mop area with soap and hot water.

CHAPTER 4 Drugs and Instruments

Mona Lisa Janarthanan, TV Ramakrishnan

QUESTIONS

Q1. **You receive a patient in cardiac arrest, cardiopulmonary resuscitation (CPR) initiated as per advanced cardiovascular life support (ACLS) protocol and started on adrenaline.**

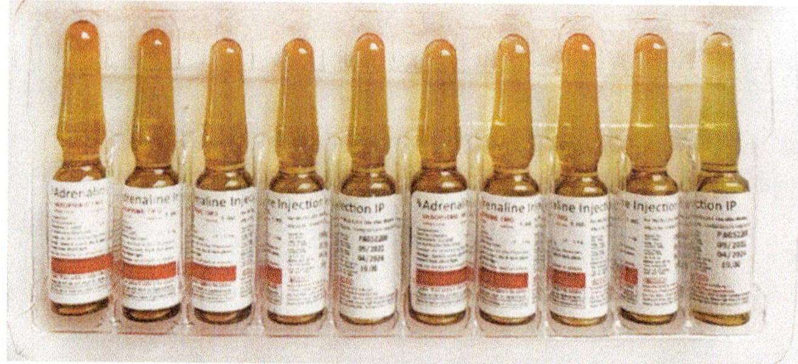

a. On what receptors does adrenaline acts?

b. What are common emergency room (ER) indications of adrenaline?

c. Comment on adverse effects of adrenaline.

Q2. **You are handling a patient with septic shock in ER, planning to start the patient on vasopressin**

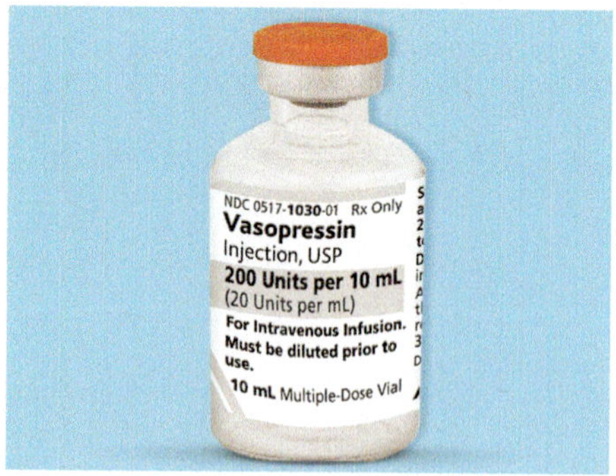

a. What is the mechanism of action of vasopressin?
b. Explain the role of vasopressin according to recent surviving sepsis guidelines.

Q3. You have received a patient, 35 years male with palpitations. Vitals—heart rate (HR): 188 beats/min and blood pressure (BP): 130/80 mm Hg. Patient is conscious, oriented with clear chest on auscultation. ECG is given in image here.

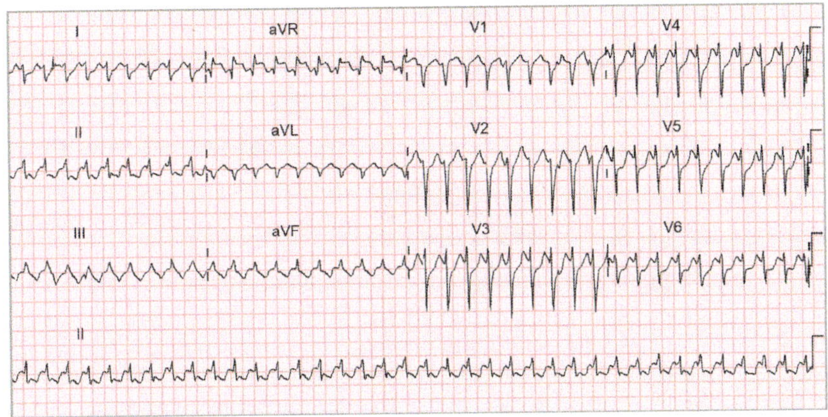

a. What is the drug of choice in stable patient?
b. How do you administer the drug?
c. What are the dosages according to ACLS guidelines?
d. What are the adverse effects of the drug?

Q4. You are planning to intubate a patient who is obese and falls under Mallampati 4 classification. Patient is in severe respiratory distress and expecting a difficult intubation. His blood gas shows hyperkalemia.

a. What is the muscle relaxant of choice for this patient?
b. What is the dosage of the drug?
c. What is the reversal agent for the particular muscle relaxant?

Q5. A 30-year-old female, who is 34 weeks pregnant, comes to emergency department (ED) with severe headache. Vitals show BP: 160/100 mm Hg. She is diagnosed as preeclampsia and prophylactically started on magnesium sulfate.

a. What are the uses of magnesium sulfate in ED?
b. What are the toxicity features of the drug?

Q6. A 5-year-old boy presented to ED with accidental ingestion of paracetamol tablets.

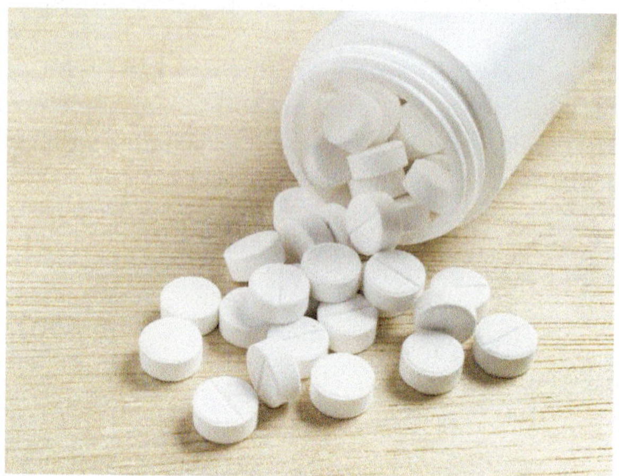

a. What is the mechanism of paracetamol toxicity?
b. Mention the features of toxicity.
c. Describe the mechanism of N-acetyl cysteine (NAC) as antidote.

Q7. A 40-year-old male presented to ED with severe ongoing chest pain. Diagnosed as ST elevation myocardial infarction and planned for primary percutaneous intervention.

a. What is the analgesic of choice for severe ongoing chest pain?
b. What is the mechanism of action of the drug?
c. What are the adverse reactions of the drug?

Q8. A 25-year-old male presented to ED with accidental injury to forehead laceration which needs to be sutured. After giving local anesthesia, patient complains of giddiness, visual disturbances, and circumoral numbness.

a. What could be the possible reason?
b. What is the maximum dosage of the drug to be administered?
c. What is the mechanism of action of the drug?
d. What is the treatment for toxicity and its mechanism?

Q9. A 36-year-old male patient presented to ED after fall from height and sustained head injury. Computed tomography (CT) brain shows intracranial bleed with cerebral edema. As antiedema measure, he is started on 3% NaCl.

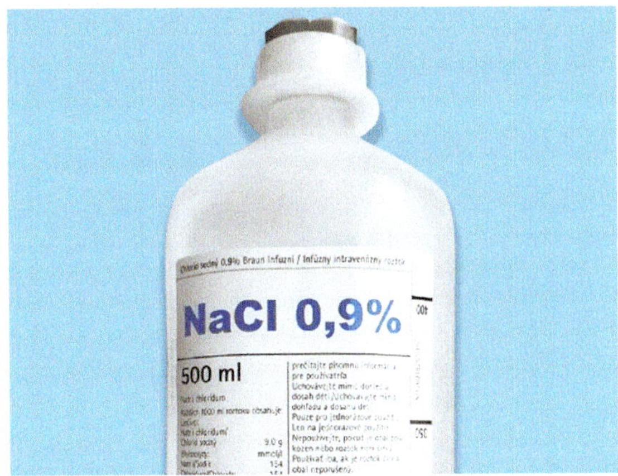

a. Mention the dosage of 3% saline to reduce intracranial pressure and in symptomatic hyponatremia.
b. What is the mechanism of action?
c. What are the precautions to be kept in mind while administering?

Q10. A 50-year-old female presented to ED with history of snake bite. Patient complains of weakness in limbs, difficulty in eye opening, and some breathing difficulty.

a. What is the drug to be initiated?
b. What is the dosage of the drug?
c. How much does one vial contain and how is it administered?
d. What venom does it neutralize?

Q11. You are handling a patient with seizures, now in postictal. There is some snoring sound heard and patient is postictal state.

a. How can you open up the airway and assist his breathing?
b. What is the contraindication for its usage?
c. How will you measure size of nasopharyngeal airway?
d. What are the complications of using nasopharyngeal airway?

Q12. You are transporting a road traffic accident (RTA) patient in ambulance, who is obese, and suspected head, and facial injury. You are in cannot intubate—cannot ventilate situation.

a. What is the airway of choice to maintain oxygenation?
b. What are the complications?
c. How to select the appropriate size?
d. What are the types?

Q13. Managing a patient with bowel obstruction in ED. You have inserted a nasogastric tube (NG).

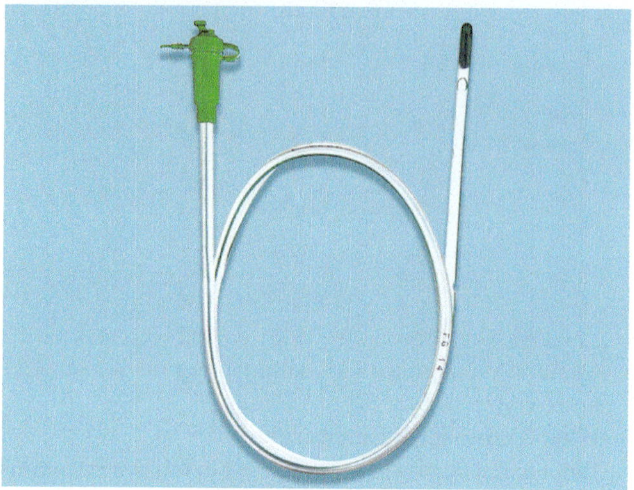

a. What are the indications for NG tube insertion in ED?
b. How do you confirm the position?
c. What can aid insertion of NG tube in intubated patients?

Q14. While admitting a patient to intensive care unit (ICU), you are advised to catheterize the patient to monitor the urine output.

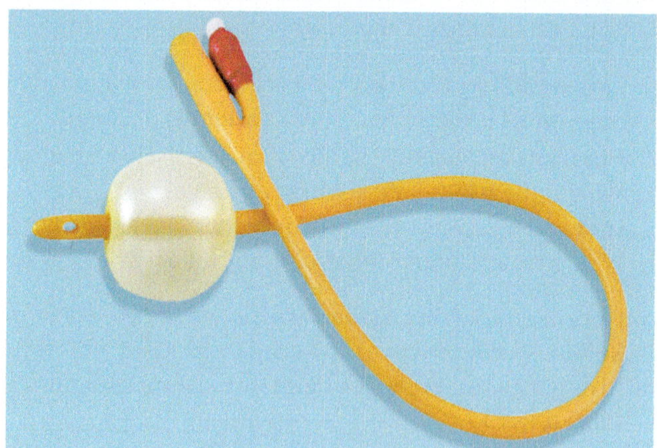

a. What is used to inflate the balloon after insertion?
b. Why in males the catheter must be fully inserted before inflating?
c. What are the types of urinary catheter?

Q15. A pediatric patient presented with acute gastroenteritis in severe shock—intravenous (IV) access could not be secured.

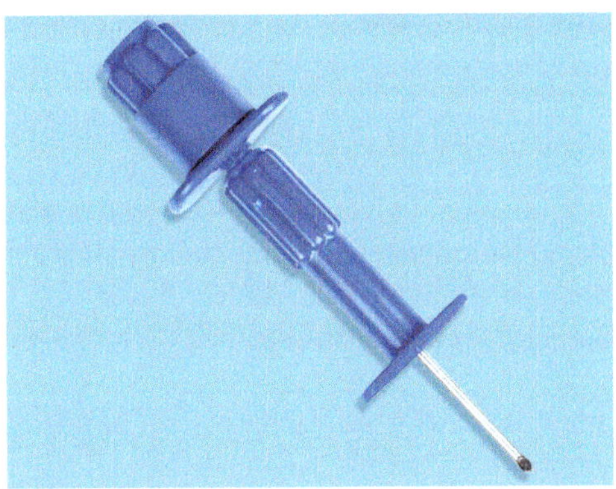

a. What is the next choice for volume resuscitation?
b. How can it be inserted?
c. How long can intraosseous (IO) access be used?
d. What medications can be given through IO access?

Q16. You are going to intubate a patient with RTA using direct laryngoscopy.

a. What are the types of laryngoscope blades used in ER?
b. What is the use of flange part of the laryngoscope?
c. Comment on classification of airway based on direct laryngoscopy.

ANSWERS

Ans. 1

a. Adrenaline acts on $\alpha 1$, $\beta 1$, and $\beta 2$ receptors
   - Indications in ER
   - Cardiac arrest
   - Anaphylaxis
   - Acute asthma exacerbations

b. Cardiogenic shock/vasodilatory shock
c. Angina, palpitations, arrhythmias, hypertension, nausea, headache, vomiting, and pulmonary edema

Ans. 2

a. Stimulates V1 receptor—vascular smooth muscle causing peripheral vasoconstriction—increases blood pressure → improves cerebral and cardiac perfusion; V2 receptor → acts on kidneys cause antidiuretic effect.

b. According to Surviving Sepsis guidelines 2021 for adults with septic shock on norepinephrine with inadequate mean arterial pressure levels, we suggest adding vasopressin instead of escalating the dose of norepinephrine.

Ans. 3

a. Adenosine is a rapid ultra-short-acting drug with half-life of <10 seconds.
b. It is always administered in left cubital—16/18 G cannula connected to 3-way cannula and administered rapidly followed by 20 mL saline chase over 1–2 seconds and limb is elevated immediately.
c. First dose—6 mg IV, Second dose—12 mg IV (can be repeated one more dose)
d. Chest discomfort, headache, flushing, nausea. Bronchospasm and atrial fibrillation can occur.

Ans. 4

a. Rocuronium
b. Dose 1.2 mg/kg (accepted range 0.9–1.2 mg/kg)
c. Sugammadex is a modified cyclodextrin antidote used for rapid reversal of rocuronium and vecuronium. Binds tightly to rocuronium in a 1:1 ratio, and this complex is excreted unchanged in the urine. This decreases free plasma concentration and establishes a concentration gradient for rocuronium to diffuse away from the neuromuscular junction back into circulation for further binding to free sugammadex.

Ans. 5

a. Uses of magnesium sulfate
   - Anticonvulsant effect
   - Preeclampsia and eclampsia, for prevention and treatment of life-threatening seizures
   - Bronchodilator effect
   - *Antiarrhythmic:* Torsades de pointes
b. *Toxicity features:* Muscle weakness, hyporeflexia, nausea/vomiting, hypoventilation, arrhythmia, neuromuscular paralysis, and coma.

Ans. 6

a. >95% conjugated by glucuronidation and sulfation. 5% undergoes metabolism via CYP2E1 pathway to form toxic metabolite NAPQI (N-acetyl-p-benzoquinone imine)
   NAPQI is irreversibly conjugated with sulfhydryl groups of glutathione.
b. Features of toxicity:
   - Nausea/vomiting
   - Abdominal pain
   - Hepatic failure
   - Renal failure (tubular necrosis)

- High anion gap metabolic acidosis
- Coma

c. Mechanism of action N-acetyl cysteine
- Increased glutathione availability (sulfhydryl donor)—glutathione substitute
- Direct binding to NAPQI
- Provision of inorganic sulfate
- Reduction of NAPQI back to paracetamol

Ans. 7

a. Morphine

b. *Mechanism of action:*
- Strong opioid agonist that acts mainly on mu receptor, as well as delta and kappa receptors
- Reduces presynaptic neurotransmission (especially glutamate)
- Central thalamic action and activation of descending inhibitory pain neurons

c. *Adverse reactions of drug:* Respiratory depression, nausea/vomiting, sedation, dysphoria, delirium, seizures, bradycardia, and hypotension

Ans. 8

a. *Lignocaine:* Local anesthetic toxicity

b. *Maximum dose:*
- 4 mg/kg plain
- 7 mg/kg with adrenaline

c. *Mechanism:* Class IB antiarrhythmic drug that shortens action potential duration; Blocks activated and inactivated Na channels with rapid kinetics

d. Lipid emulsion (20% intralipid) 1 mL/kg (over 1 minutes) q3min (repeated 3 times). Infusion 0.25 mL/kg/min

Lipid emulsion mechanism:
- Lipid sink model—draws lignocaine out of plasma
- May actually facilitate redistribution of lignocaine from target organs to fat stores
- It may overwhelm the inhibition of the translocase by mass action which increases myocardial energy supply

Ans. 9

a. *Symptomatic hyponatremia:* NaCl 3% 100 mL IV over 10 minute. May repeat up to three doses over 30 minutes. Intracranial hypertension—NaCl 3% 5 mL/kg IV bolus

b. Sodium is the principle extracellular cation. It functions in fluid and electrolyte balance. In turn, osmotic pressure control and water distribution are regulated.

c. *Precautions:* Concentrated solutions of IV sodium chloride (>1%) are irritants. The use of hypotonic saline solutions (e.g., sodium chloride 0.225%) may result in hemolysis if administered rapidly and for prolonged periods. Sodium toxicity [e.g., osmotic demyelination syndrome (ODS)] is almost exclusively related to how fast a sodium deficit is corrected; both rate and magnitude are extremely important.

Ans. 10

a. Antisnake venom (ASV)—polyvalent
b. Dose:
   - *Central nervous system (CNS) manifestations:* 10 vials given over 1 hour; 10 vials can be repeated after 2 hours if symptoms worsen
   - *Bleeding manifestations:* 10 vials given over 1 hour; 10 vials can be repeated after 6 hours if blood not clotting
c. One vial contains lyophilized powder which has to be mixed with 10 mL of distilled water administered in 5% dextrose over 1 hour.
d. Polyvalent ASV neutralizes venom of king cobra, krait, Russell's viper, and saw-scaled viper

Ans. 11

a. Head tilt chin lift with nasopharyngeal airway
b. Base of skull fracture
c. Nasopharyngeal airway of the correct size will extend from the tip of the nose to the tip of the earlobe.
d. Nasal injury/epistaxis

Ans. 12

a. Extraglottic airway device—laryngeal mask airway (LMA)
b. *Complications:*
   - Inability to ventilate (rare)
   - Inability to intubate
   - Aspiration
c. LMA insertion is weight based.
d. Intubating LMA and nonintubating LMA

Ans. 13

a. *Indications:* Decompression of stomach (e.g., obstruction or perforation), reduce incidence and risk of vomiting, monitor and evaluate upper gastrointestinal bleeding and gastric decontamination
b. Auscultation—for gush of air, X-ray confirmation
c. Magill's forceps

Ans. 14

a. Inflate the balloon with 10 mL of air or water
b. In males, any catheter must be fully inserted to the balloon inflating side-arm channel before it is safe to inflate the balloon. At the first egress of urine from the catheter, the balloon is just passing through the membranous urethra. The catheter balloon still has approximately 3–4 cm to go before clearing the bladder neck. Inflation of the Foley balloon at any point before full insertion of the catheter might result in iatrogenic urethral injury.
c. Indwelling catheter, intermittent catheter, and external (condom) catheter

Ans. 15

a. Intraosseous needle
b. Manual insertion and using devices—EZ-IO
c. Can be used until 24 hours
d. Adenosine, amiodarone, atropine, epinephrine, norepinephrine, dopamine, dobutamine, heparin, insulin, lidocaine, morphine, propofol, blood products, IV fluid (crystalloid, colloids, and Ringer's lactate), contrast

Ans. 16

a. *Miller*—straight blade, mostly for infants. *Macintosh*—curved blade, used for adults
b. Pushes tongue to the side and aids instrumentation
c. Cormack-Lehane classification

Resuscitation OSCE

Venugopalan PP

QUESTIONS

Q1. **A 38-year-old male was brought to the emergency department (ED) with a history of fever, palpitations, and chest discomfort that occurred after he went to sleep. He woke-up suddenly with agonal breathing and became unconscious. A bystander initiated cardiopulmonary resuscitation (CPR), and the patient regained consciousness within 5 minutes. The patient has a history of alcohol consumption and occasional cocaine use. Upon arrival, his initial vital signs were as follows:**

- **Heart rate (HR): 120 beats/min**
- **Blood pressure (BP): 98 mm Hg systolic**
- **Respiratory rate (RR): 28 breaths/min**
- **Temperature: 101.5°F**
- **Oxygen saturation (SpO_2): 94% in room air**

An ECG was performed and is provided below

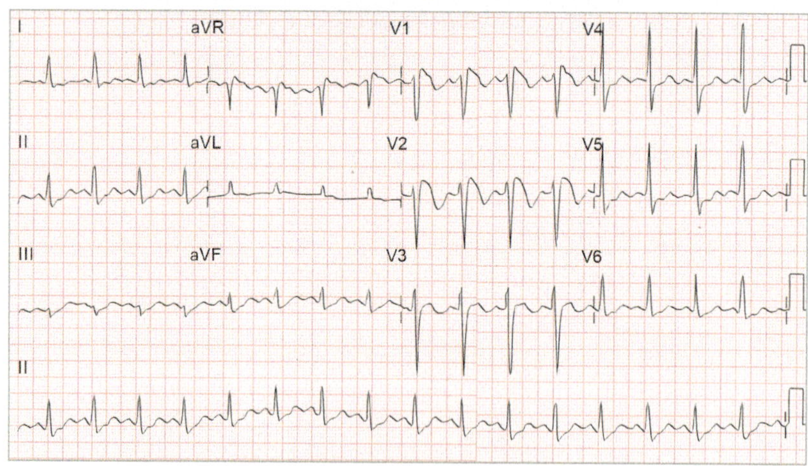

a. What are the changes seen in the ECG?
b. What is your diagnosis and differential diagnosis (DD)?
c. What are the provoking factors associated with the condition, and what are the preventive advice to the patient?

Q2. **A 56-year-old female with a history of chronic obstructive pulmonary disease (COPD), hypertension, and dyslipidemia, currently taking nicardipine, losartan, and ipratropium inhaler, underwent abdominal hysterectomy a couple of weeks ago. She presented to the ED with complaints of shortness of breath since the morning.**

Upon initial assessment, her vital signs were as follows:

- **Heart rate (HR): 140 beats/min**
- **Blood pressure (BP): 86 mm Hg systolic**
- **Respiratory rate (RR): 38 breaths/min**
- **Temperature: 98°F**
- **Oxygen saturation (SpO_2): 80% in room air**

An ED Echo was performed, and the image is provided below.

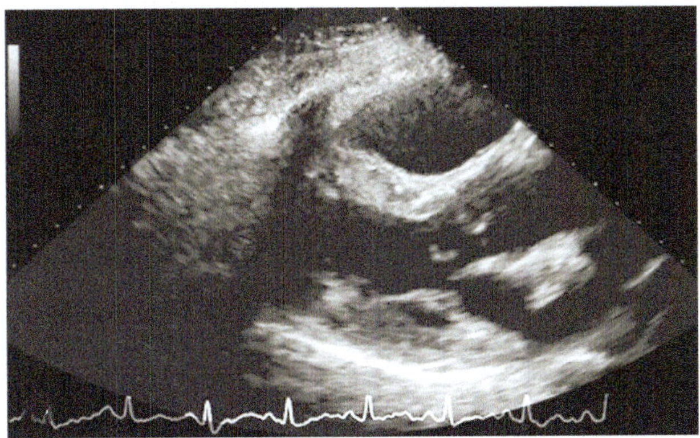

a. What is the initial management in ED?
b. What are the DDs and your possible diagnosis based on Echo?
c. What are the risk factors in this condition?
d. Enumerate treatment options.

Q3. **A 57-year-old male, known to have coronary artery disease (CAD) and diabetes mellitus, collapsed on a railway platform. A bystander initiated CPR. Meanwhile, emergency medical services (EMS) arrived with an automated external defibrillator (AED) and delivered a shock. Subsequently, return of spontaneous circulation (ROSC) attained with the first shock itself.**

a. What are the steps of AED operation?
b. AED is not automatic but automated. In which step does the automation work?
c. What are the special situations where AED use should be a special precaution?
d. What is meant by public access defibrillation (PAD)?

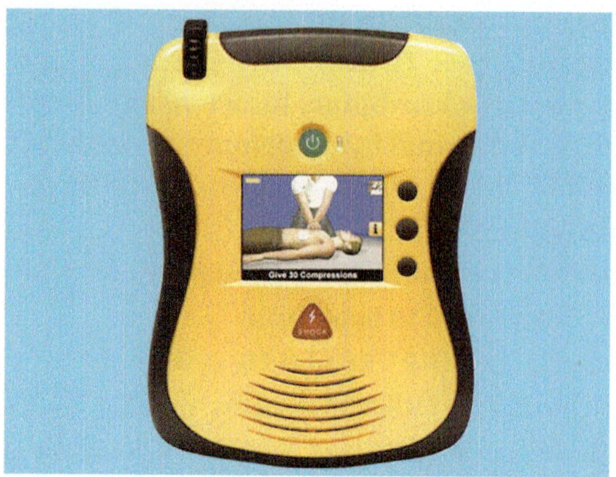

Q4. A 65-year-old male with a known history of rheumatic heart disease and mitral stenosis presented to the ED with complaints of palpitations, shortness of breath, light-headedness, and chest discomfort. On examination, he had an altered level of consciousness.

His initial vital signs were as follows:

- Heart rate (HR): 190 beats/min, irregular
- Blood pressure (BP): 88 mm Hg
- Respiratory rate (RR): 32 breaths/min
- Temperature: 98.4°F
- Oxygen saturation (SpO_2): 92% in room air

An ECG was performed and is provided below.

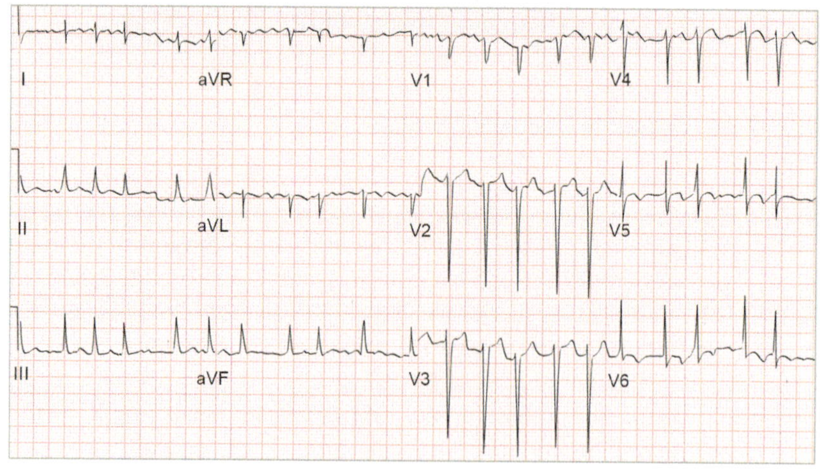

a. What are the findings of the ECG and what is your diagnosis?
b. How will you treat this patient in ED?
c. What are the management risks in this case?

Q5. A 28-year-old female presented to the ED with an altered level of consciousness, tachycardia, and tachypnea following an overdose of multiple drugs in a self-harm attempt. Her arterial blood gas (ABG) results show:

- **pH: 7.23**
- **PaO_2: 78 mm Hg**
- **$PaCO_2$: 28 mm Hg**
- **Base excess (BE): 26**

The consultant advised administering sodium bicarbonate to the patient

a. Mention the osmolality of this solution.

b. What is the class 1 indication of administrating sodium bicarbonate?

c. What is the class 3 indication of sodium bicarbonate?

d. Mention four complications of $NaHCO_2$.

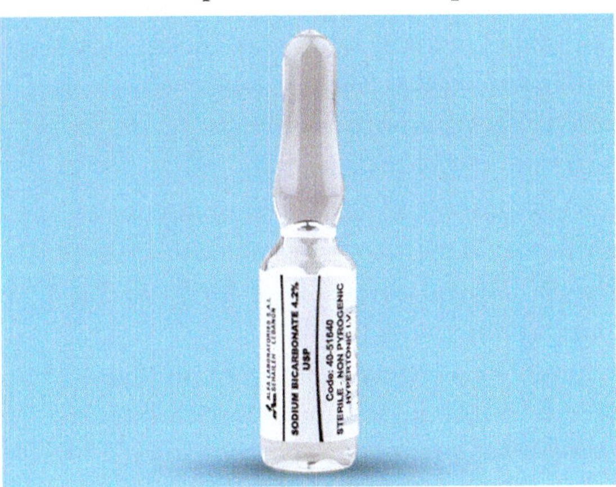

Q6. You are involved in the resuscitation of a 37-year-old male who was brought to the ED following a cardiac arrest, and you are following the advanced cardiac life support (ACLS) protocol. The initial rhythm was fine ventricular fibrillation, and you delivered two shocks and initiated CPR. However, the heart is still not responding, and you receive instructions to administer epinephrine to the patient.

a. What drug administration instructions should be given to your EMS assistant?

b. What is the mechanism of action of adrenaline in cardiac arrest scenario?

c. What are the "half-life" and "shelf life" of this drug?

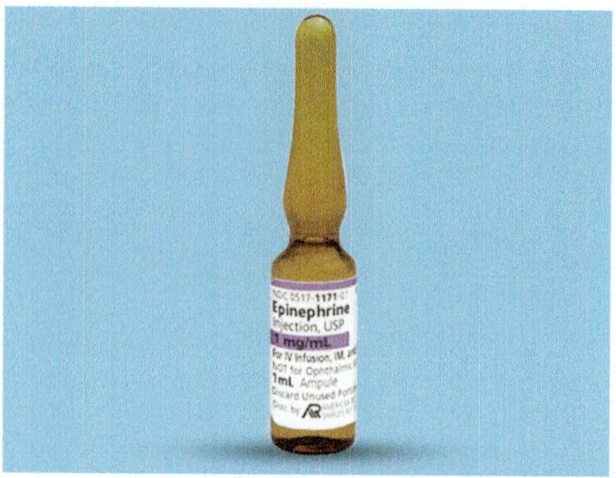

Q7. **A 28-year-old male, a nonhelmeted bike rider, was involved in an end-on collision with a truck. He was thrown from the bike and hit a tree by the roadside. He was brought to the ED in an unresponsive state with noisy breathing. Upon assessment, he was found to have sustained multiple injuries including faciomaxillary injuries (LeFort 2), a mandible fracture, and fractures of long bones.**

His initial vital signs were as follows:

- **Heart rate (HR): 130 beats/min**
- **Blood pressure (BP): 90 mm Hg systolic**
- **Respiratory rate (RR): 34 breaths/min (labored)**
- **Oxygen saturation (SpO_2): 85% on 15 L oxygen with nonrebreather mask (NRBM)**

The emergency physician attempted intubation; however, due to the severe facial and oral injuries with extensive bleeding, they were unable to visualize the vocal cords.

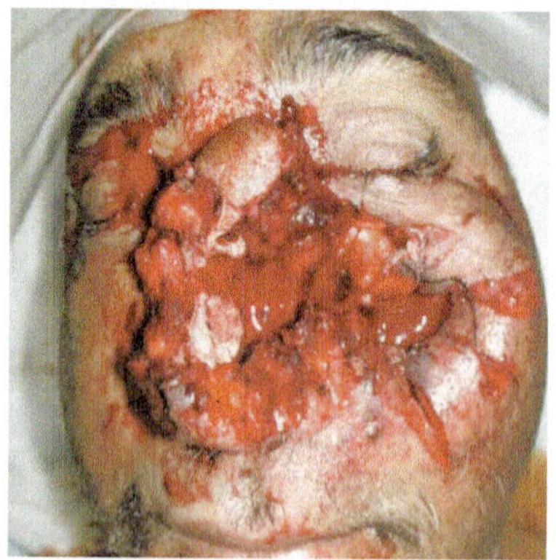

a. What are the airway management options in this case?

b. Explain steps of needle cricothyroidectomy.

Q8. **The EMS team transported a 58-year-old male from a peripheral hospital. The patient had a known history of COPD and diabetes and was experiencing shortness of breath. Upon arrival in the ED, the patient was on a (NRBM with 15 L/min oxygen flow. The patient was responsive to pressure stimuli.**

His initial vital signs in the ED were as follows:

- **Heart rate (HR): 68 beats/min**
- **Blood pressure (BP): 180/90 mm Hg**
- **Respiratory rate (RR): 32 breaths/min**
- **Temperature: 101°F**
- **Oxygen saturation (SpO_2): 100%**
- **Random blood sugar: 180 mg/dL**

An ABG analysis was performed with the following results:

- **pH: 7.2**
- **$PaCO_2$: 82 mm Hg**
- **PaO_2: 250 mm Hg**
- **Base excess (BE): -8 mEq/L**

a. Mention any four causes for COPD exacerbation.
b. Explain the reason for altered mental status.
c. What are next steps of management?

Q9. **You are attempting to resuscitate a 24-year-old female who has presented with an overdose. She is unresponsive and restless. You attempted to oxygenate with a bag valve mask (BVM) and initiated rapid sequence intubation (RSI). After multiple attempts at direct laryngoscopy, the vocal cords are not adequately visualized, making it difficult to maintain oxygenation with the BVM. You have decided to use a supraglottic airway device (SAD).**

a. Identify the SAD shown in the picture.
b. What are the advantages of this device over other SADs?
c. Explain how this device prevents air leaks upon insertion?
d. What is the disadvantage of this device?

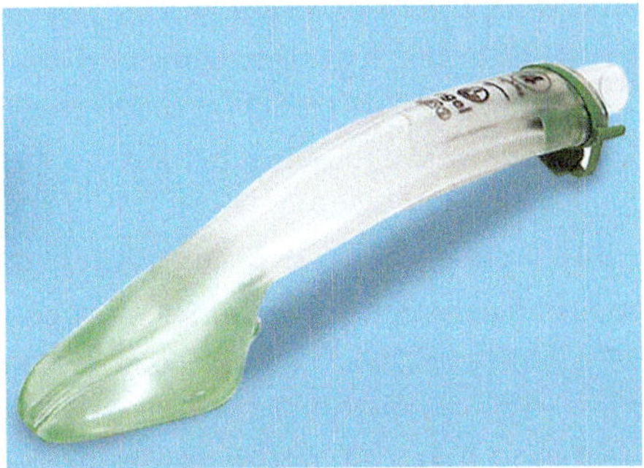

Q10. A 68-year-old male patient, known to have CAD and taking aspirin and clopidogrel, was brought to the ED following a road traffic accident. On arrival, he is speaking irrelevant words and only opens his eyes in response to pressure stimuli. When pressure is applied, he exhibits abnormal limb flexion. His right pupil is dilated and sluggishly reacting to light. His initial vital signs are HR 120 beats/min, BP 170/90 mm Hg, temperature 98.6°F, SpO_2 94% on room air, respiratory rate 32 breaths/min, and GRBS 140 mg/dL. His CT scan is shown below.

a. Calculate his Glasgow Coma Scale (GCS) score.
b. What is GCS-Pupil (GCS-P)? Calculate it for this patient.
c. How will you incorporate the patient's age and computed tomography (CT) findings, along with GCS, in the prediction of mortality and morbidity for this trauma victim?
d. Mention any four confounding factors in the GCS assessment.

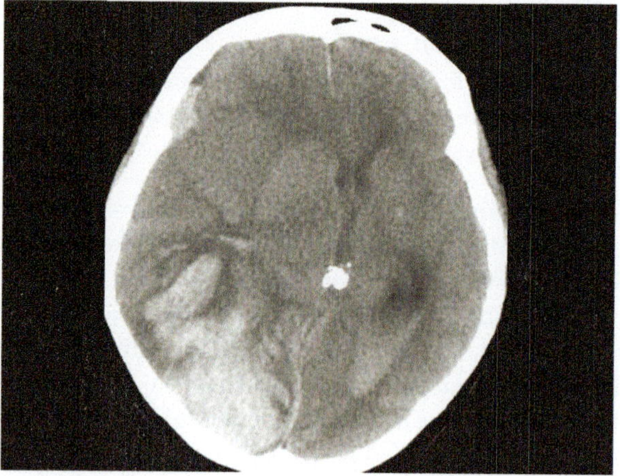

Q11. A 56-year-old male patient was brought to the ED following slurring of speech and facial deviation to the right side. He has difficulty standing up and is unable to lift his right arm. He is a known case of diabetes, hypertension, and dyslipidemia, but he has been irregular with his treatment. The entire event occurred 2 hours ago while he was having breakfast. On arrival, his vital signs are as follows: HR 78 beats/min, BP 210/120 mm Hg, RR 28 breaths/min, temperature 98.2°F, and GRBS 220 mg%.

a. Mention any three-stroke detection/assessment tools.
b. What is meant by the ASPECT score? Calculate it for this patient.
c. What are the management options for this patient?

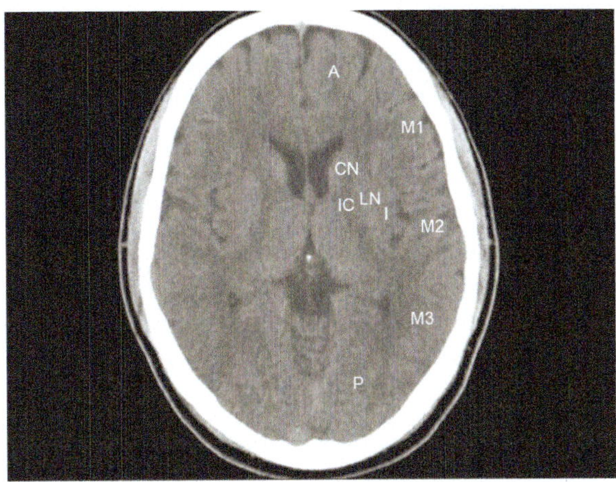

Q12. **A 13-year-old boy was brought to the ED with shortness of breath, tongue swelling, and wheezing. All of these symptoms occurred following his dinner at a restaurant where he had prawn dishes and some Chinese food. On arrival, he exhibited tachypnea and tachycardia with a blood pressure of 68 systolic. He is conscious but confused and has developed itchy rashes on his face, limbs, and trunk, which are progressing rapidly.**

a. Mention four DDs for an acutely swollen tongue.
b. What is the drug of choice for anaphylaxis? What is the dose?
c. What is meant by biphasic reaction in anaphylaxis?

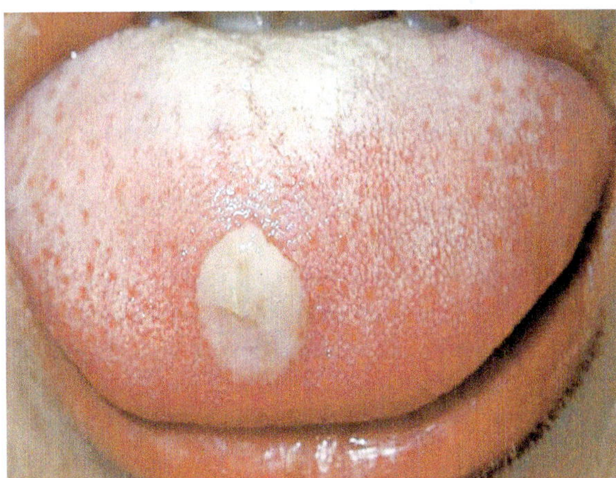

Q13. **A 25-year-old patient was brought to the ED by EMS following a road traffic accident. On arrival, he was making some sounds and only opened his eyes in response to deep pressure while**

withdrawing his limbs. His initial vitals were HR 135 beats/min, BP 82 mm Hg systolic, RR 36 breaths/min, and SpO_2 90% with 15 L of oxygen using a NRBM. You are planning to perform RSI and control the airway.

a. How will you assess the anatomic airway difficulties in this patient?
b. What physiological difficulties must you look for?
c. Which sedative/induction agents would you like to use?
d. What special precautions should be followed while intubating a patient with traumatic brain injury and raised intracranial pressure (ICP)?

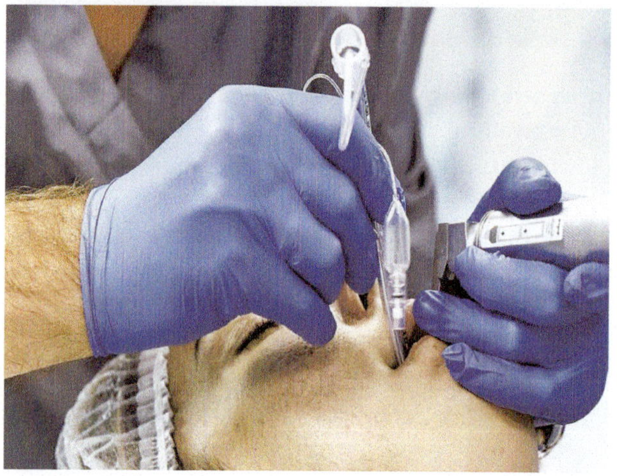

Q14. The patient shown in question 13 was intubated, and tube position was confirmed. You completed your primary survey and secondary survey, with possible injuries including traumatic brain injury, right-sided rib fractures, and a focused assessment with sonography in trauma (FAST)-positive result with a collection in Morrison's pouch. The patient became stable. The neurosurgeon was consulted, and he advised a CT head before review. You shifted the patient to CT on a transport ventilator. On the CT table, the patient's blood pressure fell to 70 mm Hg, SpO_2 dropped to 80% at FiO_2 of 1, and absent breath sounds were noted on the left side of the chest. The X-ray of the chest from the CT console is provided below.

a. What are the possibilities that you must rule out in a crashing patient on a ventilator during and after transport?
b. What are the steps of management in this case?

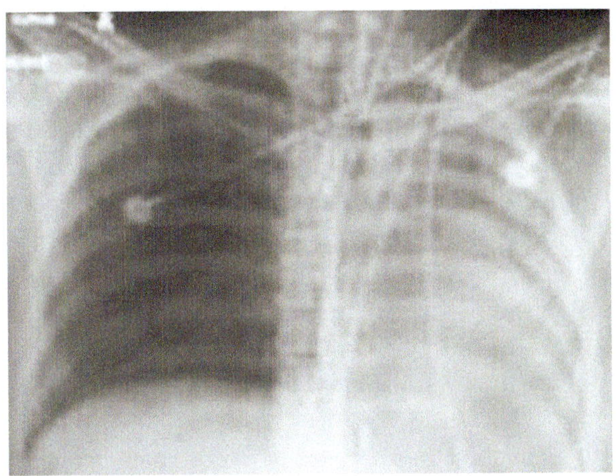

Q15. **You are resuscitating a 25-year-old female involved in a road traffic accident. She was a pillion rider, thrown out of the bike onto the road, and subsequently hit by a car, running over her hip on the same lane. On arrival, her HR is 140 beats/min, BP is 78/50 mm Hg, RR is 36 breaths/min, and SpO_2 is 90% on room air. You initiated the primary survey, inserted two large-bore intravenous (IV) cannulas, infused 1,000 ml of warmed saline, and activated the massive transfusion protocol (MTP). Her pelvic X-ray is provided below.**

a. What are the major immediate complications expected in this case?
b. Classify pelvic fractures.
c. Explain the steps of the MTP protocol practiced in your institution.

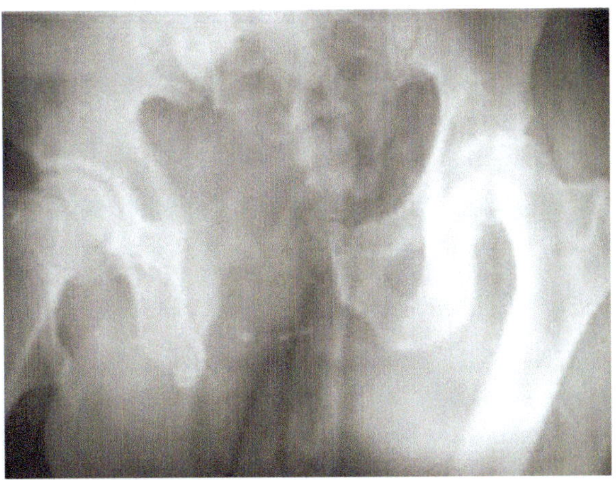

ANSWERS

Ans. 1

a. *Prominent J wave* down sloping ST-segment elevation in leads V1, V2, and V3 and QRS morphology resembling a right bundle branch block.
b. *Brugada syndrome:* Many of the conditions that may be mistaken for Brugada syndrome also cause syncope as a common symptom. A 12-lead ECG is important to evaluate for many of such diseases that may resemble Brugada syndrome. These diseases include QT prolongation, Wolff-Parkinson-White syndrome, pulmonary embolism, sick sinus syndrome, early repolarization syndrome, electrolyte abnormalities, and atrial fibrillation.
c. *Brugada syndrome is a genetic heart condition* characterized by abnormal electrical activity in the heart, which can lead to life-threatening arrhythmias, particularly ventricular fibrillation; several triggering factors can provoke arrhythmias in individuals with this condition. Fever, sodium channel blockers, antiarrhythmic drugs, excessive alcohol consumption, cocaine, and amphetamines can trigger arrhythmias in individuals with Brugada syndrome. In some cases, people with Brugada syndrome may receive an implantable cardioverter-defibrillator (ICD) to help manage the risk of sudden cardiac arrest.

Ans. 2

a. *Initial management* in ED includes primary survey and stabilizes the patient. Oxygen therapy should be initiated with Venturi mask in the view of COPD. Possible DDs are pulmonary embolism, acute coronary syndrome (ACS), acute exacerbation of COPD, and pneumothorax. Initial testing is focused on ruling out these.
b. *Echo shows* right ventricular (RV) dilatation, possibility of pulmonary embolism to be considered.
c. *Risk factors for pulmonary embolism:* Surgery (especially joint replacement surgery). Certain medical conditions including cancers, heart diseases, lung diseases, a broken hip or leg bone or other trauma, hormone-based medicines, pregnancy immobility, obesity, family history, and genetics changes.
d. *Treatment options: Anticoagulants*—heparin and warfarin; Thrombolytics—streptokinase, alteplase, and tenecteplase; Catheter-assisted thrombus removal; and Vena caval filter

Ans. 3

a. *Steps of AED operations:* A—Power on; B—Attach paddles; C—Analyze rhythm; D—Deliver shock

b. AED is not fully automatic. It recognizes a shockable rhythm. So, automation is required at either analyze rhythm or deliver shock. Press a button in these phases as equipment manual advices.
c. Special situation in which AED should be used with precaution, e.g., drowning, permanent pacemaker
d. PAD: A public access defibrillation (PAD) program aims to reduce deaths from sudden cardiac arrest in public places. PAD programs include AEDs placed in strategic locations to increase the likelihood of being nearby if someone is experiencing cardiac arrest. CPR and AED use are taught to trained employees and available for use by lay bystanders.

Ans. 4

a. The ECG rhythm strip shows variable RR intervals, tachycardia, and absent P wave, suggesting atrial fibrillation. Patient is a known case of rheumatic heart disease. Atrial fibrillation could be due to atrial enlargement.
b. This patient is unstable, has hypotension, and has an altered level of consciousness. The treatment of choice is electrical cardioversion. But always rule out the atrial clots. Do an Echo before cardioversion, preferably transesophageal echocardiography (TEE). If clots are there, start anticoagulation before cardioversion. Pharmacological cardioversion can be tried. Medication used for rate control β-blockers calcium channel blockers, digoxin, anticoagulants include warfarin, apixaban, dabigatran, edoxaban, and rivaroxaban.
c. *Complication:* Embolic stroke, atrial fibrillation (AF) with fast ventricular rhythm may lead to malignant arrhythmia and even cardiac arrest

Ans. 5

a. 2,000 mOsmol/L
b. Hyperkalemic and cardiac arrest
c. Hypercarbic acidosis
d. Tissue hypoxia due to shift of oxygen dissociation curve to left, venous irritation and phlebitis, intracellular acidosis, and intraventricular bleed in infants

Ans. 6

a. Dilute drug to 1/10,000 by adding 9 mL 0.9% NaCl, inject as bolus and administer the chaser 20 mL saline. Elevate limb to 90° to enhance the administration. Loudly tell that 1 mg epinephrine has been "given".
b. High-dose epinephrine in cardiac arrest acts through α-stimulation and results in intense peripheral vascular stimulation. The intense peripheral vasoconstriction leads to the preferential diversion of blood circulation to vital circulation like coronary and cerebral. Epinephrine may cause β-stimulation and the effectiveness and beneficial effect of this action is doubtful. The third action, epinephrine may convert a fine to coarse

ventricular fibrillation which is more amenable to defibrillation therapy. Parenterally administered, epinephrine has a rapid onset but a short duration of action fewer than 5 minutes. It is metabolized in the liver, kidneys, skeletal muscle, and mesenteric organs.

c. *Shelf life:* Limited evidence suggests that syringes filled with 1 mg/mL epinephrine are stable and sterile for 90 days. Prefilled syringes with the 1 mg/mL concentration most commonly used in anaphylaxis. More research is required for assessing its stability and sterility in different storage conditions.

Ans. 7

a. When facing a CICO (Cannot intubate, Cannot Oxygenate) scenario, the optimal choice is front-of-neck access (FONA). The utility of video laryngoscopy and fiber-optic intubation is not advisable in a crashing patient experiencing rapid desaturation and profuse bleeding in the airway.
b. *Needle cricothyroidotomy is* intended to provide a temporary measure to oxygenate the crashing patient, rather than being sustainable for an extended period. Position the patient supine. Extend the neck (except in trauma patients). Locate the cricoid cartilage and the cricothyroid membrane just above it. Take a 10-cc syringe loaded with normal saline and attach it to a wide-bore cannula (16G or 14G). Stabilize the trachea by holding the thyroid cartilage with your nondominant hand. Pierce the skin and advance the cannula-syringe assembly with negative pressure initially perpendicular to it. Once you enter the cricothyroid membrane, pierce it and confirm placement by aspiration of air. From this point onward, advance the cannula assembly caudally. Once it is fully inserted, remove the cannula stylet and connect the cannula to an oxygenation device.

Ans. 8

a. *Causes of COPD exacerbation:* Infection, pneumothorax, noncompliance of therapy, and nonsteroidal anti-inflammatory drug (NSAID)
b. The patient received high-flow oxygen therapy, which resulted in ventilatory suppression. In COPD patients, respiratory drive depends on hypoxia. Treating hypoxia can lead to hypoventilation, exacerbating preexisting carbon dioxide retention and leading to hypercapnia, which can cause narcosis.
c. An exacerbation of COPD is classically treated with titrated oxygen therapy using a Venturi mask. If the patient does not respond adequately to this treatment, biphasic positive airway pressure (BiPAP) ventilation support may be initiated. If the patient fails to improve with a BiPAP trial, invasive ventilation should be considered.

Ans. 9

a. An i-gel is a SAD that consists of a mask and a tube. It is used for general anesthesia with spontaneous ventilation or positive pressure ventilation. It is also used during CPR for short surgical procedures and as a conduit for endotracheal tube insertion.

b. I-gel is a simple device which is easy to insert without much of manipulations rapidly. It has a potential advantage of effective seal pressure which is less as compared to laryngeal mask airway (LMA) Proseal, but is enough to prevent aspiration and maintain effective ventilation and oxygenation.

c. Upon insertion, when the i-gel comes into contact with the pharyngeal mucosa, the noninflatable thermoplastic elastomer conforms to the mirror-imaged shape of the laryngeal inlet, effectively preventing air leaks.

d. I-gel is not a definitive airway. The potential for airway aspiration still exists. It will not be tolerated in patients with gag reflexes.

Ans. 10

a. The GCS is scored between 3 and 15, score 3 is considered worst and 15 is the best. GCS is based on three parameters: best eye response (E), best verbal response (V), and best motor response (M). In this case, patient is open eye on pressure/Pain - E2, producing inappropriate words -V3 and showing abnormal flexion M3, a total of 8/15.

b. *GCS-P:* Combine assessment of "conscious level" and "brainstem" function. The GCS-Pupils (GCS-P) score. The *pupil reactivity score* (PRS) **(Table 1)** summarizes information about loss of pupil reactivity to light and is calculated as follows. The GCS-P is calculated by subtracting the PRS from the GCS total score: *GCS-P = GCS – PRS.*

TABLE 1: Pupil reactivity score.

Pupils unreactive to light	*Pupil reactivity score*
Both pupils	2
One pupil	1
Neither pupil	0

c. Age and CT finding along with GCS-P will predict 30 days, 6-month mortality, and morbidity more precisely **(Table 2)**

TABLE 2: Numbers of abnormal findings and mortality.

Number of abnormalities	*Mortality rate*	*Favorable outcome*
0	10%	77%
1	24%	57%
2 or more	45%	38%

- *Age:* Outcome worsens progressively with increasing age
- *CT scan findings:* The severity of structural brain damage shown by the CT scan is categorized by the presence or absence of three main findings: a hematoma, subarachnoid hemorrhage, or absence of the basal cisterns. As the number of abnormal findings increases, mortality rises and the rate of favorable outcomes falls.

d. Confounding factors in assessing GCS are anesthesia drugs, alcohol intoxication, opioid or opioid overdose, stroke, and stroke mimics

Ans. 11

a. Stroke assessment tools—FAST (Face, Arm, Speech, Test), BE-FAST (Balance, Eyes, Face, Arm, Speech, Time), and NIHSS (National Institutes of Health Stroke Scale)
b. *ASPECT score: The Alberta stroke program early CT (ASPECT) score* 1 is a 10-point quantitative topographic CT scan score used for middle cerebral artery (MCA) stroke patients. It has also been adjusted for the posterior circulation. An ASPECT score ≤7 predicts a worse functional outcome at 3 months as well as symptomatic hemorrhage.
c. Revascularization therapy with tenecteplase or alteplase. Mechanical thrombectomy is another option.

Ans. 12

a. *Differential diagnosis:* Allergy, anaphylaxis, autoimmune disease—Sjögren's syndrome, hypothyroidism, lichen planus, trauma, vitamin deficiency like B_{12}, folate, yeast reaction
b. *Epinephrine is the drug of choice in acute anaphylaxis:* Start with 0.5 mg IM injection, repeat 2 or 3 times if not responding within 5–10 minutes. If patient is unstable give IV epinephrine 100 µg titrated doses or initiate IV infusion.
c. *A biphasic reaction* is the recurrence of anaphylaxis symptoms within 72 hours of the initial anaphylactic event, without reexposure to the trigger. Biphasic reactions are uncommon and unpredictable, and risk factors for biphasic reactions are poorly understood. Skin and mucosal symptoms occur in 90% of episodes. Respiratory symptoms and signs occur in up to 70% of episodes. Gastrointestinal (GI) symptoms such as nausea, vomiting, and diarrhea occur in 45% of episodes. Cardiovascular symptoms such as syncope, dizziness, and tachycardia can occur in 45% of episodes. The most significant risk factor for experiencing a biphasic anaphylactic reaction is a severe initial anaphylactic reaction or the need for >1 dose of epinephrine.

Ans. 13

a. *Airway assessment for anatomical difficulties:*
    - *Bag mask ventilation:* MOANS (Mask seal, Obstruction-Obesity, Age, No teeth, Stiffness and Snoring)

- *Intubation:* LEMON (Look externally, Examine 3-3-2 rule, Mallampati, Obstruction-Obesity, Neck stiffness)
- *SAD insertion:* RODS (Restricted mouth opening, Obstruction-Obesity, Disrupted or distorted anatomy, Stiff lung/cervical spine injury)
- *Front-of-neck airway (FONA):* SMART (Surgery, Mass or hematoma, Obstruction-Obesity, Radiation and Tumor)

b. *Physiological difficulties:* Hypoxia, hypotension, severe metabolic acidosis, right ventricular failure, and raised ICP

c. *Ketamine would be the first choice.* Cardiovascular stable—drugs like etomidate should also be considered.

d. *During RSI* in patients with raised ICP, it is crucial to avoid drugs and maneuver that could exacerbate existing ICP elevation. This includes management of hypoxia, hypotension, and hypercapnia during intubation. Maintaining normocapnia is essential for optimal outcomes. To optimize laryngoscopic response and minimize fasciculation due to succinylcholine, it is advisable to pretreat with LOD (Lignocaine, Opioids, and Defasciculating agents). Etomidate, propofol, thiopentone, and nowadays, ketamine, are recommended induction agents due to their favorable profiles in patients with raised ICP. During intubation, gentle maneuver is key. It is important to avoid multiple attempts, bucking, biting, and obstruction. By adhering to these principles, we can improve the safety and efficacy of intubation in patients with raised ICP.

Ans. 14

a. An intubated patient, if deteriorated like hypotension or drop in saturation at any point, must rule out the following DOPE (Displacement, Obstruction, Pneumothorax, and Equipment failure).

b. In this case, the X-ray indicates the absence of an air bronchogram on the right side with the tube appearing to be displaced more toward the right. Additionally, there is a homogenous opacity on the left side, suggesting possible right endobronchial tube displacement. Immediate management steps include increasing the oxygen flow to 100%. Auscultating the chest to assess for air entry. Ruling out a right pneumothorax. Adjust the tube position by withdrawing it in millimeters while auscultating the chest on the right side until equal air entry is heard on both sides. By following these steps, proper tube placement can be ensured, and any potential complications, such as pneumothorax, can be promptly addressed.

Ans. 15

a. The X-ray of the pelvis reveals an open book fracture, a severe injury that can result in significant blood loss, leading to hemorrhagic shock if not managed properly. This type of fracture involves a separation of the pubic symphysis and the sacroiliac joints, causing the pelvis to open up like a book. The open book fracture can lead to concealed blood loss, injury to internal organs located within the pelvic cavity. In males, this may include the urethra and bladder, while in females, it may involve the uterus and surrounding structures. Overall, prompt recognition and appropriate management of an open book fracture is crucial to prevent severe complications and ensure the best possible outcome for the patient. This typically involves early stabilization of the pelvis, aggressive fluid resuscitation, and prompt surgical intervention if indicated.

b. Pelvic fractures can be classified based on various criteria including mechanism of injury, stability, and specific fracture patterns. Here is a common classification system based on the fracture pattern:
   - Stable pelvic fractures
   - Unstable pelvic fractures
   - Complex pelvic fractures

c. A massive transfusion protocol (MTP) is a set of guidelines and procedures designed to rapidly provide blood products and manage coagulopathy in patients experiencing massive blood loss, typically due to trauma, major surgery, or obstetric hemorrhage. The goal of an MTP is to rapidly provide lifesaving blood products in a balanced manner to prevent or mitigate the consequences of massive hemorrhage, such as hypovolemic shock and coagulopathy. General outline of a typical MTP involves:
   - Activation criteria
   - Notification and communication
   - Blood product availability
   - Transfusion ratios
   - Coagulation monitoring
   - Temperature control
   - Continued assessment and adjustment
   - Documentation and quality improvement

6 CHAPTER

Cardiovascular Emergencies OSCE

Maitha Almazrouei, Omar Ghazanfar

QUESTIONS

Q1. **A 38-year-old male patient presents to the emergency department (ED) complaining of fever, chest pain, and shortness of breath with known history of IV drug abuse. Physical examination reveals a painful lesion as shown in image below.**

a. Name the clinical sign shown in the image.
b. Name two other clinical manifestations seen in this disease.
c. Mention two microorganisms which can be seen in this disease.

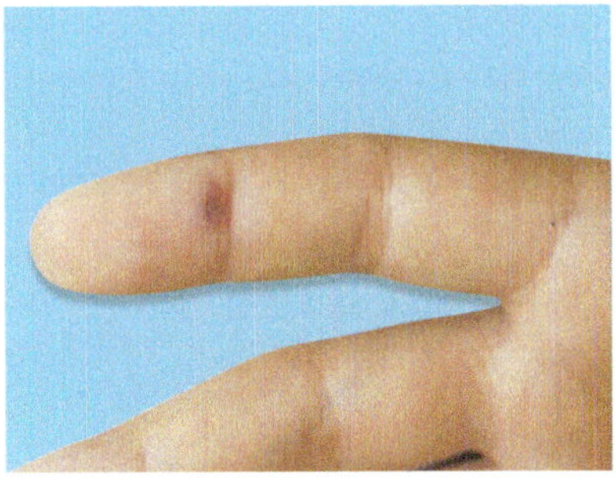

Q2. **A 25-year-old male presents to ED complaining of sharp left-sided chest pain and shortness of breath since last 1 day, the pain is worse on deep breathing. Past surgical history includes, recent left femur frature, post ORIF 3 weeks ago, chest X-ray shown below.**

a. Name the finding seen in the chest X-ray.
b. Mention three risk factors seen in this disease process.
c. Mention three abnormal physical findings seen in this disease.

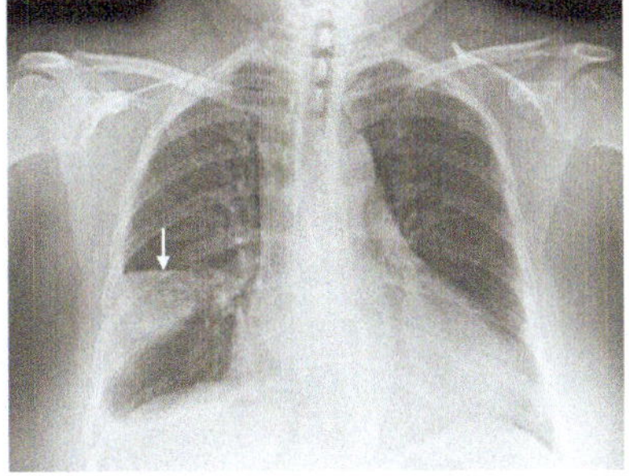

Q3. A 61-year-old male with history of hypertension and smoking presented to the ED with sudden onset of severe chest pain radiating to the back. Chest X-ray is shown in image below.

a. Describe the finding in (1) and (2) shown in the chest X-ray.
b. Mention two risk factors from this condition.
c. Outline the treatment option of this disease process.

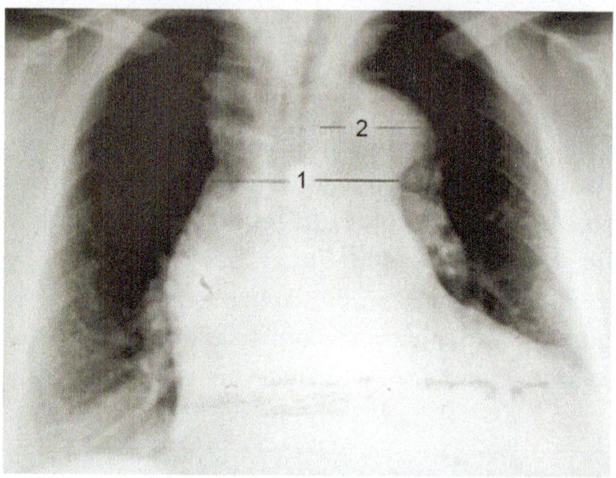

Q4. Mention the three indications for the procedure shown in this image.

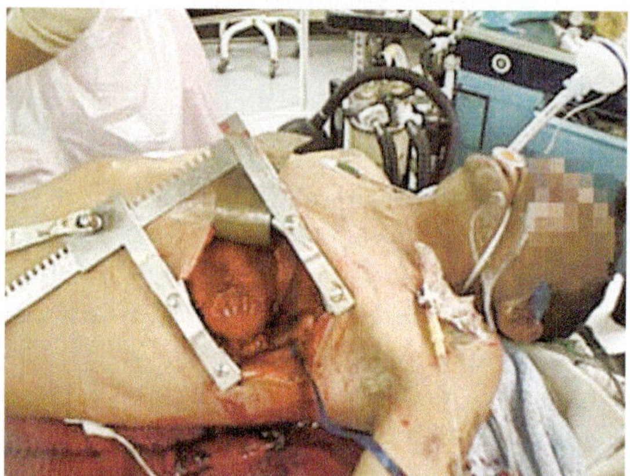

Q5. A 32-year-old male patient was brought to the ED after sustaining a gunshot wound in the midchest region. Bedside US image is shown in image below.

a. Name the view and describe the finding seen in this US image.
b. Outline the treatment done in the ED.
c. Mention the three elements of a triad that can be seen in this pathology.

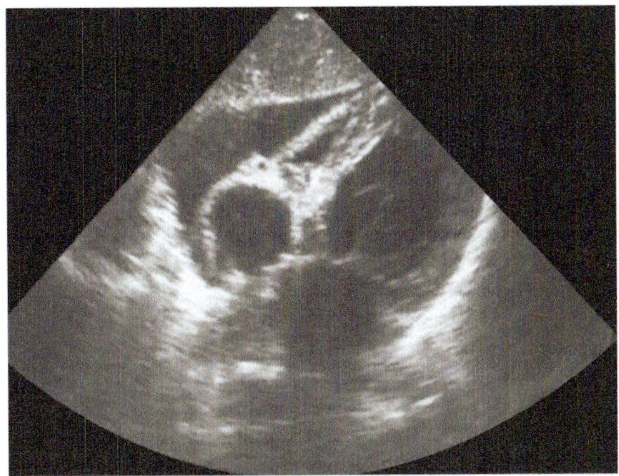

Q6. **A 65-year-old with a past medical history of hypertension and 30 pack-year smoking history is brought to the ED with a chief complaint of lower back pain.**

Vital signs are blood pressure (BP): 81/45 mm Hg, heart rate (HR): 112 beats/min, respiratory rate (RR): 22 breaths/min, O_2: 94% on room air (RA).

a. Describe the finding seen in the US.

b. Mention three risk factors of this condition.

c. Outline two treatment elements for this patient.

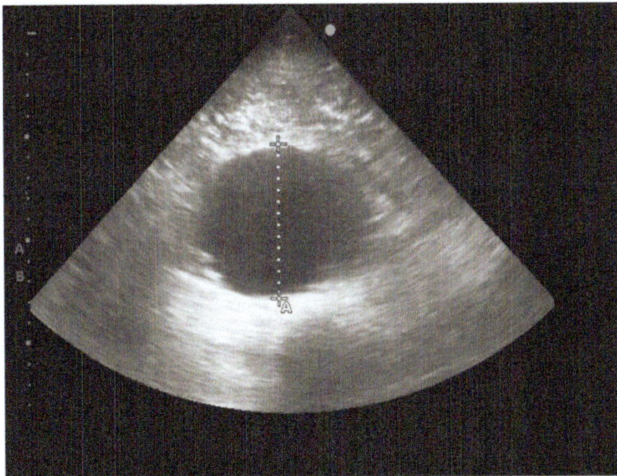

Q7. **A 55-year-old male presents to ED with history of chest pain, diaphoresis, shortness of breath, and orthopnea for 4 hours. Monitor was attached which shows vital signs: HR: 60 beats/min, RR: 22 breaths/min, BP: 97/60 mm Hg, O_2: 92% on RA. The ECG is shown in image below.**

a. Describe the finding seen in the ECG.
b. Mention one laboratory test you would send in the ED.
c. Outline the definitive therapy.

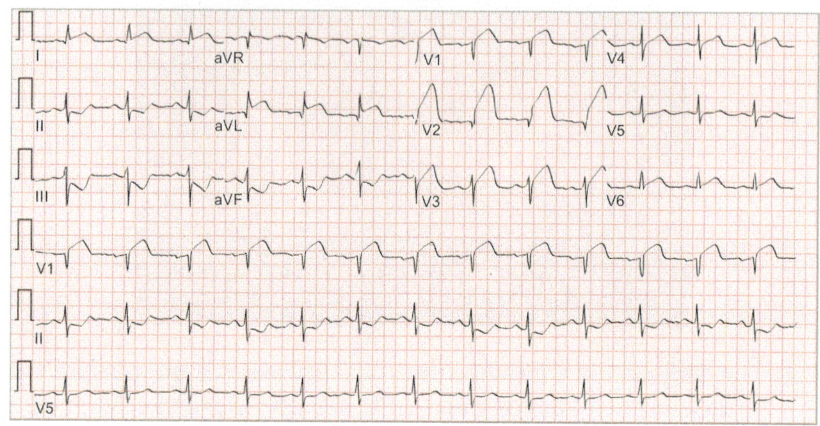

Q8. **A 1-week-old infant is brought to ED by his parents with complaint of central cyanosis. Oxygen saturation by pulse oximetry is 84% on maximal oxygen therapy, and chest X-ray is performed:**

a. Describe the finding seen in the chest X-ray.
b. Outline the drug treatment for this condition.

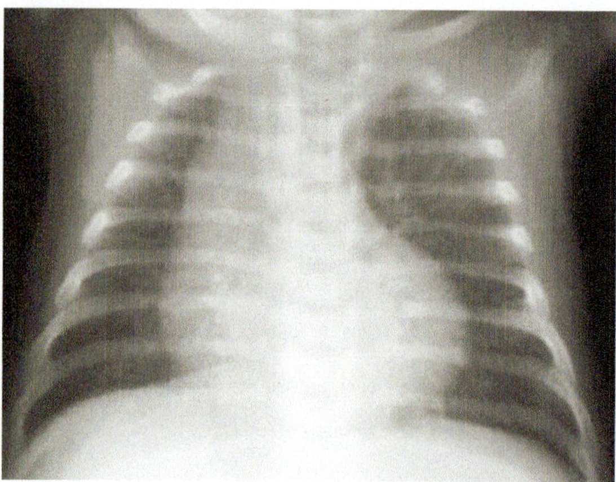

Q9. **A 55-year-old male presents to ED with long-standing hypertension and renal failure with complaints of generalized body and weakness fatigue. ECG is performed:**

a. Describe two findings seen in this ECG.
b. Outline the cause of his condition.
c. Mention three treatment options for this patient.

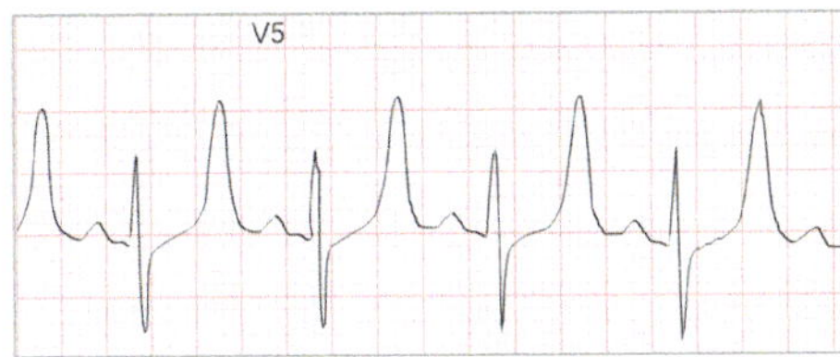

Q10. An 83-year-old man with previous coronary artery bypass grafting (CABG) and multiple percutaneous coronary interventions (PCIs) now presenting with breathlessness on exertion, three-pillow orthopnea, and bilateral lower limb edema. Interpret chest X-ray:

a. Describe the finding marked by the arrows in the chest X-ray.
b. Describe two other radiological findings.
c. Mention three treatment options for this patient.

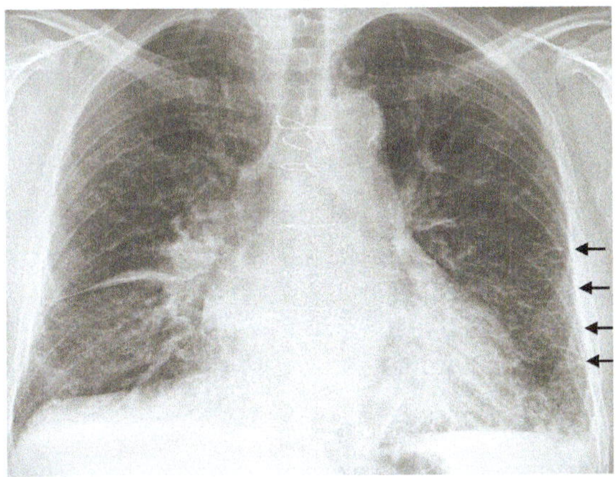

Q11. A 1-month-old infant is brought to ED by his parents with complaints of fast breathing and irritable difficulty feeding. His vital signs are RR: 56 breaths/min, BP: 90/60 mm Hg, and HR: 200 beats/min. His skin is pink and capillary refill is about 2 seconds. The ECG is shown below.

a. What is the diagnosis of this condition?
b. Mention two treatment options for this patient.

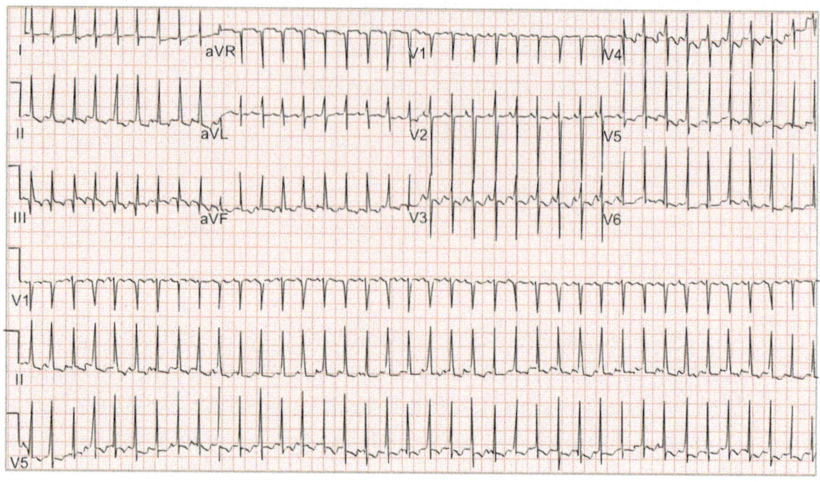

Q12. A 22-year-old male patient presents to the ED with complaints of palpitations 1 hour ago. The ECG is shown below.

a. Describe the finding seen in this ECG.

b. What is the management of this patient?

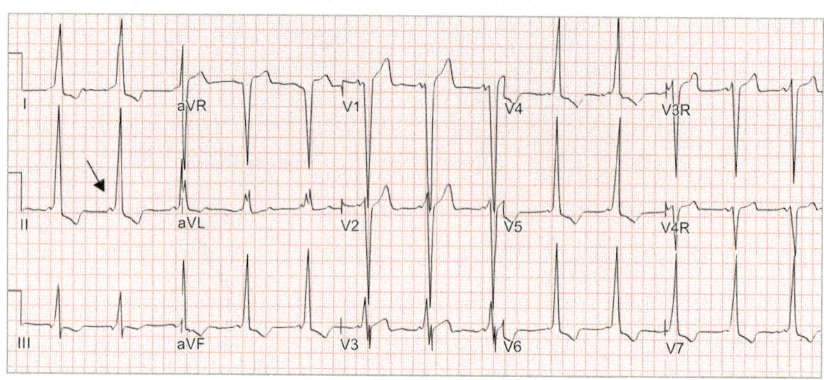

Q13. A 64-year-old female presents with lightheadedness in ED. No chest pain or shortness of breath.

Vital signs are HR: 170 beats/min, RR: 22 breaths/min, BP: 144/75 mm Hg, and O_2: 96% on RA.

a. Based on the case and ECG findings, what is the diagnosis of this condition?

b. Outline the treatment of this condition.

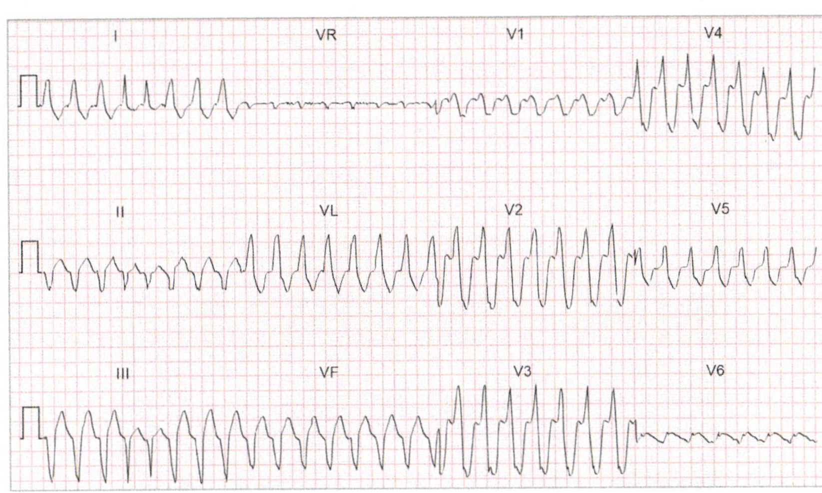

Q14. A 55-year-old male with past medical history of hypertension and type 2 diabetes presents to the ED with complaint of chest pain. The ECG is shown below.

a. Describe the ECG finding seen.

b. What is the anatomical distribution of this pathology?

c. Name the diagnosis.

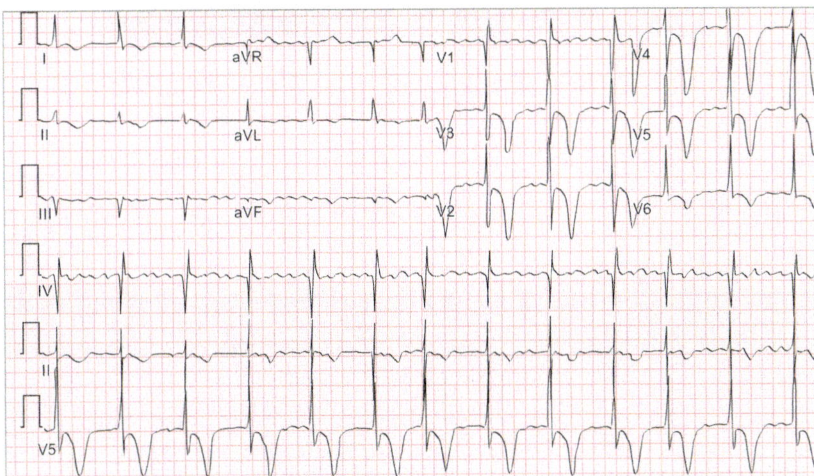

Q15. A 55-year-old male smoker presents to the ED with right-sided pleuritic chest pain, shortness of breath, and left leg pain without trauma.

Vital signs are RR: 24 bmp, P: 115 bmp, BP: 88/40 mm Hg, and SaO_2: 94% on 4 L by nasal cannula (NC).

A computed tomography (CT) lung scan is performed and reveals the image as shown below:

a. What is the name of a risk stratification tool that would help you in the diagnosis?
b. Mention two treatment options that can help in this disease process.

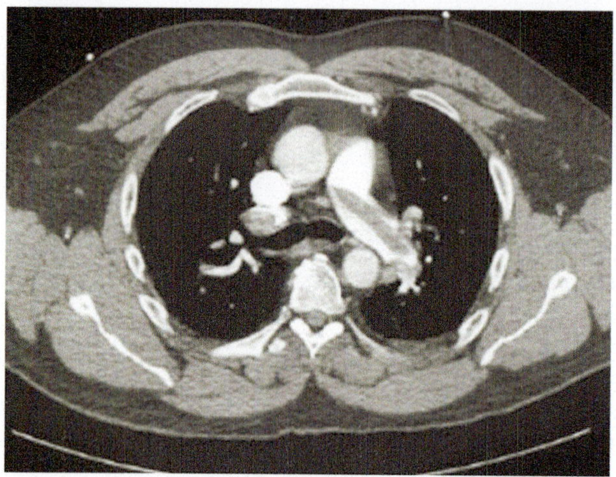

ANSWERS

Ans. 1

a. Osler's nodes
b. Other clinical manifestations are Janeway lesions, splinter hemorrhage, and Roth spots.
c. Two microorganisms for this this disease are *Staphylococcus aureus* and *Streptococcus viridans*.

Ans. 2

a. A Hampton's hump is seen in the right peripheral lower lung field. Hampton's hump represents focal intraparenchymal hemorrhage due to infarction of lung parenchyma. A peripheral, homogenous, wedge-shaped, and pleural-based opacity with the apex pointing to the hilum.
b. *Risk factors:* Active cancer, trauma/surgery within past 4 weeks, recent travel, deep vein thrombosis (DVT), prior pulmonary embolism (PE), and pregnancy.
c. *Physical signs:* Tachycardia, tachypnea, hypoxia, and unilateral leg swelling.

Ans. 3

a. (1) Widened mediastinum and (2) Prominent aortic knob
b. First connective tissue disease (Marfan and Ehlers-Danlos) and second patients older than 50 years with hypertension, bicuspid aortic valve, and pregnancy.
c. *Stanford type A dissection* involves the ascending and descending aorta and requires surgical repair. Aggressive blood pressure control and pulse control are needed to prevent on going dissection as surgical repair is planned.

Ans. 4

1. *Some indications:* Penetrating chest trauma with cardiac arrest and massive chest tube drainage
2. *Cardiac arrest following penetrating chest trauma:* Systolic blood pressure below 50 mm Hg after fluid resuscitation. Patient showing clinical signs of cardiac tamponade.
3. *Blunt trauma:* Cardiac arrest in the ED following blunt trauma of chest

Ans. 5

a. This subxiphoid view of the heart reveals a large pericardial fluid collection and compression of the right ventricle (RV) suggesting tamponade physiology.
b. Emergent pericardiocentesis
c. *Beck's triad:* Hypotension, muffled heart sounds, and jugular venous distension (JVD)

Ans. 6

a. An infrarenal abdominal aortic aneurysm (AAA), >5 cm around 7.47 cm in diameter.
b. Smoking, hypertension, male gender, family history, and dyslipidemia (DLP)
c. Resuscitate, transfuse blood products, and admit to operation room (OR) for surgical repair

Ans. 7

a. ST-segment elevation in the anterior lateral leads (V2-V6) acute ST myocardial infarction (STEMI)
b. High-sensitivity troponin
c. Immediate percutaneous transluminal coronary angioplasty

Ans. 8

a. X-ray chest showing enlarged, boot-shaped heart, consistent with tetralogy of Fallot.
b. *Treatment:* Prostaglandin E1; Stepwise approach should be adopted to manage tetralogy of Fallot; Oxygen, fluid resuscitation, morphine, and

α-agonist therapy. Neonates may be benefited by prostaglandin E1. The major adverse effects of prostaglandin E1 are apnea and hypotension.

Ans. 9

a. This patient's ECG showing peaked T waves, a widened QRS interval.
b. Hyperkalemia
c. Calcium gluconate, insulin and dextrose, albuterol, Kayexalate, and dialysis

Ans. 10

a. Kerley B lines
b. Cardiomegaly, dilated pulmonary blood vessels, and mild right pleural effusion
c. Supplemental oxygen, noninvasive ventilation, diuretics, digoxin, angiotensin-converting enzyme (ACE) inhibitors, and β-blockers

Ans. 11

a. Supraventricular tachycardia (SVT)
b. Carotid sinus massage for 30 seconds Valsalva maneuver. If fails to convert, use adenosine

Ans. 12

a. δ delta wave; Shortened PR interval, and a delayed QRS upstroke
b. *Admission and pacemaker placement:* Procainamide is the treatment of choice in stable antidromic or irregular tachycardias in Wolff-Parkinson-White (WPW) patients, while amiodarone is considered a second-line agent. Unstable patients require cardioversion.

Ans. 13

a. The ECG shows a wide-complex, regular tachycardia, which is ventricular tachycardia (VT).
b. Amiodarone, procainamide, or lidocaine may be used to treat stable VT. Although cardioversion may be necessary for patients with hemodynamic instability.

Ans. 14

a. The ECG showing deeply inverted T waves in the anterior leads
b. Anatomical distribution of this pathology corresponds to left anterior descending (LAD) artery distribution. When, these inverted T waves associated with unstable angina indicate stenosis of the proximal LAD.
c. Diagnosis—Wellens syndrome

Ans. 15

a. Wells criteria
b. Tissue plasminogen activator (tPA) and surgical or catheter-based embolectomy

7 CHAPTER Respiratory Emergencies OSCE

Bhawana Sharma

QUESTIONS

Q1. **A 12-year-old child was brought to the emergency department with coughing and signs of respiratory distress—tachypnea, dyspnea, choking sensation, grunting, labored breathing, hypoxic, and cyanosis. The history of accidental ingestion of kerosene was given by patient's parents. X-ray chest was provided to emergency physician for evaluation.**

a. Interpret the chest X-ray.

b. What is the management of kerosene ingestion?

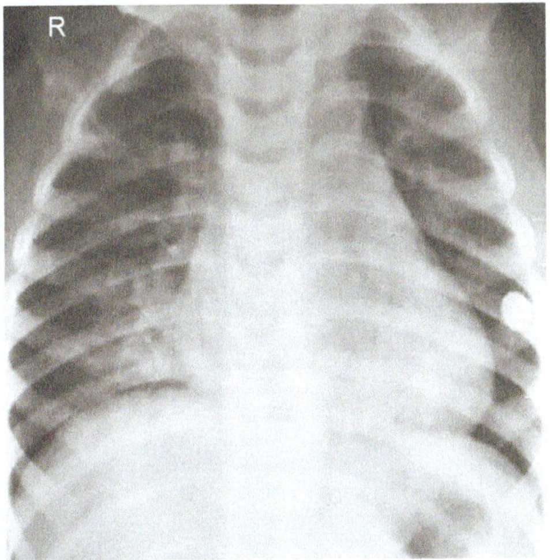

Q2. **A 52-year-old male patient was brought to the emergency department with hemoptysis-associated comorbid condition is type 2 diabetes mellitus. Patient gives history of prolonged fever (evening rise), productive cough, night sweats, weight loss, fatigue, and malaise. Chest X-ray provided to emergency physician for interpretation.**

a. Interpret chest X-ray.

b. What is the management of this condition?

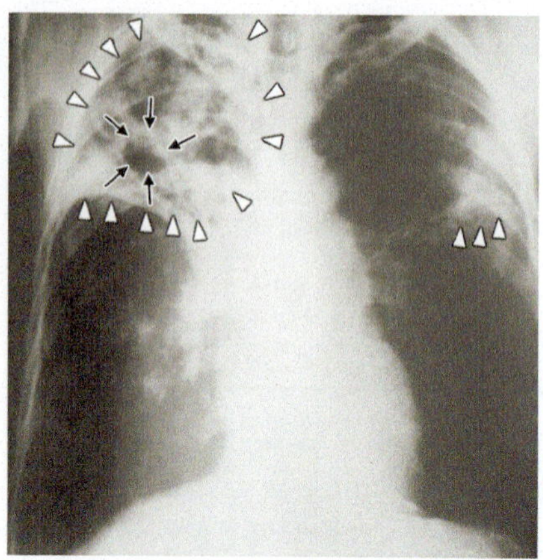

Q3. **A 28-year-old male was brought to the emergency department with chief complaints of severe shortness of breath, persistent cough, and fatigue. Patient gives history of hiking trip, where he ascended rapidly to an altitude of >11,000 feet without acclimatization. And symptoms develop soon after reaching the heights. Chest X-ray provided to emergency physician for interpretation.**

a. What is the provisional diagnosis on the basis of clinical presentation and chest X-ray?
b. Outline the management.

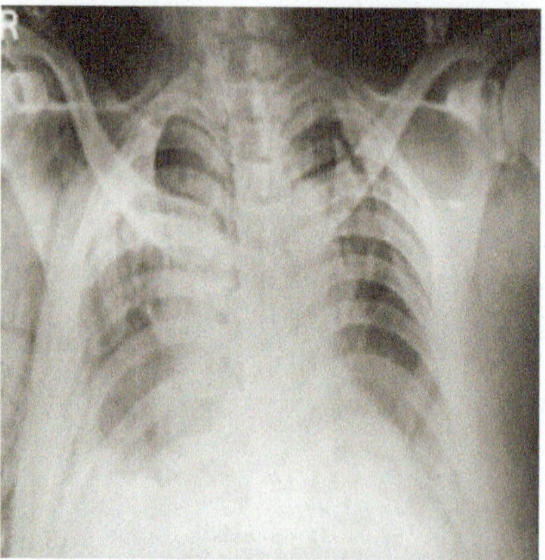

Q4. **A 65 years elderly male smoker with chronic obstructive lung disease presented to the emergency department with excessive coughing acute chest pain radiating to back. Examination of the patient reveals tachycardia and tachypnea. ECG shows sinus tachycardia and no ST-T changes. Troponin I result is negative and X-ray film is available for interpretation.**

a. Interpret the findings in X-ray chest mention the risk factor in this condition.
b. Outline the management of this condition.

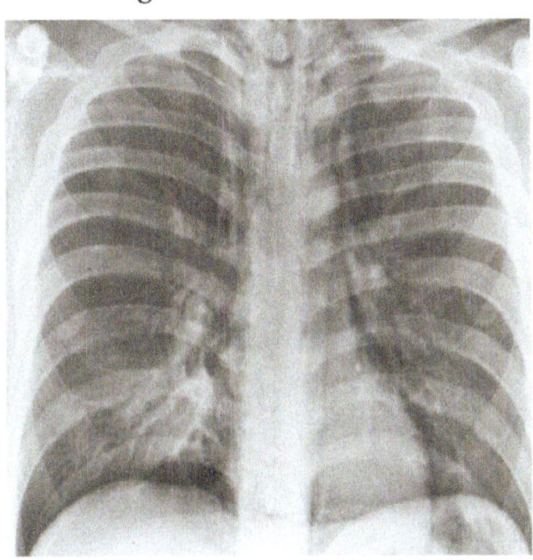

Q5. A 68 years elderly male presented to the emergency department with history of fever cough expectoration since last 4 days. Vital parameters are temperature 102°F, respiratory rate (RR): 30 breaths/min, heart rate (HR): 120 beats/min, and blood pressure (BP): 100/60 mm Hg. Patient looks drowsy, lethargic, and toxic. X-ray chest available for interpretation for emergency physician.

a. What is the interpretation of chest X-ray?
b. What are the relevant investigations?
c. Outline the initial management of the condition.

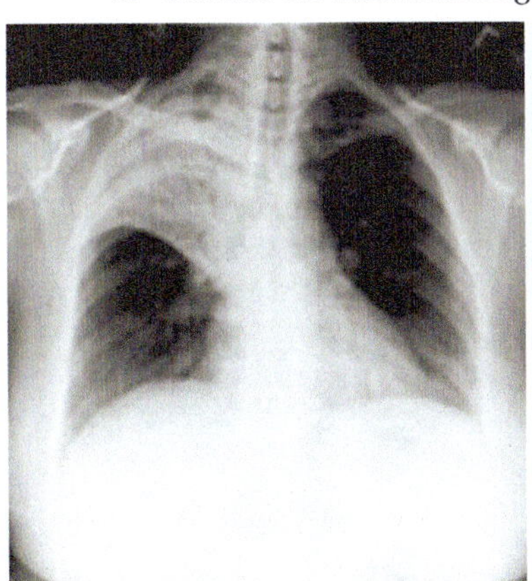

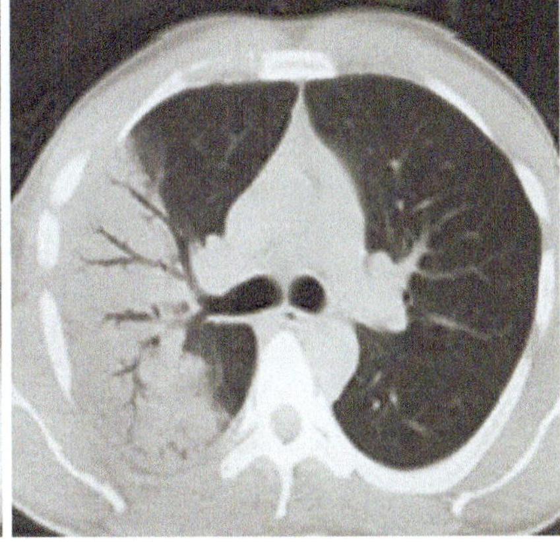

Q6. A 68-year-old male chronic smoker known history of chronic obstructive lung disease was brought to the emergency department with history of breathlessness. Initial saturation on presentation

is 86% on room air and oxygen therapy was initiated. Patient gave history of long air travel recently. Patient handed over the chest X-ray which was done in some other healthcare facility.

a. Interpret the X-ray finding.
b. What is the investigation for this situation?
c. Outline the management in brief.

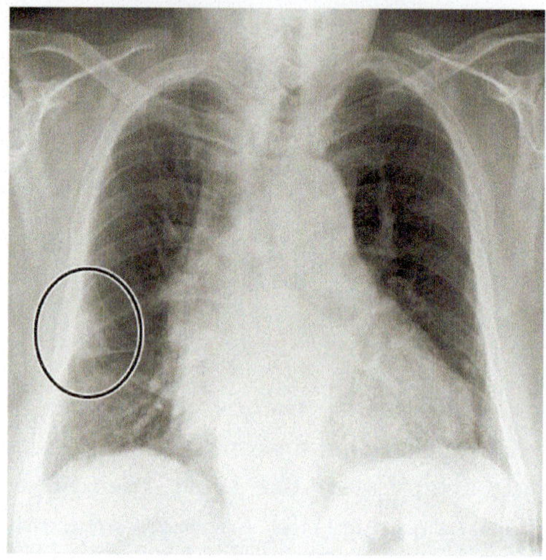

Q7. A paramedic transferring a hypoxic patient on 3 liters oxygen by nasal cannula, but patient became further hypoxic and saturation drops to 92%. Paramedic uses the device as shown in the figure to improve the oxygen saturation.

a. What is the device shown in the image?
b. Mention the uses.

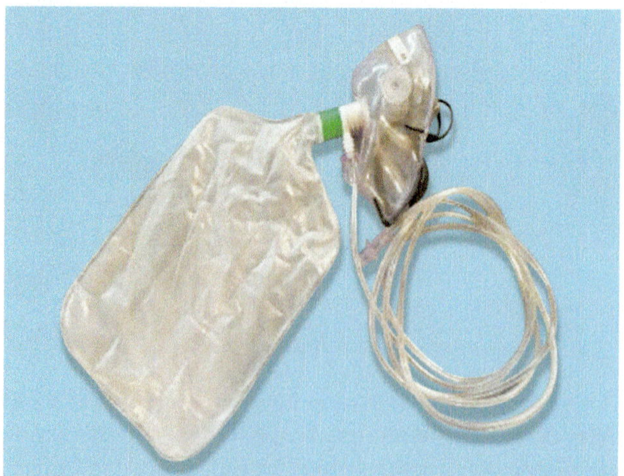

Q8. **With the above scenario, oxygen saturation did not improve after using the above device. Paramedic choose to use the below given device to improve the oxygen saturation.**

a. Identify the image.

b. Mention its uses and mechanism of action.

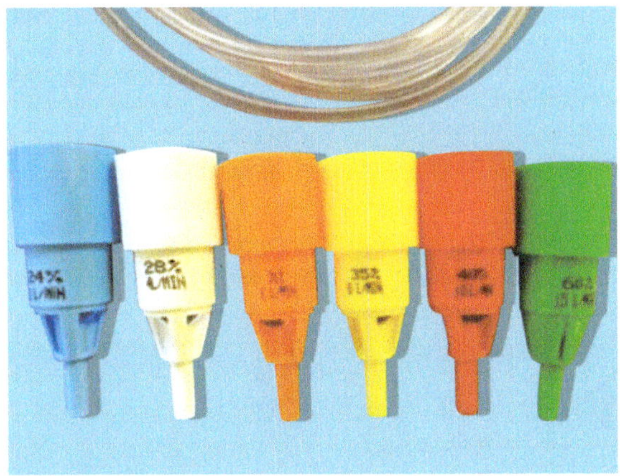

Q9. **A paramedic transferring the polytrauma patient with facial injury and low GCS and oral cavity is full of thick secretion and blood. He uses the suction cannula as shown in picture.**

a. Identify the equipment shown in the image.

b. List its uses.

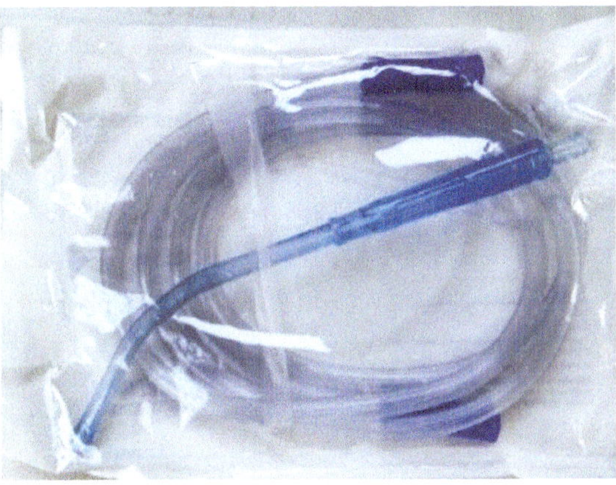

Q10. **A 21-year-old female was brought to the emergency department with sudden onset breathlessness with hypoxemia, tachypnea, tachycardia, accessory muscle use, wheezing, and impending respiratory arrest. She has a history of using bronchodilator intermittently and had been using since last 2–3 days regularly**

but her condition deteriorated. Emergency physician found few investigations performed previously.

a. What is the provisional diagnosis?
b. Interpret the investigation reports.
c. What is the management in emergency department for this condition?

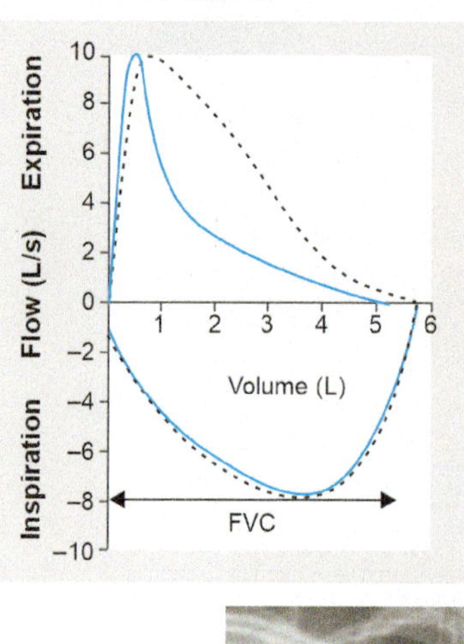

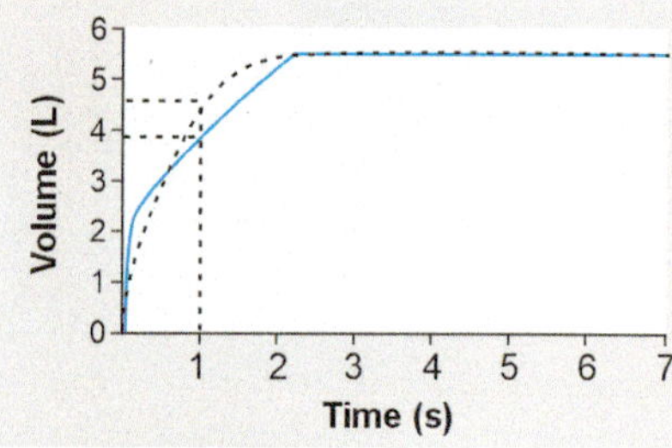

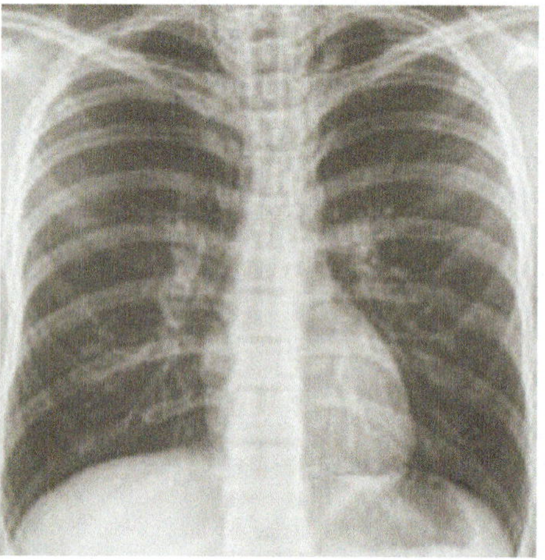

ANSWERS

Ans. 1

a. Aspiration pneumonia due to kerosene
b. Management of a patient of suspected hydrocarbon poisoning would depend upon the ingested or inhaled poison with associated organ involvement and radiological finding encountered. There is no specific antidote available for hydrocarbon poisoning.

- Start oxygen if the SpO_2 is <94% and get intravenous (IV) line secured.
- Begin with an assessment of the airway and need for airway management including the placement of advance airway.
- Any oral or oropharyngeal swelling, hoarseness of voice would warrant an early definitive airway. Assessment of breathing should include the rate, effort, respiratory distress, development of cyanosis, low SpO_2, noisy breathing, audible wheezes, and finding consistent with pneumothorax and consolidation. This would require oxygenation and ventilation.
- Nebulization with β-agonists, intercostal drain placement for pneumothorax, and prevention of secondary infection with use of appropriate antibiotics.
- Poisoning due to ingestion of hydrocarbons with no symptoms should not be lavage and activated charcoal use should be avoided as this could increase the risk of aspiration and pneumonitis.
- Early use of surfactant in aspiration could help in improving the oxygenation and prevent the development of pneumonitis in cases where the oxygen index is high.
- Use of corticosteroids not of much benefit in cases of hydrocarbon pneumonitis
- Management of pneumonitis along with respiratory distress would require mechanical ventilation.

Ans. 2

a. X-ray finding suggestive of pulmonary tuberculosis (PTB) include cavitary lesions that are most common in upper lobes. Chest X-ray showing fibrosis in upper lobes suggest old healed PTB. Prolonged fever (evening rise), productive cough, hemoptysis, night sweats, weight loss, fatigue, and malaise support the diagnosis.

b. A quick history and physical examination. Maintain airway, breathing, and circulation. All patients with massive hemoptysis must be monitored in intensive care unit (ICU).
   - Patency of the airway should be the first priority to prevent exsanguination. To achieve immediate control of the airway, patients should be intubated with large single lumen endotracheal tube for proper suctioning; it will also help in initial diagnostic and therapeutic bronchoscopy.
   - A large bore IV cannula or central venous line should be inserted, and IV fluid started. Intra-arterial catheter is necessary for more accurate monitoring of blood pressure. If the general condition of the patient is rapidly deteriorating, O-positive packed cell volume (in childbearing women O-negative) should be transfused while waiting for blood

grouping—crossmatching. Arterial blood gas (ABG) should be sent immediately.
- Multidetector computed tomography (MDCT) angiography is more useful in localizing the site, source of bleeding, and underlying lung pathology.
- The ideal time for bronchoscopy is controversial; however, general consensus is to perform it early in rapidly deteriorating patients, delayed bronchoscopy, that is within 24–48 hours of admission can be done in stable patients.
- On the basis of history, physical, and laboratory examination, specific therapy should be started to correct the cause.

Ans. 3

a. Provisional diagnosis, high-altitude pulmonary edema (HAPE)
b. Steps in management of this condition are:
   - Supplemental oxygen via portable oxygen concentrator or high-flow oxygen to alleviate hypoxia.
   - Noninvasive ventilation (NIV) or mechanical ventilation if required
   - Nifedipine, a calcium channel blocker to reduce pulmonary artery pressure
   - Corticosteroids may be considered to reduce inflammation.
   - Adequate bed rest to minimize physical exertion and reduce the workload on the heart and lungs
   - Adequate hydration

Ans. 4

a. Plain anterior chest film, suggestive of pneumomediastinum, showing lucent streaks, bubbles of air outlining mediastinal structures, and visible mediastinal pleura. Risk factors in this patient is smoking chronic obstructive pulmonary disease (COPD) and coughing.
b. Pneumomediastinum is generally known as a benign clinical condition with a good prognosis. Once the significant pathology is excluded, the pneumomediastinum treatment is directed toward symptom relief. After diagnosis, the patient can be hospitalized for next 24 hours for observation. Strict bed rest is advised with symptomatic treatment for pain. Antianxiety drugs and coughing suppressant, antitussives can be added. Oxygen administration should be added as this increases the gas absorption. Any underlying pathology such as asthma or COPD should be treated and controlled adequately.

Ans. 5

a. Consolidation, suggestive of typical pneumonia
b. Chest X-ray, computed tomography (CT) chest, microbiology—sputum Gram stain and cultures are advice for all admitted patients. The sputum

Gram stain is very useful for directing the choice of initial therapy but needs to be performed on a good quality sample and by a skilled microbiologist.

c. Assessment of the severity of illness is important for diagnostic and treatment decisions for pneumonia. To assess the severity of pneumonia, there are various scoring systems (CURB-65, CRB-65, SMART-COP, and ATS-IDSA criteria) which can help us to decide regarding admission (ICU or ward) and OPD management. The most used is CURB-65 [***C***onfusion, ***U***rea >7 mmol/L, ***R***espiratory rate >30 breaths/min, ***B***lood pressure (systolic <90 mm Hg or diastolic <60 mm Hg), Age >**65** years]. The first and foremost treatment of pneumonia is antibiotic but other supportive care also needs to be addressed like:
   - Antipyretics
   - Clear the airway.
   - Oxygen therapy if needed.
   - Adequate hydration and nutrition
   - Evaluate for ICU care
   - Need to be seen for requirement of ventilator (non-invasive or invasive)

Ans. 6

a. *Chest X-ray is suggestive of Hampton hump,* which is a wedge-shaped, pleural-based, apex central pulmonary opacity suggestive of pulmonary embolism (PE) that is uncommon and has a sensitivity and specificity of 22% and 82%.
b. *Investigations*
   - *D-dimer* is a fibrin degradation product that indicates the presence of intravascular fibrin deposition and is usually increased in thromboembolic disease.
   - Echocardiographic abnormalities are present in approximately 30–40% of patients with PE.
   - *CT pulmonary angiography* sensitivity for central clots is 100% and 90% for peripheral clots. It is 91% specific.
   - *V/Q scan:* A normal V/Q scan essentially rules out PE with an negative predictive value (NPV) of 97%. A high-probability scan has a positive predictive value of 85–90% with a sensitivity and specificity of 41% and 97%, respectively
   - *Compression ultrasonography (CUS)* can be used at various points in the investigation of PE.
   - *Pulmonary angiography* has long been considered the gold standard for the diagnosis of PE.

c. Management:
   - Systemic anticoagulation is the mainstay of the treatment for venous thromboembolism (DVT + PE). Unfractionated heparin and low molecular weight heparin (LMWH) are the two most common options.
   - Percutaneous mechanical thrombectomy by interventional radiology
   - Surgical thrombectomy

Ans. 7

a. Nonrebreathing mask
b. Do not permit mixing of exhaled gases with fresh gas supplied. The remaining exhaled air exits through vents. The presence of one-way valve ensures a fresh oxygen supply with minimal dilution from the entrainment of room air. It provides a higher FiO_2 than partial rebreathing mask provided the mask fits correctly. Minimum flow rate required is 10 L/min. Delivered FiO_2 of this system is 60–80% at flow rates of 12–15 L/min.

Ans. 8

a. Venturi device
b. Oxygen concentration is determined by the Venturi principle: oxygen passing through a small orifice entrains air to a predictable dilution. The Venturi principle depends on the Bernoulli's effect. When fluid flows through a narrow constriction, it accelerates gaining kinetic energy from the surrounding potential energy; thus a negative pressure surrounding it is created which entrains the surrounding fluid through the constriction. The FiO_2 is adjusted by changing the Venturi "valve" and setting the appropriate oxygen flow rate. The larger orifice results in the system behaving like a simple mask. However, a fixed delivery system is possible at a lower FiO_2, higher the FiO_2 required, lower the oxygen flow rate. The correct flow rate/FiO_2 of oxygen is varying with specific color of mask and written on the mask.
   - *Blue:* 2–4 L/min oxygen 24% FiO_2
   - *White:* 4–6 L/min oxygen 28% FiO_2
   - *Yellow:* 8–10 L/min oxygen 35% FiO_2
   - *Red:* 10–12 L/min oxygen 40% FiO_2
   - *Green:* 12–15 L/min oxygen 60% FiO_2

Ans. 9

a. Yankauer suction cannula
b. The upper airway may be obstructed by material in the airway such as blood, blood clots, vomitus, foreign bodies, etc. In such situations, it is Imperative to remove the material from the oropharynx. This requires a properly functioning suction usually with a Yankauer cannula. In case the material is very thick and viscid, it may have to be removed by detaching the tip of the suction cannula and using the tubing directly.

Ans. 10

a. Status asthmaticus; Status asthmaticus *or acute severe asthma (FEV1 or PEFR <25% of predicted)* is clinically characterized by hypoxemia, tachypnea, tachycardia, accessory muscle use, wheezing, impending respiratory arrest, and usual dose of bronchodilators and steroid does not improve the clinical conditions.

b. *Spirometry suggestive of restrictive lung disease:* Chest X-ray hyperinflated lung fields, and marked air bronchogram

c. Management of status asthmaticus:
   - Magnesium—1-2 g IV over 30 minutes. Nebulized magnesium is also added along with aggressive bronchodilators and inhaled corticosteroid therapy and effective in improving the pulmonary functions. Doses for nebulization magnesium sulfate 95 mg in four divided doses 20 minutes apart.
   - If the patient's condition further deteriorates (persistent respiratory distress, inability to maintain oxygen level above 90%, persistent hypercapnia, abnormal ABG -PaO_2 <60 mm Hg and/or $PaCO_2$ >60 mm Hg, alteration of mental status, acute confusion, and drowsiness) even after abovesaid measures then he can be shifted to ICU and noninvasive positive pressure (NIV) should be tried.
   - Nasal intermittent positive pressure ventilation (NIPPV) is the most popular mode of providing NIV in combination with continuous positive airway pressure (CPAP) with pressure support ventilation (PSV)
   - Mechanical ventilation: Intubation can be considered in patients with the following:
     - *NIV failure:* Worsening of ABG and/or pH in 1-2 hours; lack of improvement in ABG and/or pH after 4 hours.
     - *Severe acidosis* (pH <7.25) and hypercapnia ($PaCO_2$ >60 mm Hg).
     - *Tachypnea* >35 breaths/minute
     - *Other complications:* Metabolic abnormalities, sepsis, pneumonia, PE, barotrauma, and massive pleural effusion

CHAPTER 8 Gastrointestinal Emergencies OSCE

AN Venkatesh

QUESTIONS

Q1. Mr Ramesh is a 45-year-old male presented with worsening abdominal pain. His heart rate (HR) is 96 bpm, respiratory rate (RR): 16 breaths/min, afebrile, and blood pressure (BP): 136/82 mm Hg. On examination, he is pale and jaundiced.

a. Name at least three other general inspection findings noted in chronic alcoholic liver disease patients.

b. Patient is also noted to have clubbing. What are abdominal causes for clubbing?

c. Name three features to distinguish between spleen and kidney.

Q2. A 56-year-old male presented to the emergency room (ER) with history of vomiting fresh blood. He is conscious and oriented. He has been started on oxygen with facemask. He has IV cannula. He has a history of esophageal varices. His vitals are HR: 128 bpm, RR: 2 breaths/min, SpO_2: 98%, glucose random blood sugar (GRBS): 106 mg/dL, and BP: 86/44 mm Hg.

a. List the next three important steps in immediate management of this patient.

b. List four features specific to examination of hand that would suggest chronic liver disease.

c. Name scoring system which is used to risk stratify patients with upper gastrointestinal (GI) bleed.

Q3. A 36-year-old female presents to ER with history of having taken 15 paracetamol 650 mg tablets yesterday. Her liver functions show deranged liver function tests (LFTs). She is diagnosed as having acute liver failure due to paracetamol poisoning.

a. List at least three other idiosyncratic drug reactions causing this presentation.

b. Name some illicit drugs causing acute liver failure.

c. Name complications of pregnancy causing acute liver failure.

Q4. A 52-year-old male who is known to have alcoholic liver disease presents to ER with history of confusion and irrelevant talk.

a. List clinical features of hepatic encephalopathy.
b. List components of Child–Pugh grading of liver disease.
c. What is Wernicke's encephalopathy triad?

Q5. A 42-year-old male, who has been drinking almost one bottle of alcohol every day, has been brought to ER by his family as he has not been drinking for last 3–4 days. Since today morning, he has become agitated, confused, and disoriented. You also note that he is tachycardic also having tactile hallucinations.

a. What is the diagnosis?
b. What is ER management of this patient?
c. Your junior doctor asks you, as the patient is currently not having any seizures and maintaining his airway, what fluids to start first?

Q6. A 6-year-old boy is brought in the ER by his parents with a history of right lower abdominal pain, vomiting, and refusing any food since today morning. On examination, he is having right lower abdominal tenderness, HR: 110 bpm, temperature: 99.6, and dry tongue. His growth and development has been unremarkable. He is up to date with his immunization.

a. What is most possible diagnosis?
b. What is scoring system used to aid in the diagnosis of this condition? List the components.
c. What is immediate ER management of this patient?

Q7. A 36-year-old man presents with a 5-hour history of severe epigastric pain radiating to his back. He has vomited numerous times since the onset of the pain. He has no significant past medical history and is taking no regular medication.

a. What is the diagnosis?
b. What are common causes of this condition?
c. Give one biochemical marker and radiological test which would help in diagnosis?

Q8. A 75-year-old lady presents with acute abdominal pain which started after 15 minutes after her lunch. Pain is central, aching to gripping type of pain. She has also has two episodes of vomiting. She also gives history of passing fresh blood in stool. Her HR is 110 bpm irregular, RR: 20 bpm, SaO_2: 94%, afebrile. On examination, she has diffuse abdominal tenderness. She has had analgesia with no relief.

a. What is most likely diagnosis?
b. Which is most common anatomical location of above?
c. What is immediate ER management of this patient?

Q9. A 3-month-old child was brought in the ER by her parents with history of intermittent abdominal pain since yesterday evening, vomiting, and right upper abdominal pain. They also inform about fresh blood in stool since this morning. They have got an X-ray done. Child is currently quiet, refusing any feeds, dry mucosa, and afebrile. You discuss with pediatrician who ask for USG abdomen. You get a USG done which shows in the below image.

a. What is the diagnosis?
b. What is the most common anatomical location of this condition?
c. What is the investigation of choice for this condition?

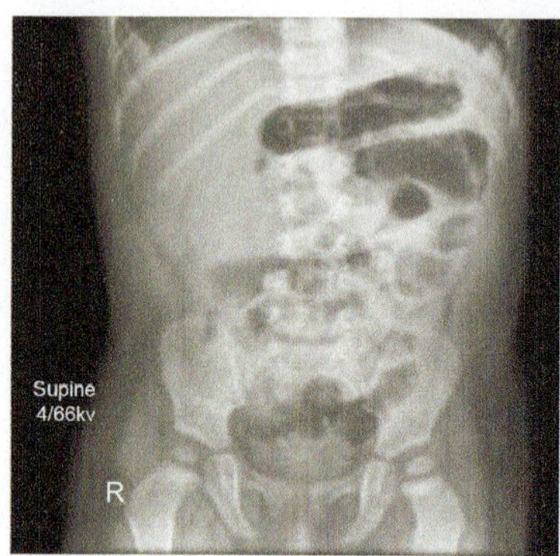

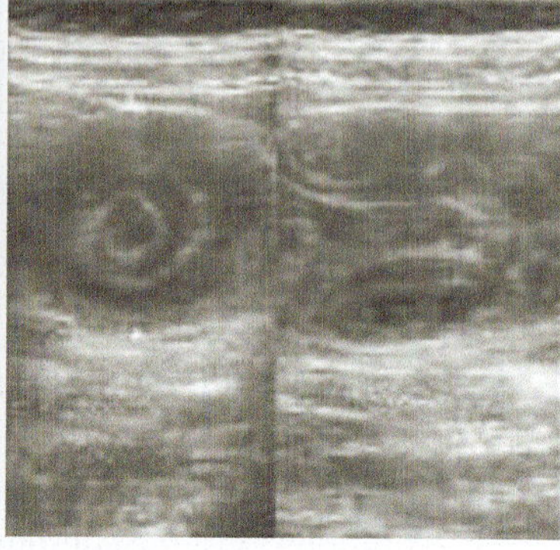

Q10. A 75-year-old lady presents with history of abdominal pain since last night after she had her dinner. She has been taking laxatives for her constipation for last 5 days. She has had one episode of stool blood stained this morning. She has been vomiting 4–5 times. Now feels tired and weak.

a. What is the first investigation recommended for this patient?
b. What is seen on the X-ray? What is the diagnosis?
c. What is treatment of this condition?

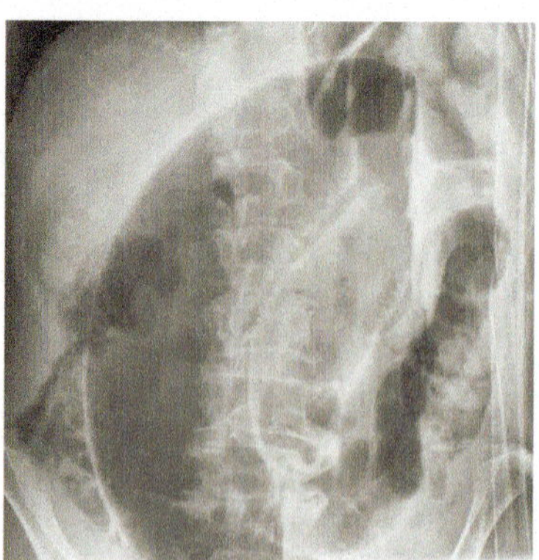

Q11. A 66-year-old female presents with severe watery diarrhea and a fever of 38.5°C. She is currently on a day 5 of a 10-day course of clindamycin for leg cellulitis.

a. What is most likely cause of diarrhea?
b. What is treatment of choice for this condition?
c. What are other steps in management of these patients?

Q12. A 67-year-old female patient presents with abdominal pain and vomiting. She tells you she has not opened her bowels in 5 days. You suspect bowel obstruction and request a plain abdominal X-ray.

a. Give three features on X-ray that would help you differentiate between small bowel and large bowel obstruction.
b. Give two features you might expect on examination in a patient with bowel obstruction.
c. Give two possible complications of bowel obstruction.

Q13. A 4-week-old child has been brought in by parents with history of recurrent vomiting, especially after feeds. Parents also state that child is always crying with hunger. Childbirth was unremarkable, but has not been putting on weight for the last 2 weeks. Child is up to date with immunization.

a. Your junior doctor asks you what is best way to examine this patient.
b. What is likely diagnosis of this patient?
c. What is management of this patient in emergency department?

Q14 A 75-year-old lady presented to the ER with history of collapse while at home. She had complained of abdominal pain for few minutes before collapse. She is regained consciousness soon after, since then she has been drowsy, tired, and pale. On examination, she is hypotensive, tachycardic and has a palpable pulsatile mass in abdomen just above the umbilical region.

a. What is most likely diagnosis?
b. What investigation can you do in ER to aid in diagnosis?
c. What is ER management of this patient?

Q15. A 35-year-old male presents to ER with history of intermittent epigastric and retrosternal chest discomfort for last few months. He also complains of occasional bloating sensation and usually has symptoms 15–20 minutes after food, sometimes relieved by drinking water. He is otherwise well. He has had a recent cardiac evaluation, which was normal.

a. Name two most likely diagnoses.
b. What is the diagnostic investigation of choice for this condition?
c. Name two class of medication, which would be beneficial for this patient?

ANSWERS

Ans. 1

a. Spider naïve, gynecomastia, dilated abdominal wall veins, and abdominal distension
b. Cirrhosis, inflammatory bowel disease, GI malignancy, and malabsorption
c. Spleen is nonballotable. Spleen moves with respiration. Spleen has a notch on the lower medial border

Ans. 2

a. IV fluids, crossmatch 4–6 units, fresh frozen plasma (FFP), vasoactive drug (e.g., terlipressin), IV antibiotics, and urgent endoscopy
b. Palmar erythema, leukonychia, liver flap, Dupuytren's contracture, and clubbing
c. Blatchford score and Rockall score

Ans. 3

a. Isoniazid, amitriptyline, and nonsteroidal anti-inflammatory drugs
b. Cocaine and ecstasy
c. Acute fatty liver of pregnancy and HELLP syndrome

Ans. 4

a. Fetor hepaticus, asterixis, constructional apraxia, ascites, and jaundice
b. Ascites, albumin, bilirubin, encephalopathy, and INR
c. Ataxia, ophthalmoplegia, and confusion

Ans. 5

a. Delirium tremens
b. IV fluids, airway maintenance, seizure control/prevention, hypoglycemia monitoring, and parenteral thiamine
c. Parenteral thiamine before glucose

Ans. 6

a. Appendicitis
b. Alvarado score, components of Alvarado are: migratory pain, anorexia, nausea, tenderness in the right lower quadrant, rebound tenderness, elevated temperature, leukocytosis, shift of WBC to left
c. IV fluids, analgesia, NPO, urgent surgical referral

Ans. 7

a. Acute pancreatitis
b. Gallstones, alcohol, other causes: "I GET SMASHED"
    - Idiopathic
    - Gallstones
    - Ethanol
    - Trauma
    - Steroids
    - Mumps
    - Autoimmune (pan)
    - Scorpion stings
    - Hyperlipidemia/hypercalcemia
    - ERCP drugs (including azathioprine and diuretics)
    - DKA
c. Serum lipase (not amylase, as lipase is more specific) and CT abdomen with contrast

Ans. 8

a. Mesenteric artery ischemia
b. Superior mesenteric artery
c. IV fluids, nil orally, analgesia, IV antibiotics, urgent surgical referral, CT abdomen with contrast

Ans. 9

a. Intussusception
b. Ileocolic region
c. Fluoroscopy with contrast enema

Ans. 10

a. X-ray abdomen
b. Coffee bean appearance and intussusception
c. Air insufflation (colonoscopy)

Ans. 11

a. *Clostridium difficile* infection
b. Metronidazole 400 mg, three times a day (or vancomycin 125 mg, four times a day) for 10–14 days
c. Barrier nurse in side room where possible. Stop antibiotics where possible. Avoid starting antibiotics where possible. Stop all laxatives. Commence stool chart. Daily examination of abdomen for tenderness or distension (indicative of colitis). Regular blood tests to check potassium, white cell count, and albumin.

Ans. 12

a. Central versus peripheral bowel loops, size of dilation, haustra (lines not seen across whole width) versus valvulae conniventes (lines seen across whole width of bowel).
b. Abdominal distension and high-pitched tinkling bowel sounds
c. Perforation, bowel ischemia, peritonitis, sepsis, intra-abdominal abscess, and fluid and electrolyte imbalance

Ans. 13

a. Abdominal palpation while the mother is breastfeeding the child. We can feel the swelling below the epigastric region.
b. Pyloric stenosis
c. NPO, IV fluids, bloods—GRBS, electrolytes, full blood count (FBC), USG abdomen, surgical referral

Ans. 14

a. AAA—abdominal aortic aneurysm
b. USG—aortic scan
c. Two large IV cannulas, IV fluids, crossmatch 4–6 units of blood (activate major hemorrhage protocol), urgent vascular/surgical referral, transfer to operation theater

Ans. 15

a. GERD—gastroesophageal reflux disease, dyspepsia
b. EGD—esophageal gastroscopy
c. Antacids and prokinetics

CHAPTER 9 Renal and Genitourinary Emergencies OSCE

Devendra Richhariya

QUESTIONS

Q1. A 28-year-old young man brought to emergency medicine department with severe right lower abdominal pain radiating to urethra and nausea. He has history of burning micturition and also red color urine. Ultrasound KUB (kidney, ureter, and bladder) is available for interpretation.

a. Identify the clinical situation.

b. What are the steps in management?

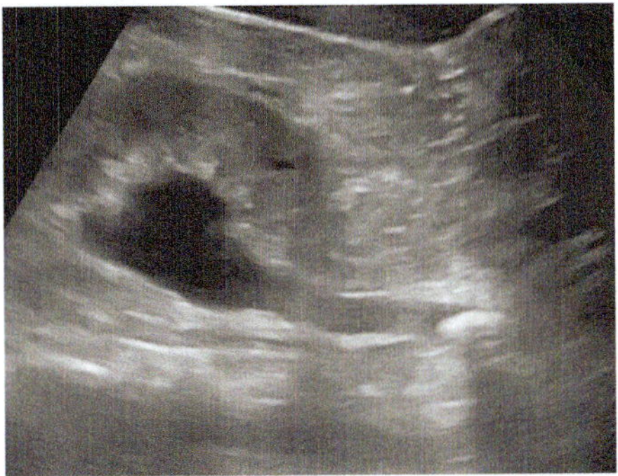

Q2. A 1-year-old baby brought to the emergency department.

a. Identify the clinical situation.

b. Name types of this condition.

c. What is the management?

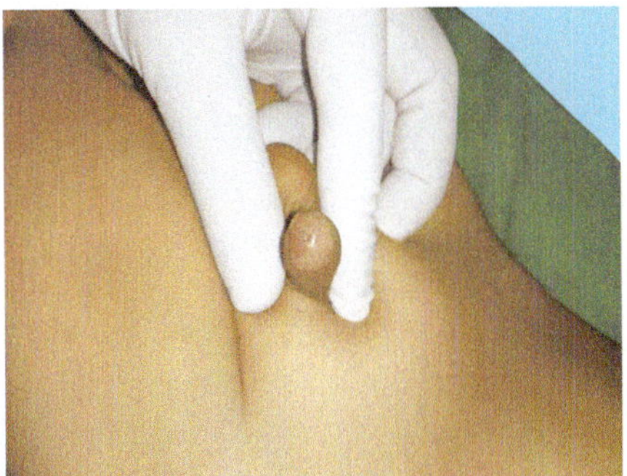

Q3. **A 5-year-old male child presented to the emergency department with sever pain and crying. Emergency physician examined him and emergency situation is described below.**

a. Identify the condition in a child presented to emergency department.
b. Name the complication of this condition.
c. What is the management?

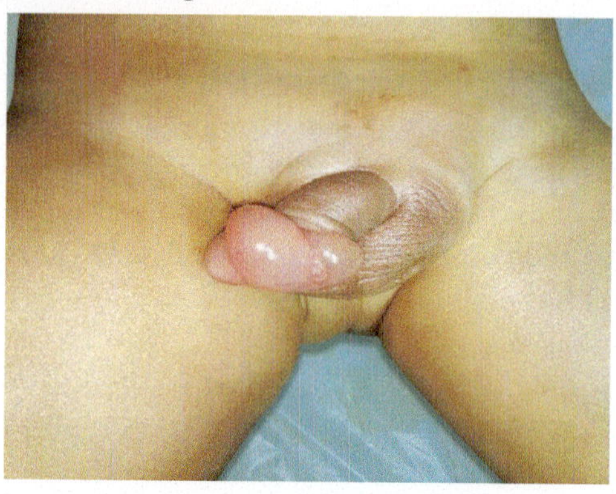

Q4. **A 28-year-old male brought to emergency department at midnight with history of a cracking or popping sound in an erect penis during intercourse followed by immediate detumescence and development of pain and swelling in penis and pain and acute retention of urine.**

a. Identify the clinical condition.
b. What is the name of the appearance?
c. What is the name of the sign?
d. What is the significance of acute retention of urine in this condition?
e. Name the complications in this condition.
f. What is the management?

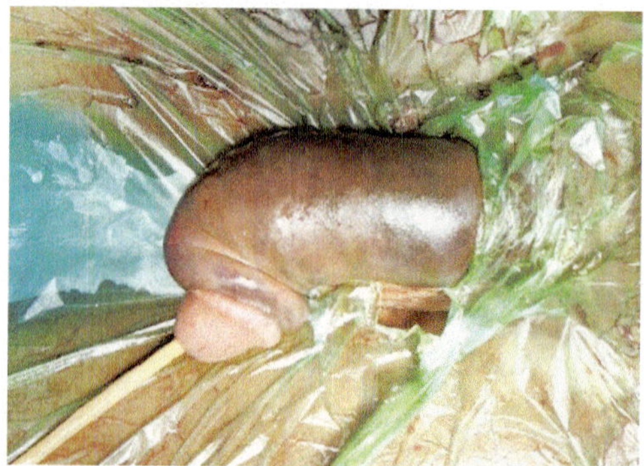

Q5. A 68-year-old male brought to emergency department with complaint of hematuria.

a. Define hematuria.
b. Name the possible etiology in this age group.
c. How do you classify hematuria?
d. How to approach hematuria?

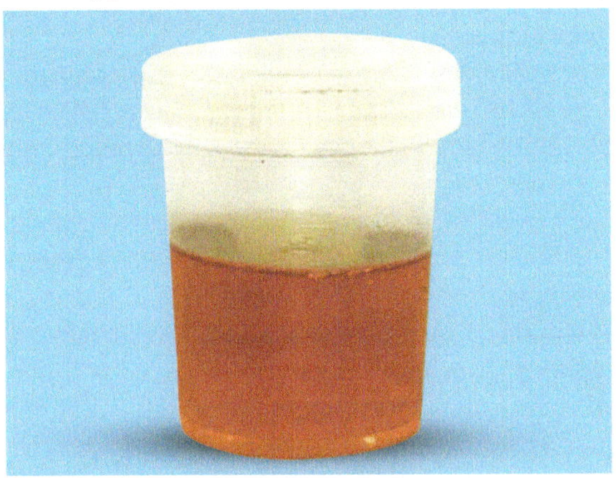

ANSWERS

Ans. 1

a. A proximal ureteric calculus on gray scale ultrasound seen as echogenic foci
b. Pain management, intravenous fluid, urologist opinion, and CT KUB if required

Ans. 2

a. Phimosis in a child
b. Phimosis can be divided into physiological and pathological (true) phimosis.
c. Treatment of phimosis can be divided into nonsurgical or conservative and surgical treatment.

Ans. 3

a. *Paraphimosis:* Paraphimosis is a urological emergency in which foreskin is left retracted due to its entrapment behind the glans penis.
b. Paraphimosis leads to strangulation of glans and lymphovascular compromise of the prepuce leading to venous engorgement, inflammation, pain, and even necrosis, further impending the reduction of foreskin.
c. The main aim of treatment of paraphimosis is reduction of preputial and glans edema and restoration of prepuce to its original position. There are

many different methods of reduction of paraphimosis, such as manual retraction, pharmacological therapy, minimally invasive therapy, and surgical therapy.

Ans. 4

a. Penile fracture; penile fracture is rupture of tunica albuginea due to trauma to penis in a tumescent state.
b. Eggplant appearance
c. *Aubergine sign*; the deviation of swollen penis is opposite to the side of tear, because of the mass effect of hematoma. This defect can sometimes be palpable with a blood clot over it and can be rolled under the fingers known as *"rolling sign"*
d. Acute urinary retention gives the hint of associated urethral rupture
e. Complications such as corporeal fibrosis, delayed chordee with resultant shaft deformation
f. Treatment can be conservative or surgical. Conservative approach may be advocated in cases of intact tunica on imaging but strong clinical suspicion. It includes cold fomentation, anti-inflammatory agents, fibrinolytics (trypsin and streptokinase) and antiandrogens (like stilboestrol, to prevent erections). However, conservative approach is not recommended because of the long-term complications.

Ans. 5

a. "Hematuria" in simple term means "blood in urine". In normal urine, <3 RBCs/HPF (red blood cells/high power field) can be present. Any hematuria with >3 RBC/HPF is marked as significant and needs further investigation and management.
b. Regarding this given age benign prostate hypertrophy (in males), malignancy, and urinary tract infections
c. Hematuria may be classified as *gross* (macroscopic hematuria or which is visible to naked eyes) or *microscopic hematuria* (detected only on urine examination)
d. *Approach:* Confirmation of hematuria (urine examination), rule out benign causes, baseline renal function, urological evaluation (urine cytology imaging, CT urography, MR urography, intravenous pyelography, ultrasonography, and cystoscopy)

10 CHAPTER Neurological Emergencies OSCE

Gouri Ranade, Sakthi Muthalraju

QUESTIONS

Q1. **A 65-year-old woman with history of type 2 diabetes comes into emergency room (ER) with sudden onset weakness in her right leg. Also, she described a sudden transient loss of vision in right eye. These symptoms lasted for about 1 hour.**

a. What is the diagnosis and list two differentials?
b. What is the phenomenon with her eye called?
c. What is ABCD2 score and describe its significance?

Q2. **A 27-year-old male came to ER with history of difficulty in swallowing, painful contraction of neck muscles, and involuntary tongue protrusion. He was taking metoclopramide tablets for vomiting for a day.**

a. What is the diagnosis and list two differentials?
b. Name four medications associated with this condition.
c. Name the medications used to treat this condition.

Q3. **A 50-year-old female, past medical history of chronic kidney disease (CKD) and hypertension, was brought to ER by her family with history of altered behavior since last 6 hours. Also, she has been having headaches and vision problems for 2 days. Her vitals were taken heart rate (HR): 91 beats/min, blood pressure (BP): 230/110 mm Hg, respiratory rate (RR): 17 breaths/min, SpO_2: 100%. While she was being examined in ER, she had a generalized tonic-clonic seizure (GTCS) (seizure) episode. Her magnetic resonance imaging (MRI) is shown below.**

a. What is the most likely diagnosis?
b. List four differential diagnoses.
c. What are the findings seen in the MRI image given below?
d. List the ER management of this condition.

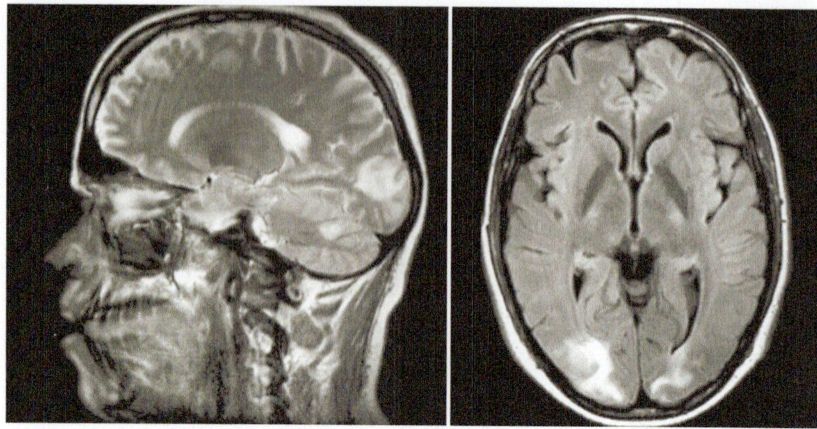

Q4. **A 48-year-old man is brought into the ER by the police and bystander after being found wandering in the streets. He is irritable, agitated, and confused. You note a strong smell of alcohol on his breath.**

a. Describe the features of Korsakoff psychosis
b. Describe the classic triad of Wernicke's encephalopathy.
c. What is the drug to be prescribed to treat Wernicke's encephalopathy?
d. Describe delirium tremens and its drug of choice in ER.

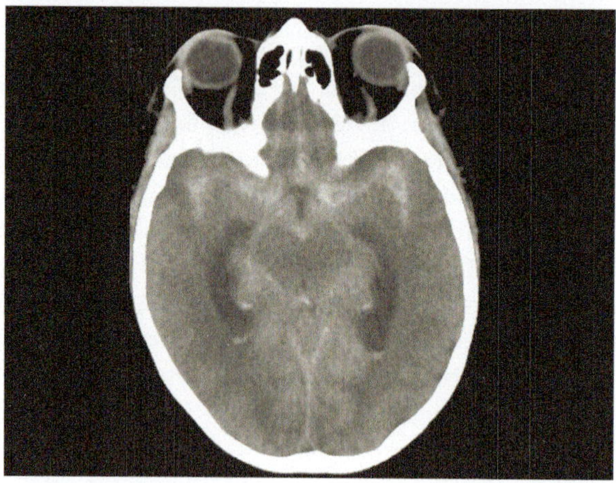

Q5. **A 65-year-old woman is brought to ER with acute onset weakness of her left side which started 2 hours back. She has weakness over the left face and arm associated with slurred speech. A computed tomography (CT) scan is performed and available for interpretation.**

a. Describe the findings present in the undermentioned CT image and what is the artery involved in this condition?
b. Describe ROSIER 7 (recognition of stroke in the emergency room) score and BE-FAST score?
c. What is NIHSS (National Institutes of Health Stroke Scale) score and its importance?
d. Describe four stroke mimics.
e. What are the contraindications for thrombolysis?

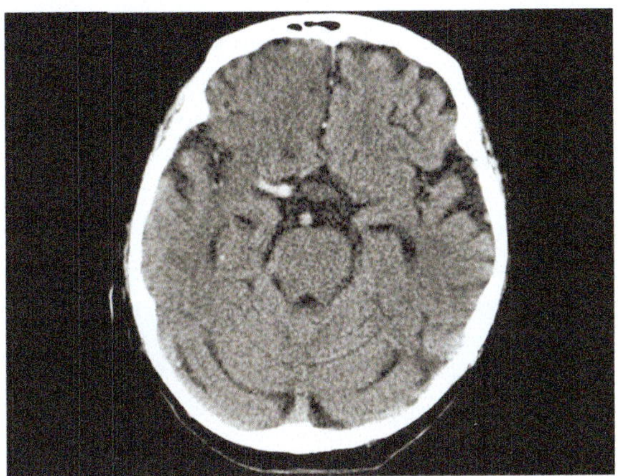

Q6. A 70-year-old man presents to ER with a 4-hour history of a severe and sudden onset occipital headache associated with photophobia and vomiting. Patient has neck rigidity on examination. A CT scan was performed.

a. Describe the finding in the CT image.
b. What is the ER management of subarachnoid hemorrhage (SAH)?
c. Give three complications of SAH.
d. How would you have proceeded with further management of this patient if the CT would have been normal?

Q7. A 55-year-old woman presents to ER with complaints of multiple episodes of sudden, severe, and stabbing pain over the cheek and upper lip on the right side which lasts for about 2 minutes, every day since last 1 week. It happens mostly when she is washing her face or brushing her teeth.

a. What is the most likely diagnosis?
b. What is the ER management of this patient and first-line drug used for this condition?
c. What anatomical structure is responsible for this condition?
d. Mention four differential diagnoses.

Q8. A 40-year-old male presents to ER with right-sided isolated facial palsy which he noticed since today morning. He is unable to wrinkle his forehead or fully close his eye.

a. What is the most likely diagnosis?
b. Describe its ER management and discharge advice.
c. Mention four differential diagnoses.

Q9. You perform a fundoscopic examination on a patient presented with sudden onset headache, vomiting, and altered sensorium. The fundoscopic image is shown below.

a. Describe the findings are seen in this image.
b. Describe other signs you might see on examination in addition to the above finding.
c. What is the clinical management of this patient in emergency department?
d. What investigation is contraindicated in this patient?

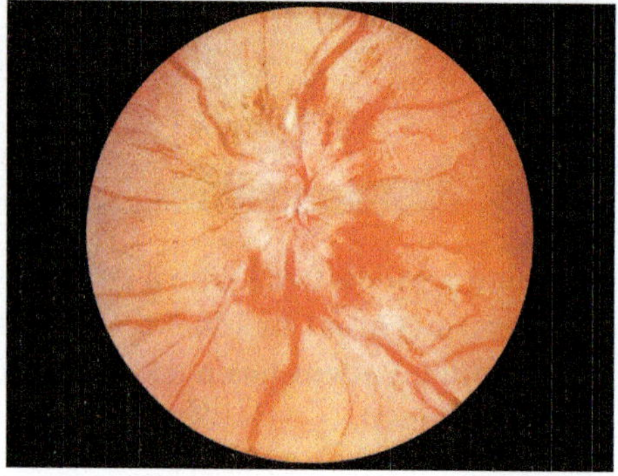

Q10. A 55-year-old woman presents with a 2-hour history of continuous spinning sensation, nausea, and persistent vomiting. Her symptoms worsen on changing posture, but it has even at rest. She gives a history of recent viral illness.

a. Describe the causes of acute vestibular syndrome.
b. What is HINTS examination?
c. Mention two drugs that could ease her symptoms.
d. Describe four clinical features that points toward a central cause of vertigo.

Q11. A 55-year-old woman presents to ER with a progressive headache in the left temporal region for 3 hours associated with blurring of vision in the left eye and tenderness over her left temporal/ scalp region. Her bloods are normal except an erythrocyte sedimentation rate (ESR) of 70 mm/hour.

a. What is the most likely diagnosis?
b. Describe the ER management and investigations.
c. Mention four differential diagnoses.

Q12. A 25-year-old female presents to ER with a severe pulsatile headache over right forehead and temporal region associated with nausea and vomiting. She prefers to stay in dark and silent room. She had similar episodes in the past.

a. What is the most likely diagnosis?
b. Name a precipitating factor for this condition.
c. Describe the emergency management.

Q13. A 28-year-old man is brought in by his family after they witnessed a shaking episode while he is asleep.

a. Give two features in this kind of presentation that may suggest seizure activity.
b. Give two differential diagnoses for seizures.
c. Give two features that would warrant an urgent CT brain.

Q14. A 78-year-old man is brought to the ER with an occipital headache and vomiting and instability on walking for 3 hours. His past medical history includes diabetes mellitus/hypertension (DM/HTN). Patient is alert, conscious, and oriented. His BP was high—210/110 mm Hg. An image from his CT brain scan is shown below.

a. Describe the CT scan findings.
b. Describe the management of this patient.
c. You are called to review this patient. His conscious level has dropped and now he does open his eyes, even to pain, moaning incomprehensibly but can localize painful stimuli. What is his Glasgow Coma Scale (GCS) score?
d. Give two reasons that could have caused his deterioration.

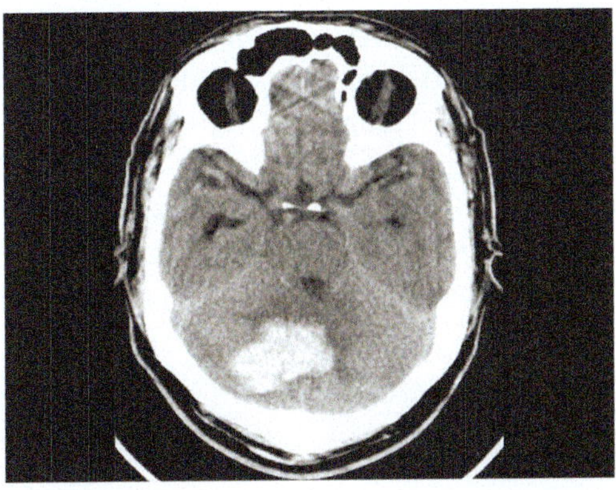

Q15. A 35-year-old male was brought to ER with severe headache, lethargy, and vomiting for 1 day. He denies any history of fever or travel. CT head that was done on arrival was normal. Lumbar puncture was done. Results as follows:

- **White cell count—870/mm^3**
- **Predominant cell type—lymphocytes**
- **Organisms—none**
- **Protein—0.8 g/dL**
- **Glucose—3/4 plasma concentration**

a. Give three organisms most commonly associated with bacterial meningitis.
b. Describe clinical signs of raised intracranial pressure.
c. Identify the abnormalities in the cerebrospinal fluid (CSF) obtained. What is the diagnosis based on this result?
d. What further test could be performed on CSF from this patient to investigate another possible cause of acute severe headache?

Q16. A 65-year-old man with alcohol dependence is found having generalized tonic-clonic seizures in his home and is brought by family to emergency department, still actively seizing. His airway is controlled, and he is on 15 L of oxygen/min via nonrebreathing mask.

a. What is the definition of status epilepticus?
b. What in a chronic alcoholic predisposes them to fitting?
c. What are your three management priorities?
d. If the fitting does not stop, what would your management be?

ANSWERS

Ans. 1

a. Transient ischemic attack (TIA) [anterior cerebral artery (ACA) territory]; Differential diagnoses (DDs): Stroke, Todd's paralysis, retinal/vitreous hemorrhage, and temporal arteritis
b. Amaurosis fugax
c. *ABCD2 score: A*ge > 60 years = 1. *B*lood pressure > 140/90 mmHg = 1. *C*linical features (Unilateral weakness = 2. Speech disturbance without weakness = 1). *D*uration of symptoms (>1 hour = 2. 10–59 minutes = 1). *D*iabetes = 1.

It calculates risk of stroke after TIA, score of 6 or more strongly predicts a stroke and needs urgent specialist referral.

Ans. 2

a. Acute dystonic reaction; DDs: Hypocalcemia and hypomagnesemia
   Primary neurological cause: Temporal lobe epilepsy, meningitis, stroke, Wilson's disease, and tetanus.
   Strychnine poisoning, anticholinergic agents
a. Haloperidol, selective serotonin reuptake inhibitor (SSRI), metoclopramide, droperidol, prochlorperazine, promethazine, and ranitidine
b. Procyclidine 5–10 mg (IV/IM) or benztropine 1–2 mg (IV/IM) are the drugs of choice

Ans. 3

a. Posterior reversible encephalopathy syndrome
b. Reversible cerebral vasoconstriction syndrome (RCVS)
   - Cerebral venous thrombosis/demyelination
   - Progressive multifocal leukoencephalopathy (PML)
   - Autoimmune or paraneoplastic encephalitis
   - Viral encephalitis
   - Toxic leukoencephalopathy
c. Hyperintensity over parietal-occipital regions on T2/FLAIR (fluid-attenuated inversion recovery)
d. BP control—mean arterial pressure (MAP) should be lowered by ~20–25% within 1–2 hours. Seizure management—treat hypomagnesemia/fluid overload, if present

Ans. 4

a. Amnesia, memory problems, confabulation, and lack of insight
b. Confusion, ataxia, ophthalmoplegia; Other features include nystagmus, memory disturbance, hypothermia, hypotension, and coma
c. Intravenous (IV) thiamine
d. Delirium tremens is one of the presentations of acute alcohol withdrawal. It can present as agitation, confusion, paranoia, visual, and auditory hallucination, seizures, hyperthermia dehydration, electrolyte imbalance, and shock.

Ans. 5

a. Right-sided hyperdense MCA sign. Middle cerebral artery is involved.
b. Both scores are used for easy recognition of stroke in emergency department and prehospital setting.

ROSIER score

Has there been loss of consciousness or syncope?		
	Y (–1) ☐	N (0) ☐
Has there been seizure activity?		
	Y (–1) ☐	N (0) ☐
Is there a *new acute* onset (or on awakening)?		
I. Asymmetric facial weakness	Y (+1) ☐	N (0) ☐
II. Asymmetric arm weakness	Y (+1) ☐	N (0) ☐
III. Asymmetric leg weakness	Y (+1) ☐	N (0) ☐
IV. Speech disturbance	Y (+1) ☐	N (0) ☐
V. Visual field defect	Y (+1) ☐	N (0) ☐
		*Total score ______ (–2 to +5)
Provisional diagnosis:	☐ Stroke	☐ Nonstroke (specify) ______

*Stroke is likely if total scores are >0. Scores of ≤0 have a low possibility of stroke but not completely excluded.

BE-FAST score

Is the patient having a stroke?	✓	Check if yes
Balance • Perform bilateral index finger-to-nose test and bilateral heel-to-shin test • Does the patient have sudden loss of balance or coordination, trouble walking, or dizziness?		B
Eyes • Assess four quadrants of visual field by having patient locate your index finger. • Does the patient have trouble seeing out of one or both eyes or sudden double vision?		E
Face • Ask the patient to smile or show their teeth. • Does the patient's face look uneven, have sudden drooping, or numbness on one side?		F
Arms • Ask the patient to raise and extend both arms with their palms up. • Does one arm drift downward? • Does the patient have sudden numbness or weakness of the arm on one side of the body?		A

Contd...

Contd...

Speech • Ask the patient to say, "you cannot teach an old dog new tricks." • Does the patient have slurred speech, trouble speaking, understanding, or seem confused?	S
Time • What time did the symptoms start? _____:____ • What time was the patient last known well (last appear normal)? _____:____	T
Glucose level = __________	

If these criteria are met, the patient qualifies for qualifies for a stroke alert:
- Patient received one or more check marks (√); and
- Glucose is over 80 mg/dL; and
- Last known well time is under 4.5 hours

c. The National Institutes of Health Stroke Scale (NIHSS) is a systematic and quantitative assessment tool to measure stroke-related neurological deficit.

Score	***Stroke severity***
0	No stroke symptoms
1–4	Minor stroke
5–15	Moderate stroke
16–20	Moderate-to-severe stroke
21-42	Severe stroke

d. Hypoglycemia, migraine, labyrinthine disorders, global ischemia due to hypotension, vasovagal syncope, sepsis (may exacerbate old neurological signs); Other neurological disease (e.g., Bell's palsy), mass lesions (e.g., subdural hematoma, cerebral abscess, cerebral tumors), postictal states, focal seizures and generalized seizures, hyponatremia, and hepatic encephalopathy

e. *Absolute contraindications:* Prior intracranial hemorrhage, known cerebral arteriovenous malformation, known cerebral neoplasm (primary or metastatic), ischemic stroke within 3 months, suspected aortic dissection, active bleeding or bleeding diathesis (excludes menses) Significant trauma within past 3 months

   Relative contraindications: Severe uncontrolled HT on presentation [systolic blood pressure (SBP) > 180 mm Hg or diastolic blood pressure (DBP) >110 mm Hg], prolonged (>10 minutes), cardiopulmonary resuscitation (CPR), history of prior ischemic stroke >3 months, major surgery <3 weeks, recent internal hemorrhage (within 2–4 weeks), noncompressible vascular punctures, pregnancy, active peptic ulcer, and current use of anticoagulants

Ans. 6

a. Hyperdense signal in the subarachnoid space suggestive of SAH
b. Urgent neurosurgery referral; Oral nimodipine (60 mg four-hourly) to prevent delayed cerebral ischemia due to vasospasm. Manage hypertension (nitroprusside and labetalol). If intracranial pressure (ICP) is raised; raise the head of the bed, analgesia and sedation, hyperventilation, and hypertonic saline/mannitol.
c. *Complications:* Rebleeding, hydrocephalus, and ischemia secondary to cerebral vasospasm. syndrome of inappropriate antidiuretic hormone secretion (SIADH), neurogenic pulmonary edema, seizures, myocardial ischemia, or left ventricular (LV) dysfunction
d. If the CT is negative, but the history is strongly suspicious for SAH, lumbar puncture should be performed, ideally 12 hours after the onset of the headache and examine the CSF for the detection of xanthochromia.

Ans. 7

a. Trigeminal neuralgia
b. Analgesics, neurology referral, and carbamazepine
c. Maxillary and mandibular division of the trigeminal nerve
d. *Differential diagnoses:* Dental pain, sinusitis, and atypical facial pain. Cluster headache, postherpetic neuralgia, temporomandibular joint (TMJ) disorders, and giant cell arteritis.

Ans. 8

a. Right-sided lower motor neuron (LMN) facial palsy—Bell's palsy
b. Oral prednisolone 25 mg twice daily for 10 days, or giving 60 mg daily for 5 days followed by a daily reduction in dose of 10 mg (for a total treatment time of 10 days). Reassure patients that the prognosis is good and most people with Bell's palsy make a full recovery within 9 months. Advise the person that they should keep the affected eye lubricated with drops during the day and ointment at night, and that if they are unable to close the eye at night, they should tape it closed using microporous tape.
c. Differential diagnoses: Bell's palsy, Ramsay Hunt syndrome, cholesteatoma, and parotid tumor. Malignant otitis externa, otitis media, Lyme disease, Guillain-Barré syndrome, and sarcoidosis

Ans. 9

a. Papilledema
b. *Clinical signs of raised ICT:* Reduced consciousness, pupillary signs, focal neurological deficit, abnormal posturing, Cushing's triad hypertension, bradycardia and irregular breathing, and abnormal "doll's eye" movements.

c. Raise the head of the bed, analgesia, and sedation hyperventilation, hypertonic saline/mannitol.
d. Lumbar puncture

Ans. 10

a. Migraine, acute vestibular neuritis, labyrinthitis, and posterior circulation stroke
b. HINTS examination
c. Prochlorperazine, cinnarizine, cyclizine, promethazine, and betahistine
d. Persistent, severe, or prolonged vertigo/vomiting; new onset headache, focal neurological signs and symptoms, central type of nystagmus, abnormal response to Hallpike maneuver
   Prolonged, severe imbalance, no other ENT symptoms such as hearing loss, tinnitus, or aural fullness

Ans. 11

a. Giant cell arteritis
b. Steroids, if visual involvement and aspirin (75 mg daily). Urgent referral for temporal artery biopsy.
c. *Differential diagnoses:* Cervicogenic headache, primary headache syndromes including tension headache, migraine, cluster headache, hemicrania continua, and trigeminal neuralgia; TMJ dysfunction

Ans. 12

a. Migraine
b. *Precipitating factors:* Combined oral contraceptive pill, alcohol missed meals or drinks, fatigue, menstruation stress (bright lights, loud noise, and extremes of weather). Certain foods, e.g., cheese and chocolates
c. Triptans + nonsteroidal anti-inflammatory drug (NSAID) or paracetamol

Ans. 13

a. *Any two of:* Urinary or fecal incontinence, bitten side of tongue or cheek, headache and myalgia following the event, disorientation and drowsiness for a period after the event (postictal phase), amnesia of the event, head turning to one side, unusual posturing or prolonged limb jerking during event, and prodromal 'deja vu'
b. *Any two of:* Syncope (may provoke a postanoxic convulsion), TIA, hypoglycemia, complex migraine, cardiac arrhythmias, psychogenic nonepileptic seizures, rigors, and panic attack
c. *Any two of:* Persistent altered consciousness (taking into account the postictal phase), focal neurological deficit, history of trauma, known HIV or immunocompromised, known malignancy, suspected intracranial infection, e.g., fever bleeding disorders (and anticoagulants), alcoholism, and focal or partial onset before generalization

Ans. 14

a. There is an area of high attenuation in the right posterior fossa likely to represent an acute hemorrhage into the left cerebellum.
b. *Management:* Urgent neurosurgical review, BP control, raise the head of the bed, analgesia and sedation, hyperventilation, and hypertonic saline/mannitol.
c. GCS—8 (E = 1, V = 2, and M = 5).
d. *Complications:* Obstructive hydrocephalus, compression of the brain stem itself

Ans. 15

a. *Neisseria meningitidis*, *Streptococcus pneumoniae*, and *Haemophilus influenza*
b. Reduced or fluctuating level of consciousness, focal neurological signs, abnormal posturing
c. Pupillary signs [unequal, dilated, or poorly responsive pupil(s)], papilledema, abnormal dolls, eye movements, relative bradycardia, and hypotension (Cushing's reflex)
d. Abnormally high CSF, lymphocyte count with no organisms present, the values for CSF protein, and glucose are slightly elevated. This picture is consistent with a viral meningitis.
   CSF can be tested for the presence of xanthochromia to rule out subarachnoid hemorrhage.

Ans. 16

a.
   - Continuous seizure activity for 5 minutes or more without return of consciousness
   - Recurrent seizures (two or more) without an intervening period of neurological recovery
b.
   - Hypoglycemia/excess alcohol or alcohol withdrawal
   - Hyponatremia
   - Falls and intracranial hemorrhage (ICH)
   - Poor compliance to anticonvulsants
   - Hepatic encephalopathy
   - Overdose of tricyclic antidepressants (TCAs)
c.
   - Maintain airway/oxygenation
   - Thiamine 100 mg IV
   - Lorazepam 4 mg IV
d.
   - Second dose of lorazepam 4 mg IV
   - Second-line agents
   - Levetiracetam 60 mg/kg IV, maximum 4,500 mg
   - Fosphenytoin or phenytoin 20 mg/kg IV, maximum 1,500 mg

- Valproate 40 mg/kg IV, maximum 3,000 mg
- Intubation—third line
- Propofol 2-5 mg/kg IV, then infusion of 50-80 μg/kg/min (3-5 mg/kg/h)
- Midazolam 0.2 mg/kg IV, then infusion of 0.05-2 mg/kg/h
- Ketamine 0.5-3 mg/kg IV, then infusion of 0.3-4 mg/kg/h
- Lacosamide 400 mg IV over 15 minutes, then maintenance of 200 mg q12h PO/IV
- Phenobarbital 15-20 mg/kg IV at 50-75 mg/min

CHAPTER

Endocrine Emergencies OSCE

Shweta Ashok

QUESTIONS

Q1. **An 8-year-old female child was brought to the emergency room (ER) with history of (h/o) 10–15 episodes of loose watery stools for 2 days, 4–5 episodes of vomiting since morning, and some altered behavior noticed by mother since afternoon. Presenting vitals are as: E3V4M6, afebrile, heart rate (HR)—140 beats/min, blood pressure (BP)—100/70 mm Hg, blood sugar—541 mg/dL. Her arterial pH is 7.1, serum potassium—5.9 mEq/L, serum sodium—132 mEq/L, and bicarbonate—6 mEq/L.**

a. Based on the clinical presentation, what is the most probable diagnosis?
   - Gastroenteritis
   - Diabetic ketoacidosis (DKA)
   - Appendicitis
   - Urinary tract infection

b. What would be the initial management priority for this patient?
   - Administering intravenous (IV) fluids
   - Starting antibiotics
   - Monitoring blood glucose levels
   - Initiating psychiatric evaluation

c. Considering the electrolyte imbalances, what intervention is most appropriate for correcting the elevated potassium level?
   - Administering insulin and glucose
   - Administering sodium bicarbonate
   - Administering calcium gluconate
   - Administering a loop diuretic

Q2. **A 44-year-old, male known diabetic for 8 years on oral hypoglycemic agents (OHAs), was brought to ER in unconscious state at 4 AM. Attender gives h/o reduced food intake for past 1 week. He consumed dinner last night and taken his regular OHAs before bed. His recent vital signs show fasting blood sugar (FBS): 96 mg/dL and postprandial blood sugar (PPBS): 129 mg/dL. His diabetologist has altered his medications 3 days back.**

Currently, he is taking a tablet. Glycomet GP1 twice a day. In ER, central pulse +, HR: 110 beats/min, BP: 110/70 mmHg, SpO_2: 98% on room air (RA), and capillary blood glucose (CBG): 47 mg/dL.

a. What is your provisional diagnosis?
b. How will you prove the diagnosis?
c. How will you manage this patient in the emergency department?

Q3. **A 35-year-old female presented to ER with increasing shortness of breath, orthopnea, paroxysmal nocturnal dyspnea, and lower limb edema for 1 week. She has h/o unintentional weight loss +, heat intolerance, diarrhea, abdominal pain, and palpitations since 2–3 months. She has h/o childbirth 6 months back and gestational hypertension (not on medicines). O/E, morbid obesity +, E4V5M6, HR: 125 beats/min, respiratory rate (RR): 24 breaths/min, BP: 100/80 mm Hg, lower limb pitting edema +, mild exophthalmos +, and chest: bilateral crepitation +. Investigations show ProBNP (pro B-type natriuretic peptide): 2,740 pg/mL, thyroid-stimulating hormone (TSH): <0.1 mIU/L, FT4: 2.8 ng/dL, ECHO: EF 20% severe LV, and USG neck: hypervascularity of thyroid gland.**

a. What is your provisional diagnosis?
b. What are your treatment goals for this condition?
c. What are the five "B's" to manage this condition?

Q4. **An 81-year-old was found unconscious with low temperature, central pulses +, pulse rate (PR): 45 beats/min, loss of eyebrows, dry skin, and big tongue. History of thyroidectomy 2 years back.**

ECG—low voltage with bradycardia

Laboratory tests show serum Na^+: 130 mEq/L, pCO_2: 54 mm Hg, and pO_2: 68 mm Hg.

a. What is the diagnosis?
b. What is the plan of care for this patient?
c. What is the Specific treatment for this patient?

Q5. **A 30-year-old male was referred with h/o altered sensorium since 2 days, abdominal pain, and loose stools for 10 days, disturbed sleep, loss of weight, and appetite over past 6 months.**

O/E, Patient was drowsy, thin built, weak, dehydrated, drooling saliva from mouth, HR: 112 beats/min, BP: 90/60 mm Hg, RR: 22 breaths/min, chest: clear, per abdomen (P/A): soft, diffuse tenderness all over abdomen, and no neurological deficit noticed. Laboratory tests show serum Na^+: 117 mEq/L, serum K^+: 4.78, serum Cl^-: 95.8, random blood sugar (RBS): 56 mg/dL. Chest X-ray and USG abdomen were normal.

Patient was admitted in intensive care unit (ICU) where he had recurrent episodes of hypoglycemia and hypotension refractory to fluid therapy.

a. What is your provisional diagnosis?
b. What is the gold standard test for confirming the condition?
c. What is the treatment/further plan of care for this patient?

Q6. **A 35-year-old male, no comorbid condition, was brought to emergency department with sudden onset of headache and several chest pain, radiating to back since past 3 hours. Patient gives h/o consuming multiple energy drinks, but denies intake of alcohol or any other substances.**

O/E, pain score: 7/10, HR: 110 beats/min, BP: 190/120 mm Hg, SpO_2: 98% on RA, RR: 32 breaths/min.

ABG revealed significant lactic acidosis with pH: 7.14, pO_2: 15, pCO_2: 33.6 mm Hg, PO_2: 115.6 mm Hg, HCO_3: 12 mEq/L, base excess of 16 mmol/L, and lactate of 12 mmol/L.

12 lead ECG—sinus rhythm with ST depression V4-V6.

ECHO—regional wall hypokinesia in lateral area of left ventricle and EF ~ 20–30%.

Troponin T: positive, white blood cells (WBCs): 39 × 10^9/L, and normal C-reactive protein.

Computed tomography thorax and abdomen ruled out aortic dissection or large pulmonary embolism. A 6 cm large tumor in the left adrenal gland was found.

a. What is your probable diagnosis?
b. What is the diagnostic test for the condition?
c. What is the treatment in ER?

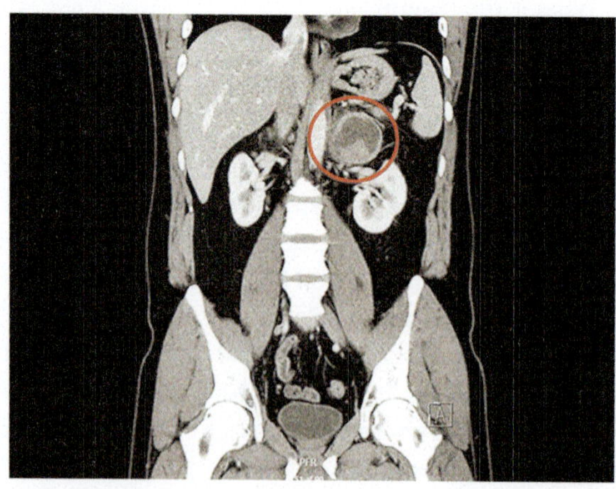

Q7. A 69-year-old male with lung cancer undergoing chemotherapy presents to the emergency department with generalized weakness and confusion. Laboratory results reveal a serum sodium level of 121 Eq/L.

a. Which of the following conditions is most likely causing the hyponatremia in this patient?
   - Dehydration due to vomiting
   - Addison's disease
   - Syndrome of inappropriate antidiuretic hormone secretion (SIADH)
   - Chemotherapy-induced electrolyte imbalance

b. In managing the hyponatremia in this patient, what is the recommended rate of correction to avoid the risk of osmotic demyelination syndrome (ODS)?
   - 12–15 mEq/L/24 hours
   - 6–8 mEq/L/24 hours
   - 2–4 mEq/L/24 hours
   - 20–25 mEq/L/24 hours

c. Aside from fluid restriction, which of the following interventions may be considered in the management of hyponatremia associated with SIADH?
   - Intravenous hypertonic saline
   - Diuretics
   - Oral rehydration solutions
   - Enteral nutrition

d. The patient's urine osmolality is found to be elevated. What does this finding suggest about the patient's renal function?
   - Decreased renal blood flow
   - Tubular dysfunction
   - Concentrated urine despite low serum sodium
   - Impaired glomerular filtration

Q8. A 60-year-old female, known diabetic, hypertensive for past 15 years, presented to ER with h/o vomiting—multiple episodes since today morning, abdominal discomfort, decreased oral intake for past 5 days and lethargy.

O/E, drowsy, arousable, dehydrated, HR: 110 beats/min, BP: 90/50 mm Hg, SpO_2: 98% on RA, CBG: 782 mg/dL, serum ketones+, chest: clear, P/A: diffuse tenderness+, and no guarding

ABG: pH: 7.32, pCO_2: 38 mm Hg, pO_2: 98 mm Hg, HCO_3: 18 mEq/L, Na^+: 132 mEq/L, serum K^+: 4.5 mEq/L, and serum Cl: 98 mEq/L

a. List a few probable differential diagnoses for this patient.
b. Calculate the net osmolarity of this patient.
c. How will you resuscitate this patient?

Q9. A 31-year-old lady has presented to you with increased urinary frequency and muscle weakness. Her past medical history includes severe depression, for which she takes sertraline.

On routine bloods, her calcium is 2.9. Chest X-ray and urinalysis are normal.

a. What is the most likely cause of the patient's symptoms and elevated serum calcium level?
   - Medication-induced hypercalcemia
   - Hyperparathyroidism
   - Renal dysfunction
   - Vitamin D deficiency
b. Upon initial assessment, the patient appears confused and disoriented. What urgent intervention should be prioritized?
   - Administer IV bisphosphonates
   - Obtain a chest X-ray
   - Start IV hydration with normal saline
   - Order urgent neuroimaging (CT or MRI)
c. Which electrolyte abnormality is commonly associated with hypercalcemia and should be monitored closely?
   - Hypokalemia
   - Hyponatremia
   - Hypernatremia
   - Hypophosphatemia
d. In the emergency department, the patient's blood pressure is elevated. What antihypertensive medication can be cautiously used in the setting of hypercalcemia?
   - Amlodipine
   - Lisinopril
   - Hydralazine
   - Metoprolol

Q10. You are a senior resident in the emergency department. You receive a 70-year-old woman, known case of type 2 diabetes mellitus, with complaints of increased thirst, polydipsia, and polyuria over past few days despite maintaining stable glycemic control. Patient denies any recent illness, trauma, or changes in medication. Her current medications are tablet glimepiride 2 mg, tablet metformin 1,000 mg, and desmopressin acetate

0.2 mg. Her urine volume is significantly high (6 L/day). Surprisingly, her urine glucose test came back negative. Her vital signs show HR: 90 beats/min, BP: 130/80 mm Hg, RR: 18 breaths/min, and temperature: 98.6°F (37°C). Laboratory tests show Na^+: 150 mEq/L, serum K^+: 4.0 mEq/L, HCO_3: 26 mEq/L, blood urea nitrogen (BUN): 20 mg/dL, creatinine: 1.0 mg/dL, low urine specific gravity (<1.005), dilute urine with low osmolality (130 mOsm/kg), and serum osmolarity of 300 mOsm/kg.

a. What is your probable diagnosis?
b. What is a water deprivation test?
c. How will you manage this patient?

Q11. **A 38-year-old, Mrs X, P2L2A1 presented to ER with complaints of severe fatigue, weakness, and confusion. The patient reports a gradual onset of weakness and fatigue over the past several weeks. She mentions a recent episode of postpartum hemorrhage during childbirth approximately 6 months ago. She also describes difficulty concentrating, weight loss, and an overall decline in her health.**

Her vital signs show BP: 90/60 mm Hg, HR: 110 beats/min, RR: 18 breaths/min, and SpO_2: 98% on RA.

Patient appears pale, fatigued, and slightly confused. Skin was cool and clammy. Chest was clear, P/A: soft and non-tender.

Laboratory tests show hemoglobin (Hb): 9.5 g/dL, serum Na^+: 135 mEq/L, serum K^+: 4.2 mEq/L, blood glucose: 85 mg/dL, creatinine: 0.9 mg/dL, thyroid function test: within normal limits, and prolactin: elevated.

a. What is the most likely cause of Mrs X's symptoms?
   - Thyroid dysfunction
   - Postpartum depression
   - Sheehan syndrome
   - Polycystic ovary syndrome (PCOS)
b. Which of the following is a common complication associated with Sheehan syndrome?
   - Hyperthyroidism
   - Hyponatremia
   - Thrombocytosis
   - Hypertension
c. What is the primary reason for Mrs X's confusion?
   - Electrolyte imbalance
   - Anemia
   - Pituitary necrosis
   - Hypothyroidism

d. What initial intervention is to be done in the ER?
- Initiation of antihypertensive medications
- Blood transfusion
- Administration of IV fluids
- Hormone replacement therapy

Q12. A 55-year-old female, known diabetic and hypertensive, on medicines, is brought to the ER by her husband due to a sudden onset of weakness, confusion, and shortness of breath. She has been feeling unwell for the past few days, complaining of fatigue, body aches, and a low-grade fever. Over the last 24 hours, her symptoms have rapidly worsened.

Her vital signs show BP: 80/50 mm Hg, HR: 120 beats/min, RR: 24 breaths/min, and SpO_2: 88% on RA.

She had undergone an elective surgery (cholecystectomy) 5 days back and had developed postoperative sepsis from the surgical site infection. She was started on broad-spectrum antibiotics and her condition initially improved. However, over the last 24 hours, there has been a sudden deterioration in her clinical status.

a. Which vital sign abnormality is commonly associated with critical illness-related corticosteroid insufficiency (CIRCI)?
- Hypertension
- Bradycardia
- Tachypnea
- Hyperthermia

b. What diagnostic test is essential for confirming the diagnosis of CIRCI in this case?
- Chest X-ray
- Blood culture
- Cortisol level measurement
- Electrocardiogram (ECG)

c. What is a common electrolyte abnormality associated with critical illness that may be present in the blood tests?
- Hyperkalemia
- Hyponatremia
- Hypocalcemia
- Hypernatremia

d. In addition to administering IV fluids and initiating supplemental oxygen, what is the next appropriate step in the management of hypotension?
- Initiate broad-spectrum antibiotic therapy
- Administer stress-dose corticosteroids
- Order a chest X-ray
- Perform a lumbar puncture

ANSWERS

Ans. 1

a. Diabetic ketoacidosis. DKA is a serious complication of diabetes mellitus, particularly in children. It occurs due to a deficiency of insulin, leading to hyperglycemia, ketosis, and metabolic acidosis. The symptoms often include polyuria, polydipsia, vomiting, altered mental status, and dehydration. The combination of gastrointestinal symptoms, altered behavior, hyperglycemia, and metabolic acidosis seen in this case points toward DKA as the most likely diagnosis.

b. Administering IV fluids. IV fluid administration is crucial for managing dehydration, restoring electrolyte balance, and initiating treatment for DKA. The child likely needs both fluids and insulin to address the hyperglycemia and correct the metabolic acidosis associated with DKA. Starting antibiotics (option 2nd) is not the initial priority in this case, as there is no clear indication of a bacterial infection at this point. Monitoring blood glucose levels (option 3rd) is important but is secondary to the immediate need for fluid resuscitation and correction of metabolic imbalances. Initiating psychiatric evaluation (option 4th) is not the primary concern at this stage; the altered behavior is likely related to the underlying medical condition, and addressing the medical emergency takes precedence. Administering IV fluids is the initial management priority to stabilize the child's condition and address the dehydration associated with DKA.

c. Administering insulin and glucose. In the context of DKA, insulin deficiency leads to a shift of potassium out of cells into the bloodstream, contributing to hyperkalemia. Administering insulin is a key component of DKA management. Insulin helps to reduce blood glucose levels, reverse ketosis, and promote the movement of potassium back into cells, thus lowering serum potassium levels. Simultaneously, glucose is administered along with insulin to prevent hypoglycemia. The insulin corrects the metabolic acidosis associated with DKA, and glucose ensures that the patient's blood sugar does not drop too low during insulin therapy.

Ans. 2

a. *Hypoglycemia:* Sulfonylurea induced

b. *Diagnosis of hypoglycemia:* Whipple's triad symptoms of hypoglycemia, documented low blood glucose, and recovery with administration of carbohydrate

c. *Management in emergency department:*
   - Secure an IV line
   - Give injection 50% dextrose (50 mL provides 25 mL of glucose) IV bolus

- Repeat dextrose (50% dextrose or 25% dextrose) after 15 minutes, if hypoglycemia persists
- IVF. 5% dextrose as maintenance fluid. Target CBG >100 mg/dL
- In sulfonylurea-induced hypoglycemia, injection octreotide 50–100 µg S/C, repeat every 6–8 hours or continuous infusion at 125 µg/hour.
- Injection diazoxide can be used in treating refractory sulfonylurea-induced hypoglycemia. It should be given as slow IV infusion (300 mg over 30 minutes in every 4 hours).

Ans. 3

a. Thyroid storm or thyrotoxicosis crisis
b. The immediate goals when treating thyroid storm are:
   - Decrease thyroid hormone synthesis
   - Prevent thyroid hormone release.
   - Decrease peripheral action of circulating thyroid hormone to reduce heart rate and support the circulation. To treat the precipitating condition.
c. When treating thyroid storm, consider the five "B's": *B*lock synthesis (i.e., antithyroid drugs), *B*lock release (i.e., iodine); *B*lock T4 into T3 conversion (i.e., high-dose propylthiouracil, propranolol, and corticosteroid), *B*eta-blocker, and *B*lock enterohepatic circulation (i.e., cholestyramine).

Ans. 4

a. Possibility of myxedema coma—a severe and life-threatening complication of hypothyroidism
b. *Treatment involves:*
   - Adequate oxygenation and ventilation; advanced airways
   - Fluid replacement and hypotension correction with isotonic crystalloids (normal saline or ringer lactate). Careful administration of 3% NaCl, if severe hyponatremia and depressed mental status.
   - Thyroid replacement therapy and steroids along with restriction of free water will correct mild hyponatremia.
   - Passive rewarming methods such as blankets are preferred. Avoid active rewarming method due to risk of cardiovascular collapse.
   - Empiric antibiotics are indicated initially in critically ill patients.
c. *Specific treatment:* Levothyroxine (T4) is most recommended for replacement as compared to liothyroxine. Some protocols suggest combination therapy as more physiologic replacement.
   - Injection levothyroxine (T4) can be considered in geriatric patients or those with cardiac disease. Loading dose: IV dose of 200–500 µg over first hour followed by 50–100 µg/day or oral dosing at 50–100 µg/day as tolerated.

- Liothyroxine (T3) may be considered in young and healthy patients. Give loading dose of 5–20 µg IV or PO followed by 5–10 µg q8h until improvement.
- Levothyroxine (T4) at 200–250 µg bolus and 50 µg PO daily and liothyroxine (T3) 10 µg IV or PO loading and 10 µg q8h
- All three methods can precipitate a cardiac event such as angina, dysrhythmia, or infarction. All patients should be on continuous cardiac monitoring during IV thyroid hormone.
- Corticosteroids are recommended as 5–10% have incidence of concurrent adrenal insufficiency. Early corticosteroid replacement is indicated. IV hydrocortisone 100 mg every 8 hours or dexamethasone 2–4 mg

Ans. 5

a. Adrenal crisis or Addisonian disease
b. Diagnosis is confirmed by cosyntropin stimulation test (CST). CST is used for evaluation of hypothalamus-pituitary-adrenal (HPA) axis in patients suspected of adrenal insufficiency. Adrenal insufficiency is best diagnosed by change in cortisol (after 250 µg cosyntropin) of <9 µg/dL or random total cortisol of <10 µg/dL.
c. Treatment in emergency department:
    - After standard stabilization of ABCDE, volume replenishment with adequate IV fluids. Treat hypoglycemia with dextrose and glucocorticoid replacement therapy with IV hydrocortisone 100 mg bolus followed by 50–100 mg q6h over the 24 hours till patients stabilize.
    - Dexamethasone 4 mg IV bolus considered in emergency when emergent steroid administration required.
    - In maintenance phase, these patients require hydrocortisone 5–25 mg/day and prednisolone 3–5 mg/day.

Ans. 6

a. Possibly pheochromocytoma with cardiovascular complications
b. The best method for diagnosing pheochromocytomas is using a 24-hour urine collection.
    - Catecholamine metabolites include metanephrine, normetanephrine, dopamine, and vanillylmandelic acid (VMA).
    - A 24-hour urine test is considered positive if the catecholamine levels exceed two times the upper limit of normal.
    - The most commonly ordered blood test for pheochromocytoma is the plasma-free metanephrine test. Though more convenient to obtain than a 24-hour urine collection, plasma-free metanephrine testing is plagued by frequent false-positive results.

c. Treatment of pheochromocytoma:
   - Acute crisis is treated medically to control the effects of excess catecholamines.
   - Phenoxybenzamine is used in the treatment of hypertensive crisis; dose 10–40 mg IV over 1 hour. It can be given orally in a dose of 10–60 mg/day in divided doses.
   - Phentolamine is given in dose of 5–10 mg intramuscularly for the control of acute paroxysmal hypertension.
   - Definitive treatment is by surgical resection of the tumor.

Ans. 7

a. *Syndrome of inappropriate antidiuretic hormone secretion (SIADH):* In patients with lung cancer, tumor cells can produce and release excessive amounts of antidiuretic hormone (ADH) or ADH-like substances. This leads to increased water reabsorption in the kidneys, dilution of sodium in the bloodstream, and subsequent hyponatremia. The elevated urine osmolality in SIADH indicates concentrated urine despite low serum sodium levels.
b. *6–8 mEq/L/24 hours:* Osmotic demyelination syndrome (ODS), also known as central pontine myelinolysis, is a serious and potentially fatal neurological complication that can occur if hyponatremia is corrected too rapidly. The brain's cells can adapt to chronic hyponatremia by adjusting their osmotic balance. If sodium levels are corrected too quickly, the rapid changes in osmolality can lead to demyelination of the neurons in the central pontine region of the brain. The recommended rate of correction for hyponatremia is generally conservative to prevent ODS. The optimal rate of correction is approximately 6–8 mEq/L/24 hours. This slow correction allows for the brain cells to adapt to the changing osmotic environment, reducing the risk of neurological complications.
c. *Intravenous hypertonic saline:* Intravenous administration of hypertonic (concentrated) saline is a therapeutic option in severe cases of hyponatremia or when there are neurological symptoms. It helps raise the serum sodium concentration more rapidly by providing a higher concentration of sodium than what is present in the body. Careful monitoring is essential to prevent overcorrection, which could lead to ODS. Diuretics are generally contraindicated in SIADH because they worsen hyponatremia by promoting additional water loss.
d. *Concentrated urine despite low serum sodium:* The elevated urine osmolality in the context of low serum sodium levels points toward the kidneys' ability to concentrate urine, which is a characteristic feature of SIADH. In SIADH, the kidneys respond to elevated levels of ADH by reabsorbing water, resulting in concentrated urine despite low serum sodium levels.

Ans. 8

a. Possible differential diagnosis for this case:
   - Hyperglycemic hyperosmolar state
   - Diabetic ketoacidosis
   - Acute kidney injury
   - Sepsis
   - Acute pancreatitis

b. Calculating osmolarity of the patient using the formula below:
   Osmolarity (mOsm/L) $= 2 \times$ *(corrected* Na^+*)* $+$ *(Glucose/18)*
   Given values, calculated $Na^+ = 132$ mEq/L, glucose $= 782$
   Hence, calculating the corrected sodium using the formula below:
   Corrected Na^+ $=$ *Calculated* Na^+ $+ [1.6 \times (glucose - 100)]/100$
   $Na^+ = 132 + [1.6 \times (782 - 100)]/100 = 142.91$
   Hence, the corrected sodium for this patient $= 142.91$
   Applying the values in the formula 1
   Osmolarity $= (2 \times 142.91) + (782/18) = 285.82 + 43.44 = 329.26$
   Hence, the osmolarity of the patient $= 329.26$ (hyperosmolar state)

c. Treatment in the emergency department:
   - *Fluid resuscitation:* Given the signs of dehydration and hypotension, IV fluids are essential. Initially, normal saline can be administered.
   - *Insulin therapy:* Insulin should be initiated to bring down the elevated blood glucose levels. Regular insulin is typically used in the treatment of DKA.
   - *Electrolyte correction:* Addressing electrolyte imbalances is crucial. Potassium replacement may be required as insulin administration can cause potassium to shift into cells.
   - *Monitoring:* Continuous monitoring of vital signs, blood glucose levels, electrolytes, and acid-base status is necessary.
   - *Addressing the underlying cause:* Identify and treat the underlying cause, such as the infection that might have triggered the episode.
   - Admission in ICU.

Ans. 9

a. *Hyperparathyroidism:* Hyperparathyroidism is a condition characterized by overactivity of the parathyroid glands, leading to excessive secretion of parathyroid hormone (PTH). In hyperparathyroidism, the increased PTH levels result in elevated serum calcium levels (hypercalcemia). Vitamin D deficiency can cause secondary hyperparathyroidism, but the patient's presentation, including muscle weakness and urinary frequency, is more suggestive of primary hyperparathyroidism. Renal dysfunction can lead to hypercalcemia, but the patient's normal urinalysis suggests that the kidneys are not the primary cause of the elevated calcium levels.

b. *Start IV hydration with normal saline:* Intravenous hydration with normal saline is an important intervention for hypercalcemia. Since the patient is confused and disoriented, urgent neuroimaging is crucial to assess for potential neurological complications.
c. *Hypophosphatemia:* Hypophosphatemia is commonly associated with hypercalcemia, and the two often coexist. Monitoring phosphate levels are important because severe hypophosphatemia can lead to various complications including muscle weakness, respiratory failure, and cardiac dysfunction.
d. *Hydralazine:* In the setting of hypercalcemia, blood pressure can be elevated due to the effects of high calcium levels on the vascular smooth muscle. Hydralazine is a direct-acting vasodilator that works by relaxing the smooth muscles in blood vessels, without affecting the calcium channels or renin-angiotensin system, leading to a reduction in blood pressure.

Ans. 10

a. Based on the clinical presentation and diagnostic results, patient may have diabetes insipidus, likely of central origin.
b. Water deprivation test or desmopressin stimulation test is a diagnostic procedure used to differentiate between central or nephrogenic type of diabetes insipidus and helps in guidance of treatment plan. Here is how the desmopressin test is typically conducted:
    - Baseline measurements of urine volume, urine osmolality, and plasma osmolality are taken to establish the patient's initial status.
    - *Water deprivation:* The patient is asked to abstain from drinking fluids for a specific period, typically overnight or for several hours. During this period, urine and blood samples are collected at regular intervals to monitor changes in urine volume and concentration, as well as plasma osmolality.
    - *Desmopressin administration:* After a sufficient dehydration period, desmopressin (also known as DDAVP, a synthetic analog of ADH) is administered either through an IV injection or intranasal spray.
    - *Monitoring response:* Post desmopressin administration, urine and blood samples are collected at intervals to observe the response. If the cause of diabetes insipidus is central (resulting from a deficiency of ADH), there should be a significant increase in urine osmolality and a decrease in urine volume.
    - *Post-test measurements:* Additional measurements of urine volume, urine osmolality, and plasma osmolality are taken to compare with baseline values.
    - *Interpretation:* A positive response to desmopressin (e.g., increased urine osmolality and decreased urine volume) suggests a central or

neurogenic cause of diabetes insipidus. This implies that the patient's pituitary gland is not producing enough ADH. A lack of response to desmopressin may indicate nephrogenic diabetes insipidus, where the kidneys do not respond appropriately to ADH.

c. *Management:*
   - *Initiation of intranasal desmopressin (DDAVP):* 10 μg in one nostril daily to maximum of 40 μg divided into two or three doses per day.
   - Continuous monitoring of fluids and electrolyte balance
   - Identification and management of any underlying causes (e.g., trauma and tumors)
   - Patient education regarding medication compliance and fluid intake

Ans. 11

a. *Sheehan syndrome:* This is the most likely cause given the patient's recent h/o postpartum hemorrhage during childbirth. Sheehan syndrome occurs when there is insufficient blood supply to the pituitary gland during childbirth, leading to its necrosis and subsequent hormonal deficiencies. The symptoms described are consistent with the hormonal deficiencies associated with Sheehan syndrome.
b. *Hyponatremia:* Due to pituitary gland injury that results in an ADH shortage, hyponatremia is a typical consequence of Sheehan syndrome. When there is not enough ADH, the kidneys cannot properly retain water. Dilutional hyponatremia is the outcome, which is an excessive loss of water through urine.
c. *Pituitary necrosis:* Mrs X's confusion is likely attributed to pituitary necrosis, a characteristic feature of Sheehan syndrome. When pituitary necrosis occurs, it can lead to a deficiency of multiple hormones produced by the pituitary gland including adrenocorticotropic hormone (ACTH), which stimulates the adrenal glands to produce cortisol. In the absence of cortisol, patients can experience symptoms, such as weakness, fatigue, and confusion.
d. *Administration of IV fluids:* In the ER setting, the initial and crucial intervention is the administration of IV fluids. This is essential for addressing hypotension and dehydration, which are likely the immediate consequences of postpartum hemorrhage and the resulting Sheehan syndrome. Hormone replacement is the long-term management for Sheehan syndrome.

Ans. 12

a. *Tachypnea:* Critical Illness-related corticosteroid insufficiency is associated with adrenal dysfunction during severe illness or stress. In cases of CIRCI, there is an inadequate physiological response of the adrenal glands to the stress, leading to a decreased production of cortisol.

This can affect various organ systems including the respiratory system. Tachypnea, or rapid breathing, is a common vital sign abnormality associated with CIRCI. The decreased cortisol levels can lead to impaired function of the respiratory muscles, resulting in increased respiratory rate. Tachypnea is a compensatory mechanism in response to the stress and metabolic demands on the body. Hypertension, bradycardia, and hyperthermia are not typically associated with CIRCI.

b. *Cortisol level measurement:* To confirm the diagnosis of CIRCI, measuring cortisol levels is essential. In patients with CIRCI, cortisol levels may be low despite the presence of a stressful situation. This test helps assess the adrenal response and guides the decision to initiate stress-dose corticosteroid therapy.
c. *Hyponatremia:* In the context of critical illness-related corticosteroid insufficiency, the dysregulation of various hormones, including cortisol, can affect the balance of electrolytes, leading to hyponatremia. Hyponatremia is often seen in conditions where there is increased secretion of ADH, which can occur in response to stress and critical illness.
d. *Administer stress-dose corticosteroids:* In CIRCI, the adrenal glands may not produce an adequate amount of cortisol in response to the stress of critical illness. This can lead to adrenal insufficiency and contribute to hypotension. Stress-dose corticosteroids, such as IV hydrocortisone, help replace the deficient cortisol and improve cardiovascular instability in patients with adrenal insufficiency.

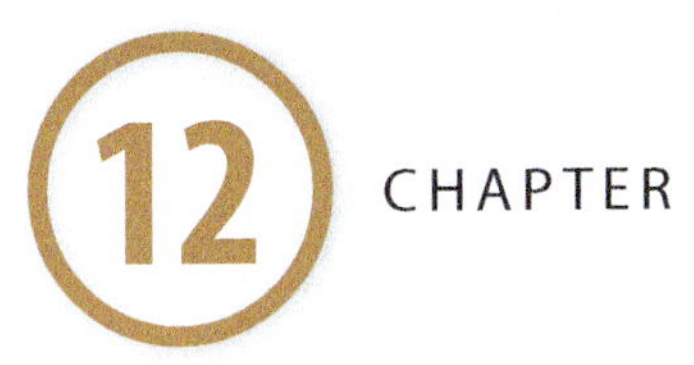

Eye, ENT, and Oral Dental Emergencies OSCE

Nilanka Mudithakumara

QUESTIONS

Q1. A 24-year-old man presented with tender reddish swollen pinna of the right ear sparing the lobule of the ear. He had a minor scratch injury 1 week back, not settled with oral cefalexin treatment.

a. What is the diagnosis?
b. What is the organism causing the above condition and what is the first-line therapy?
c. What are the anticipated complications if not treated properly?

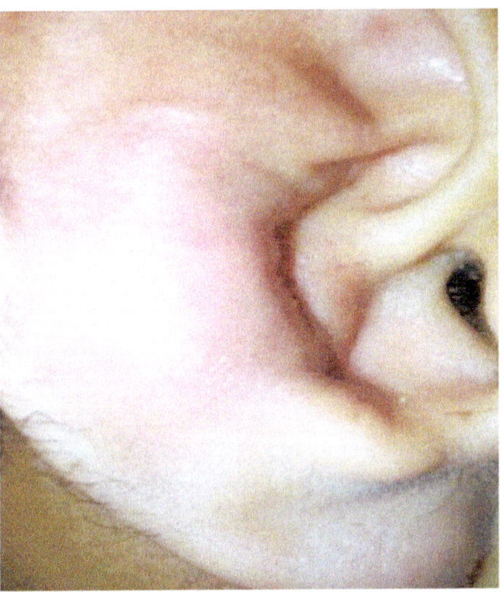

Q2. A 52-year-old male presents to emergency treatment unit with continuous flow of bleeding from nose for 5 minutes.

a. What are the history components to be asked?
b. What is the compression technique used and the duration?
c. What is the suspected area of bleeding?

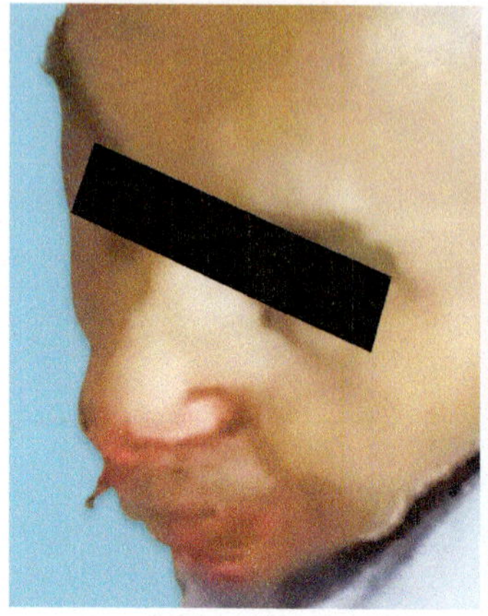
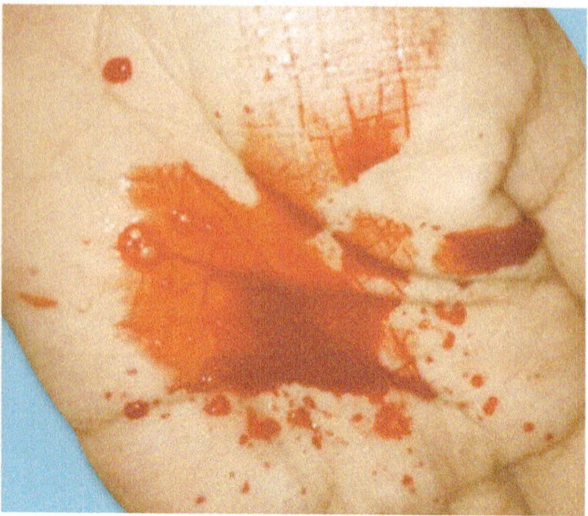

Q3. A 5-year-old male presents to emergency department with progressing dysphagia and drooling with neck swelling for past 12 hours. He has infected right lower molar teeth for past 1 week.

a. What is the possible diagnosis?
b. What is the leading cause of mortality in this condition?
c. What are the other clinical features you expect to see in this patient?

Q4. A 6-year-old boy presented with left ear pain followed by 1 week of common cold. He was diagnosed to have acute otitis media at the emergency department.

a. What are the diagnostic features of the tympanic membrane?
b. What are the red flags of acute otitis media?
c. What are the expected complications?

Q5. A-10-year-old boy presents with edema, redness, and warmth of the left eyelid and the surrounding tissues.

a. What clinical features differentiate preorbital cellulitis from orbital cellulitis from eye examination?
b. What is the anatomical margin of orbital versus preorbital cellulitis?
c. What are the complications of preorbital cellulitis and orbital cellulitis?

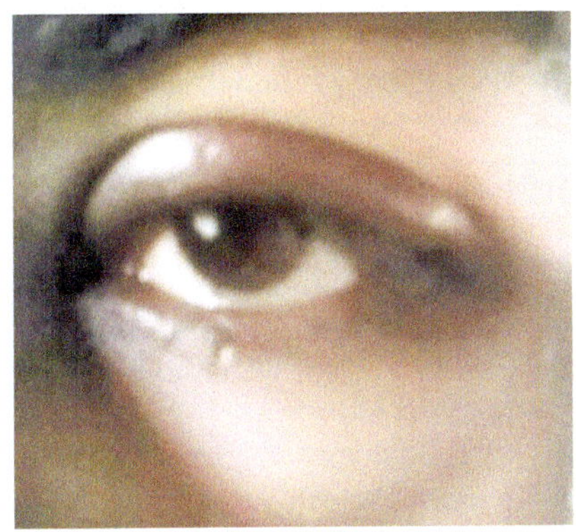

Q6. A 50-year-old man presents to the accident ward following 3 hours of trauma to the left eye with painful vision loss. Proptosis, diffuse subconjunctival hemorrhage, severe periorbital edema, and ecchymosis were present. An immediate surgical procedure was done for orbital decompression.

a. What is the name of the onsite surgery? And how is it done?
b. What are the indications for lateral canthotomy and contraindications?
c. What is the possible condition in this case requiring this procedure?

Q7. A 25-year-old male presented with severe pain of the right forehead area for last 5 days, followed by painful erythematous vesicular rash limited to right half of the forehead.

a. What is the diagnosis and the signs lead to the diagnosis?
b. What is the pathology?
c. What are the complications and management?

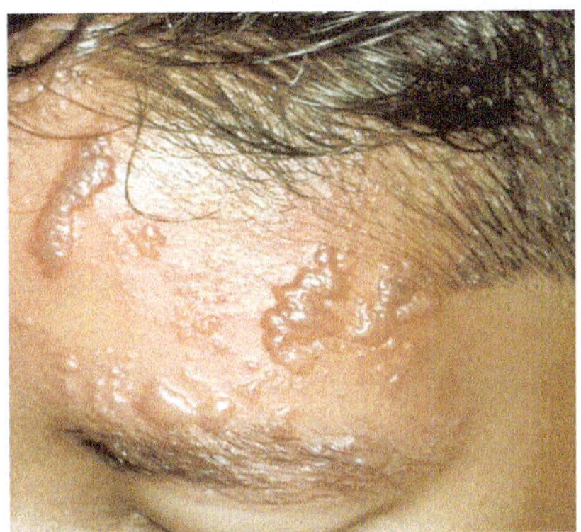

Q8. A 20-year-old male presents to the emergency department following left eye injury while using a grinding machine to cut a metal bar.

a. What clinical symptoms the patient may have?

b. What are the gross features of the above diagnosis?

c. What is the treatment option?

Q9. A 40-year-old diabetes female comes with rapidly progressive reduced vision and redness of the right eye which she had a cataract surgery 5 days ago. On examination, a level of pus was visible in the anterior chamber.

a. What is the name of the examination finding? And what is the suspected condition?

b. What is the definitive treatment?

c. What are the complications expected?

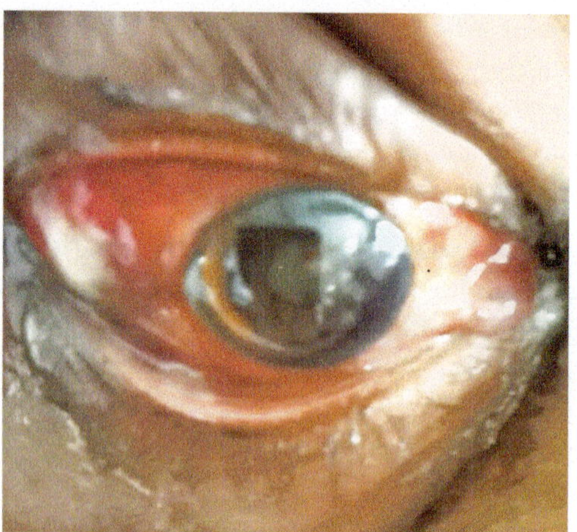

Q10. A 30-year-old man comes with acute foreign body sensation and pain of the left eye, immediately following grinding a metal rod without safety goggles.

a. What are the condition and the diagnostic test?

b. What are the examination features you expect to see?

c. What is the management if the above diagnostic test is positive?

Q11. A known patient with sickle cell disease presents with eye trauma.

a. What is the condition?

b. What are the interventions that prevent further bleeding?

c. What routine drug is contraindicated due to increasing sickling in sickle cell disease patients with this condition?

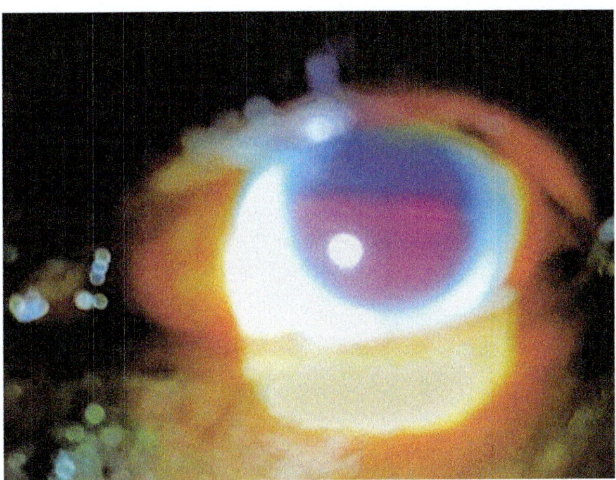

Q12. A 17-year-old girl presented with a tooth fracture of a left molar teeth while trying to open a bottle with mouth. A part of the tooth appeared red in color.

a. What is the type of the tooth fracture?

b. What are the clinical features expected in this patient?

c. What is the drug of choice in the emergency department?

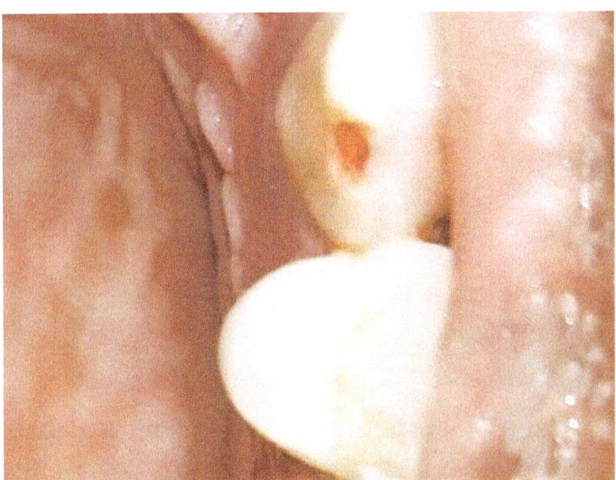

Q13. A 35-year-old man presents following nasal trauma causing nasal bone fracture.

a. What feature you do not want to miss in the patient?

b. What are the complications of the above finding, if unrecognized?

c. What are the other managements?

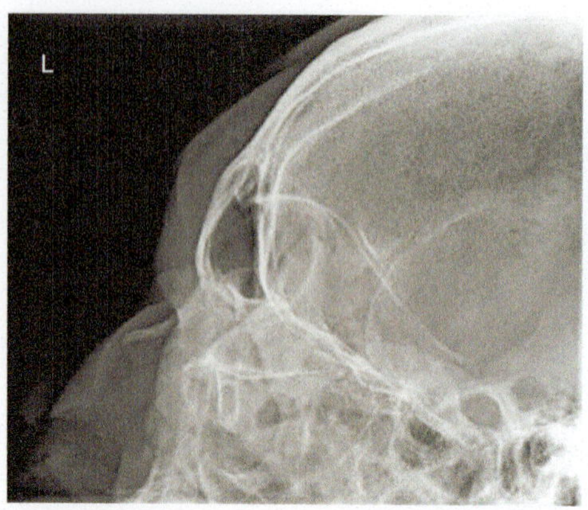

Q14. A 40-year-old male presented following a road traffic accident with facial injury. X-ray of the skull demonstrated orbital floor fracture of the left eye.

a. What clinical features you expect to see in inferior orbital floor fracture?
b. What muscle entrapment is suspected?
c. What are the complications of muscle entrapment, if the above condition is not treated as a true surgical emergency?

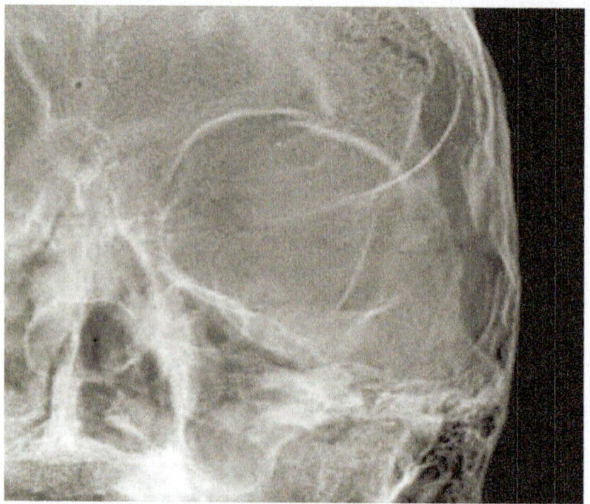

Q15. A 30-year-old female presents to emergency department with throat and neck pain, dysphagia, fever, and tachycardia. She remembers fish bone stuck in the throat 1 week back. Her oropharyngeal examination normal and the lungs are clear; saturation maintained 97% on room air, but positive for cervical lymphadenopathy.

a. What is the condition of the patient?
b. What are the predominant bacteria causing this condition?
c. How to diagnose with a lateral radiological imaging of the neck?

Q16. A 21-year-old cricket player presents with sudden onset reduction of vision following blunt trauma with the cricket ball to the right eye. His pupil's shape is changed into a "teardrop shape".

a. What are the other examination features expected to see?
b. Which examinations and investigations should be avoided in this patient?
c. What are the treatment strategies?

ANSWERS

Ans. 1

a. Perichondritis of right ear
b. *Pseudomonas aeruginosa* treat with oral fluoroquinolones
c. Abscess, liquefying chondritis cavitations of the cartilage, necrosis, and chondral deformities

Ans. 2

a. Side, duration and amount of bleeding, history of trauma, past history of similar episodes, recent upper respiratory tract infections, concomitant bleeding or bruising in the other areas, comorbidities/ongoing medications causing bleeding, history of substance use (cocaine), and alcohol use
b. *Trotter's method:* Make the patient sit up, leaning forward, firmly pinch the soft part of the nose, compressing nostrils for at least 10 minutes (with mouth open over a bowl to estimate the blood loss)
c. *Anterior bleeding:* Kiesselbach's plexus (Little's area)

Ans. 3

a. Ludwig's angina
b. Airway compromise
c. Reduced mouth opening distance, woody mouth floor, bilateral swelling of submental, sublingual and submandibular spaces and lymphadenopathy, erythema, tongue protrusion, impending compromise of airway, respiratory distress, trismus, fever, and sepsis and toxicity features

Ans. 4

a. Injected tympanic membrane, bulging and red tympanic membrane
b. <6 months old/immunocompromised/only hearing ear/cochlear implants/possible suppurative complications
c. Tympanic membrane perforation/acute mastoiditis/facial nerve palsy/intracranial spread of infection (rare)/atelectasis and cholesteatoma

Ans. 5

a. Orbital cellulitis has changes in color vision, pain with extraocular muscle movements, ophthalmoplegia, and proptosis whereas preorbital cellulitis does not. Intraorbital pressures are normal in preorbital cellulitis.

b. Preorbital cellulitis occurs anterior to the orbital septum whereas orbital cellulitis occurs posterior to the orbital septum.
c. Preorbital cellulitis can progress into orbital cellulitis and its sequelae: Cavernous sinus thrombosis, subperiosteal abscess, orbital abscess, necrotizing fasciitis, loss of vision, intracerebral abscess, and meningitis.

Ans. 6

a. Condition is orbital compartment syndrome. *Lateral canthotomy*—cutting the lateral canthus laterally 1–2 cm and the inferior crus of the lateral ligament under local anesthesia. Next to cut the superior crus if the orbital pressure remains high.
b. *Indications:* Decreased visual acuity/restricted extraocular movement/afferent pupillary defect/proptosis/increased intraocular pressure >40 mm Hg; Contraindications—globe rupture
c. Retro-orbital hematoma causing orbital compartment syndrome

Ans. 7

a. Herpes zoster/shingles of right ophthalmic nerve distribution
b. Reactivation of herpes zoster virus, which lies dormant in sensory ganglia following chickenpox (varicella) infection years ago.
c. Herpes zoster ophthalmicus—keratitis of the eye, acute retinal necrosis, retinal detachment, permanent vision loss, Ramsay Hunt syndrome, analgesics, antiviral therapy (within 72 hours of onset of clinical symptoms), early ophthalmology referral, and systemic glucocorticoids.

Ans. 8

a. Foreign body sensation, pain of the eye, tearing, light sensitivity, and vision loss
b. Fixed mid-dilated pupil, conjunctival injection, and haziness if the cornea
c. Reduce IOP IV/PO acetazolamide/mannitol (followed by mitotic agents (pilocarpine), topical β-blockers—timolol, IV analgesics and antiemetics

Ans. 9

a. Hypopyon. Right eye endophthalmitis (endophthalmitis/panophthalmitis)
b. Intravitreal antibiotics following vitreous culture (early ophthalmology involvement) and vitrectomy
c. Permanent vision loss, loss of the eye architecture, enucleation, systemic complications, panophthalmitis, corneal ulceration, and orbital cellulitis

Ans. 10

a. Left eye corneal foreign body. Test—Seidel test on fluorescence stain
b. Corneal foreign body, conjunctival injection, presence of the foreign body, and positive Seidel test

c. Computed tomography (CT) to rule out intraocular foreign body, IV antibiotics, tetanus booster, analgesia, ophthalmology referral, avoid measuring intraocular pressure if globe rupture is suspected by penetrating trauma.

Ans. 11

a. Hyphema of the left eye
b. Elevate head end/mydriasis/control of intraocular pressure (with topical β-blockers)
c. Acetazolamide

Ans. 12

a. Dental fracture; complicated dental fracture of the tooth pulp (Ellis type 3)
b. Severe pain and tooth sensitivity of the fractured tooth
c. Application of calcium hydroxide on the exposed pulp

Ans. 13

a. Nasal bone fracture and septal hematoma
b. Necrosis of the nasal cartilage, cosmetic deformities, and nasal perforations
c. Pain management and closed reduction

Ans. 14

a. Orbital floor fracture; swelling under eye, black eye, blurred vision, decreased vision pain on eye movement
b. Left inferior rectus muscle entrapment
c. Inferior rectus muscle ischemia and necrosis, permanent extraocular motility limitation, and permanent diplopia.

Ans. 15

a. Retropharyngeal abscess; fish bone injury causing retropharyngeal/parapharyngeal abscess complicated with sepsis.
b. *Streptococcus pyogenes*, *Staphylococcus aureus*, *fusobacteria*, *Prevotella*, and *Veillonella*
c. *Widened prevertebral tissues:* Anterior-posterior diameter of the soft tissues along the anterior bodies of C1-4 <40% or C2 <7 mm, <1 adjacent vertebral width C5-8 or C6 <22 mm

Ans. 16

a. Globe rupture; protruding foreign body in the eye/decreased visual acuity/afferent pupillary defect/extrusion of vitreous/external prolapse of iris or ciliary body.
b. Avoid intraocular pressure measurement/avoid eyelid retraction/avoid performing ocular ultrasound/avoid eye patch
c. Head elevation to 30°, antibiotics and tetanus prophylaxis, analgesics, and antiemetics

Dermatology Emergencies OSCE

Tejas D Patel, Nishi Trivedi

QUESTIONS

Q1. A 20-year-old female presents to the emergency department (ED) with history of eating some food from a street vendor 2 hours ago, followed by sudden swelling over her face including her lips and eyelids.

a. Identify the diagnosis and define the condition.
b. What are the types of angioedema?
c. What drugs can cause the condition?
d. What is the underlying etiology of this condition?
e. What would be the initial management of this patient in the ED?

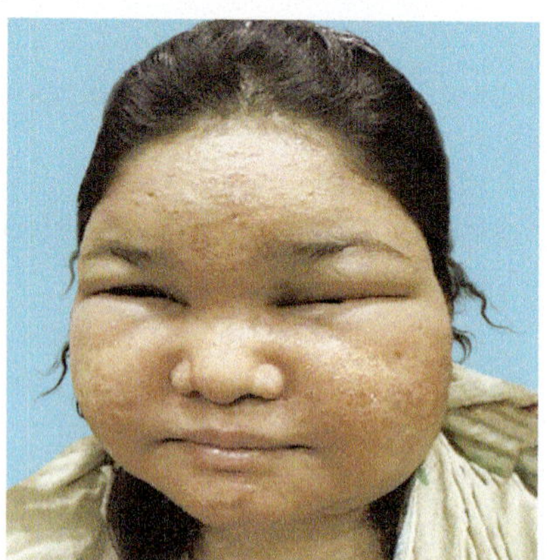

Q2. A 12-year-old girl presents to the casualty with the following itchy lesions. She has a history of fever for 2 days along with cough and cold.

a. What type of skin lesion is visible in the image?
b. What are other primary skin lesions?
c. Give the main subtypes of urticaria and the most likely diagnosis of the above case.
d. What are some important history and examination points in this case to exclude other differentials?
e. What should be the management in the ED?

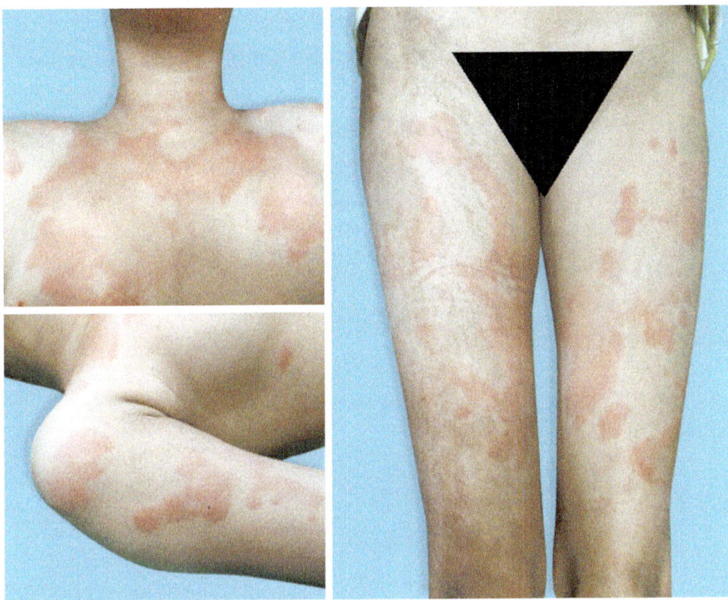

Q3. A 30-year-old male presented to the ED with a painful skin lesion on his back since 1 day. He had taken some medication from a local doctor for his diarrhea 2 days back. He reports similar complain 1 year back when he had taken some painkiller medication as well.

a. Describe the lesion. What is your differential diagnosis?
b. What is the significance of the mentioned history in the case given?
c. What is the approach to be followed in this patient?

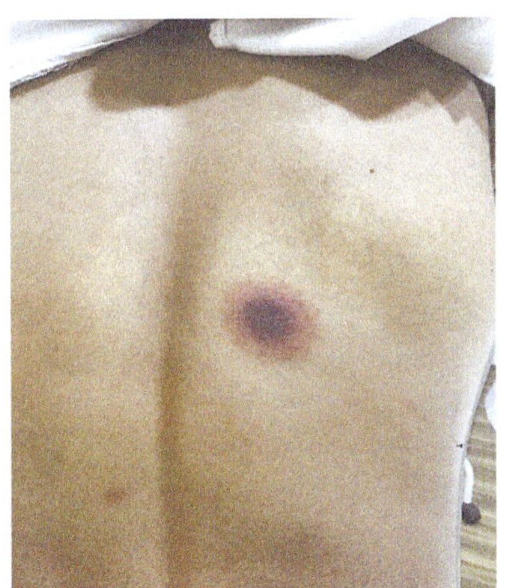

Q4. A 45-year-old female presented to the ED with skin peeling (image shown below), fever, and malaise since 1 week. She gave history of taking a medication for a seizure since 15 days.

a. What is the differential diagnosis?
b. What can be the other presentations and features of this condition?
c. What should be the management by the emergency physician at this point?
d. What are the potential complications? Is there any severity score?

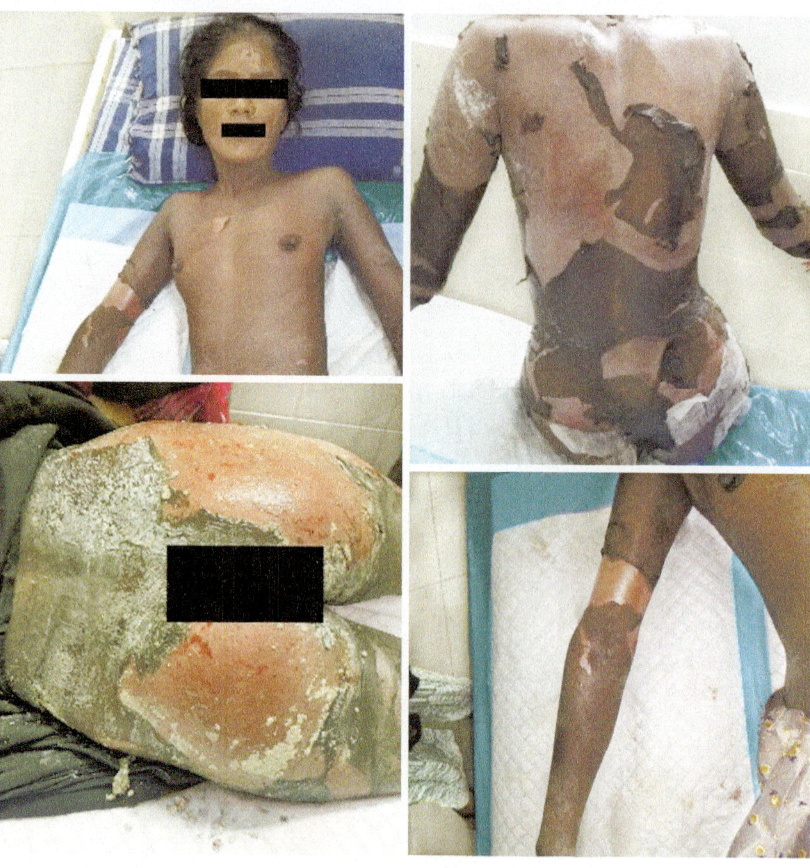

Q5. A 60-year-old woman who is a known diabetic came to the casualty with fluid-filled lesions associated with severe pain over her left side of the face since 3 days. The lesions were limited to the midline.

a. What is the diagnosis? What are the points that are in your favor?
b. What are the potential complications in this case?
c. What should be done to reduce complications?

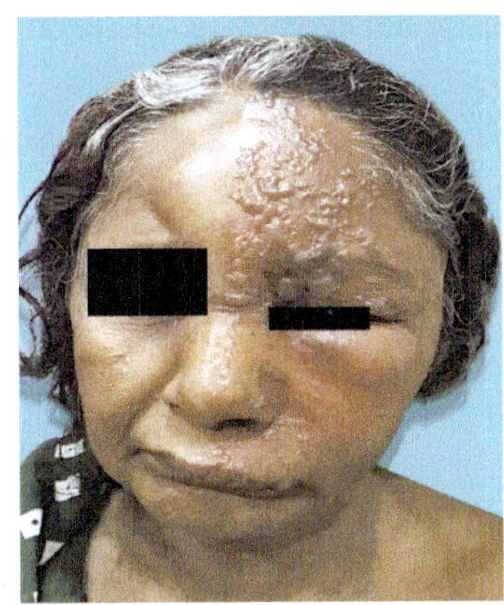

Q6. **A 23-year-old married female presented with fluid-filled lesions that ruptured spontaneously to form raw areas over her body since 3 months. Her current lesions are as shown in the below image with a foul mousy odor. She gives history of oral ulcers preceding the development of the skin lesions. Her vital signs show that her temperature is elevated.**

a. What investigations would you first like to do in the ED for this patient?
b. What is the differential diagnosis?
c. What should be the management of such patients by the emergency medicine physician?

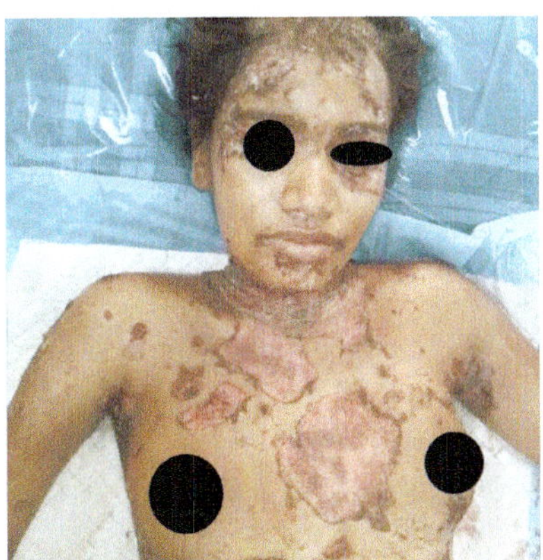

Q7. **A 45-year-old woman who is a known case of psoriasis presented to the ED with painful oral lesions and fever. She had recently been started on a new drug. On questioning her son, she revealed that by mistake she had taking the drug daily instead of once a week as had been advised by her doctor.**

a. What drug can be the cause of these symptoms? What are the other signs of the condition?
b. What are the investigations required and the reason for advising each of them?
c. What should be the management of the patient?

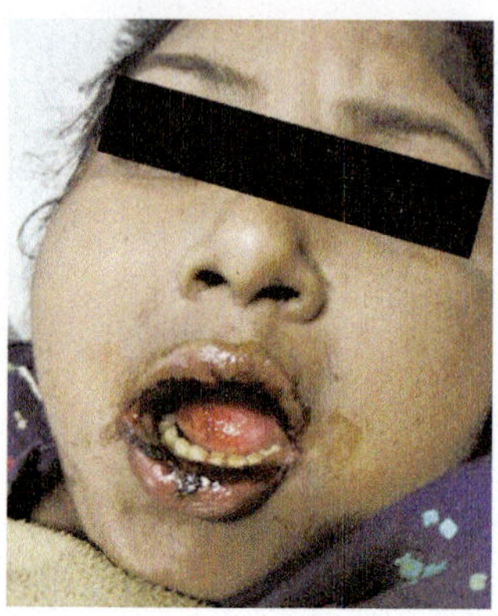

Q8. A 35-year-old female presented with below skin lesions, fever, malaise, and joint pain for 3 months. She also gave history of photosensitivity. Her vital signs were normal except for a slightly elevated temperature. Her bloodwork showed hemoglobin (Hb): 8 g/dL, red blood cell (RBC) count: 3.5/mm^3, white blood cell (WBC) count: 3,500/mm^3, and platelet count: 90,000/mm^3. Urine routine examination had albumin +.

a. What is your clinical impression from the given information? What can be the clinical features of this condition?
b. What panel of investigations are required to be performed?
c. What should be the treatment plan in this case?

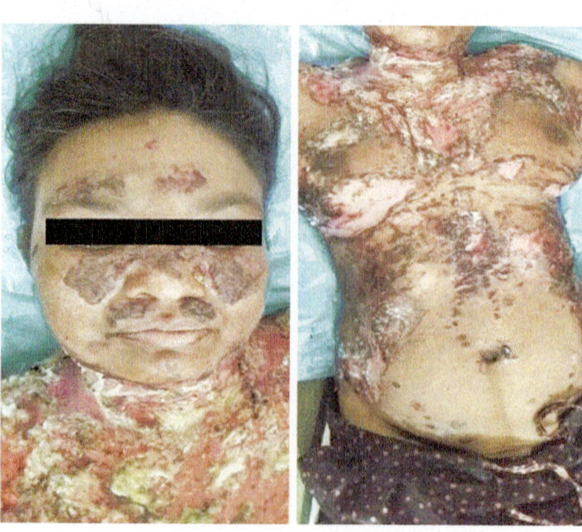

Q9. A 57-year-old male who is a known case of chronic plaque psoriasis and psoriatic arthritis for 20 years presented with fever, a tender rash on his trunk, and pus-filled lesions over the rash since a week (images shown below).

a. What is the differential diagnosis? What are the points favoring your most likely diagnosis?
b. What are the expected complications?
c. Describe the management of this patient.

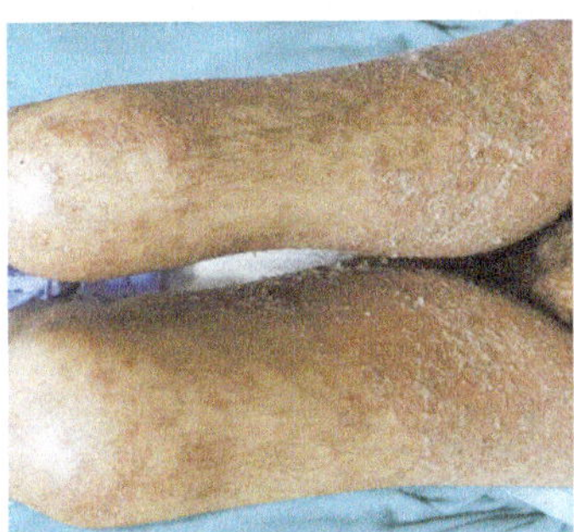
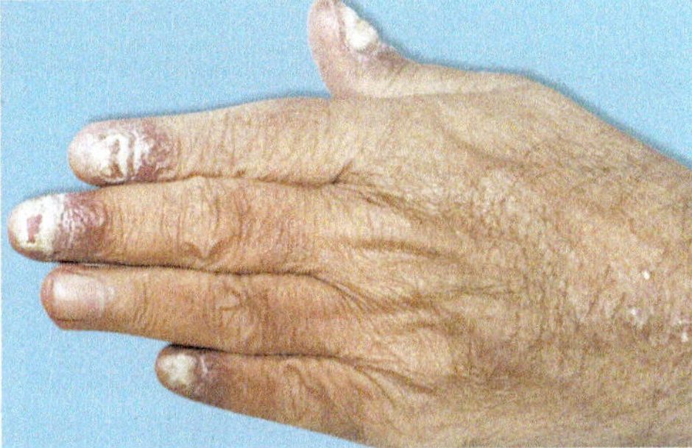
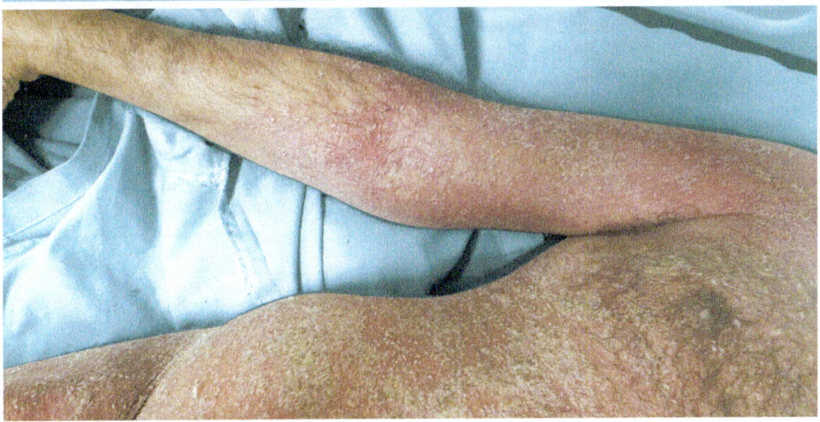

Q10. A 25-year-old girl presented to the casualty department with a limp due to pain and burning sensation in her left foot. Her image is attached below. She said her lesions appeared suddenly in the last 3 hours after some chemical solvent with which she was working in the factory fell on her foot. She has no other lesions or complains.

a. What are the primary skin lesions in this case? Define them along with a few examples where they are found.
b. What is the most likely diagnosis? What can be its other presentations?
c. What is the management?

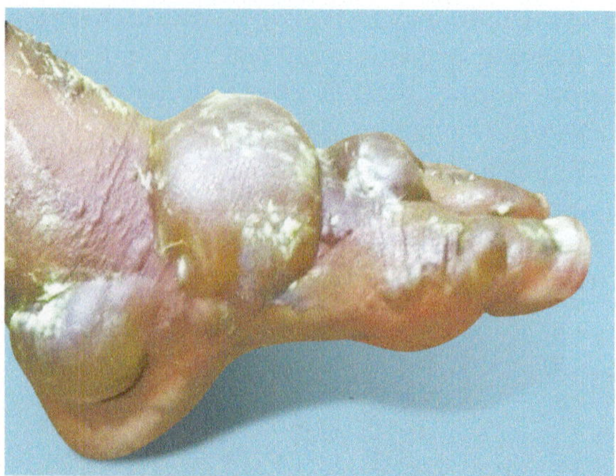

Q11. A 37-year-old unmarried male presented with generalized redness and scaling associated with pitting edema and fever for 10 days. Images are shown below.

a. Define the condition. What can be the etiology?
b. What are the complications that you anticipate in this patient?
c. Describe in brief the management of the condition.

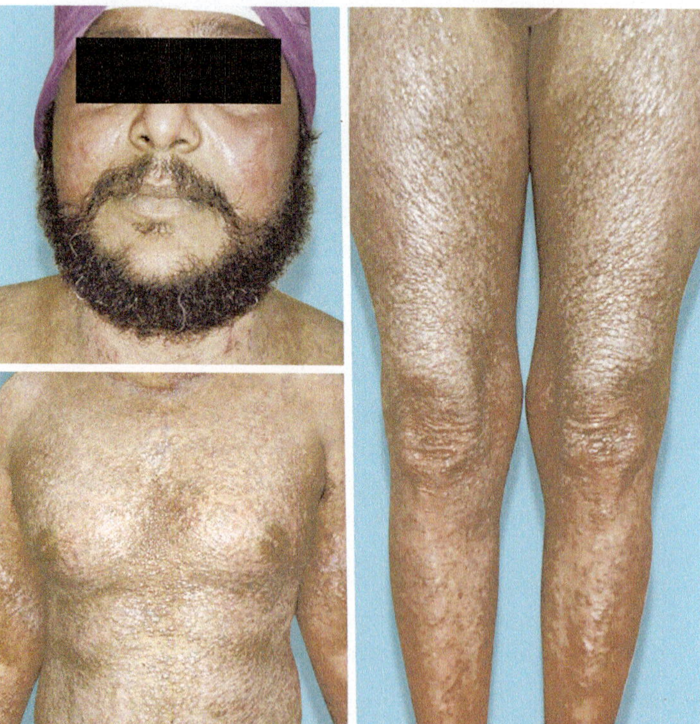

Q12. **A 53-year-old married Hindu male patient presented with complaints of intense itching on his right leg since 7 days.**

a. What is the differential diagnosis?

b. How is eczema classified?

c. What is the management of this patient?

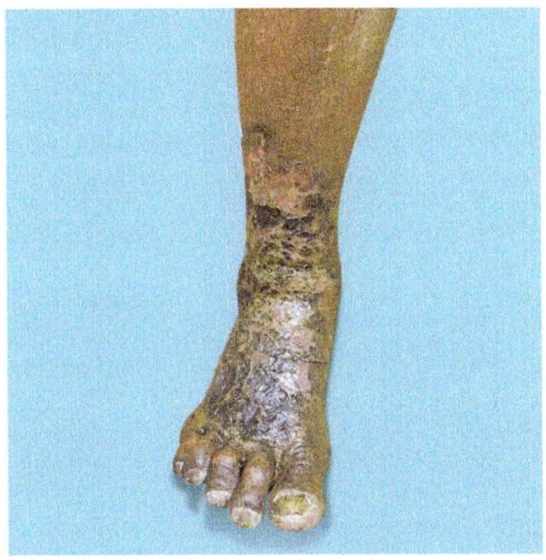

Q13. **A 62-year-old lady presented to the ED with fever and generalized lesions as shown in below image for 3 days. She reports that a week back she had been given some medication for her stomach upset. She has no other comorbidities.**

a. Describe the rash and give your differential diagnosis.

b. What are the common drugs that are implicated in acute generalized exanthematous pustulosis (AGEP)?

c. What is the management of this patient as an emergency physician?

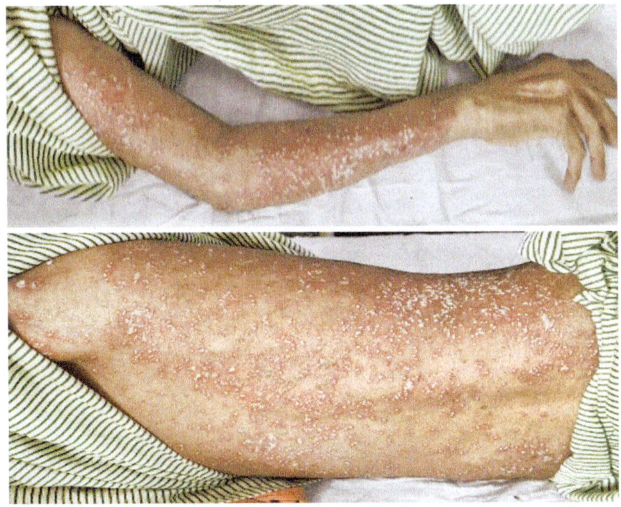

Q14. A 4-year-old boy presents to the ED with lesions as shown in the image below. He has fever, sore throat, and malaise since the last 3 days. His mother reports some ulcers in his mouth which have made him irritable.

a. Describe the rash. Enumerate causes of a maculopapular rash in a child.
b. What are the red-flag signs that indicate referral to a pediatric intensivist?
c. What is the most likely diagnosis? How should this patient be managed?

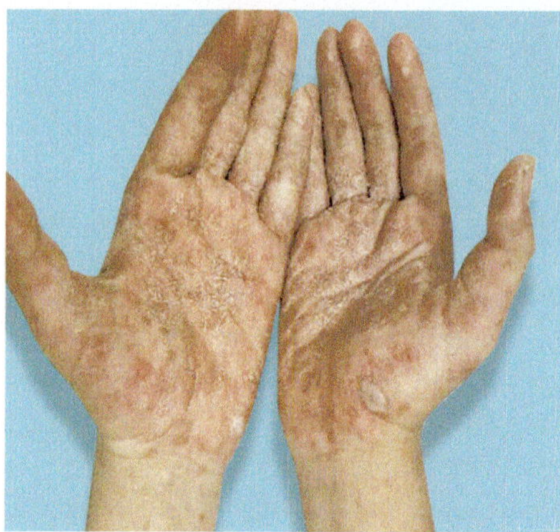

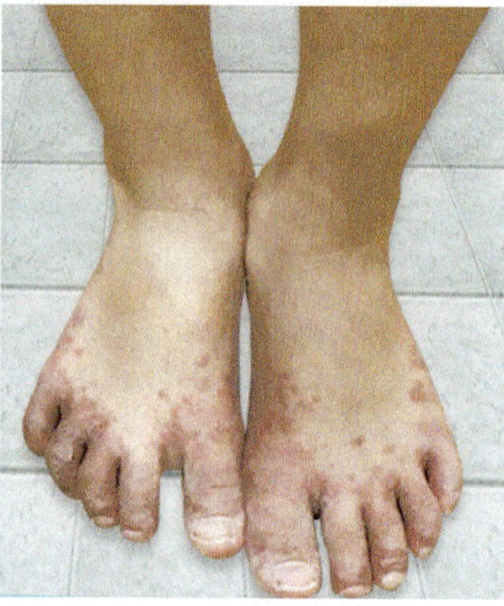

Q15. A 30-year-old male patient, resident of Bihar, presented with malaise and lesions as shown in image below. He reports that his facial lesions were skin colored earlier but have now become tender, erythematous, and swollen since a week. He complained of not being able to feel any sensations on these lesions. He also had annular "inverted saucer" shaped lesions on his trunk. He gave history of taking some medicine from a red-colored strip for 3 months 1 year ago which he stopped on his own.

a. What is the differential diagnosis for the images shown below?
b. As per the history given and images shown, what diagnosis should be suspected? How should the patient be investigated?
c. What is the management of this patient?

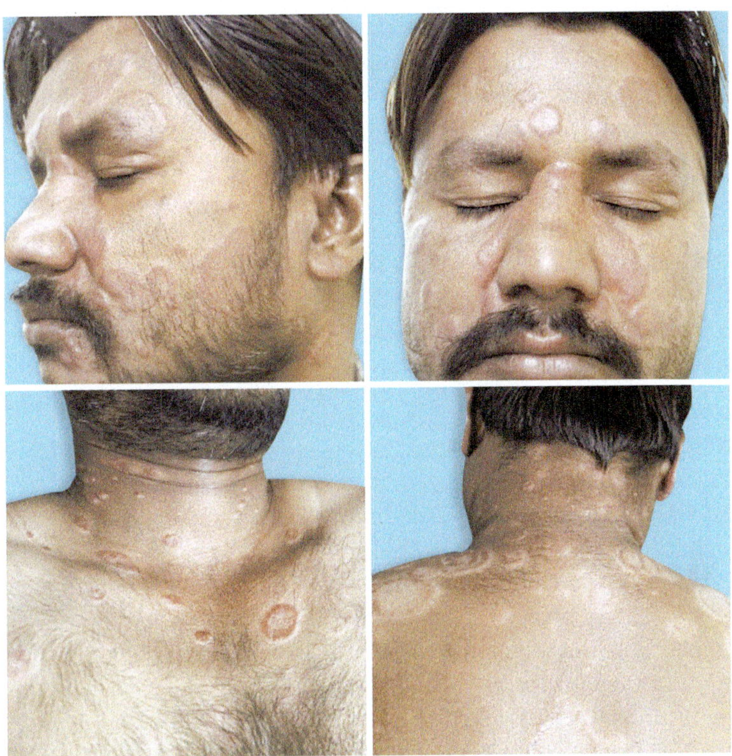

ANSWERS

Ans. 1

a. Angioedema is defined as "circumscribed nonpitting edema of the subcutaneous tissues and/or submucosal tissues affecting lips, face, neck primarily with occasional involvement of the oral cavity, larynx, and gut."
b. Acquired and hereditary. Acquired is more common, can be associated with urticaria. Hereditary type is rarer and presents as angioedema in isolation, more severe and longer lasting. It can have abdominal symptoms as well.
c. Angiotensin-converting enzyme inhibitors (ACEis), angiotensin receptor blockers (ARBs), nonsteroidal anti-inflammatory drugs (NSAIDs), and few antibiotics
d. Angioedema can be histamine mediated (more common) or bradykinin mediated. The former is a type 1 hypersensitivity reaction resulting from degranulation of mast cells and basophils. Bradykinin is a vasoactive peptide that activates endothelial cells. Several systems regulate bradykinin including the coagulation, complement, and contact

pathways. Excess bradykinin is due to production, release, or inhibition of its breakdown. This form comprises drug-induced angioedema (i.e., ACEi-mediated), hereditary angioedema, and idiopathic angioedema.

e. Emergency physicians must inquire about lip swelling, tongue swelling, and gastrointestinal (GI) symptoms (nausea, vomiting, diarrhea, and pain). Ask for prior personal or family history of angioedema, medications, and related symptoms (e.g., itching, breathlessness, syncope, and lightheadedness). The primary focus of ED management is assessment of the airway and evaluation for anaphylaxis, which is the closest differential. Patients should be treated with antihistamines and steroids. Epinephrine to be administered if airway involvement is a concern.

Ans. 2

a. Wheals are seen in this image. A wheal is a transient elevation of the skin due to dermal edema.
b. Examples of other primary skin lesions include macule, papule, plaque, nodule, vesicle, bulla, etc.
c. Spontaneous and inducible urticaria are the main subtypes. Spontaneous urticaria may be further classified into acute, episodic, or chronic. Inducible urticaria includes those urticarias in which a specific stimulus induces a reproducible wheal formation. For example, dermographism, cold urticaria, cholinergic urticaria, contact urticaria, etc. The case is most likely to be of acute spontaneous urticaria (infection induced).
d. History of recent infection, drug intake, food intake, and lip/ears/eyelids swelling (angioedema) are important to find the cause of urticaria. History of wheals lasting longer than 24–48 hours, pain/tenderness, healing with pigmentation can suggest urticarial vasculitis. On examination, diascopy can be done to look for any purpuric lesions which are not blanchable. Purpura can be a sign of vasculitis as well.
e. Since the patient has symptoms of upper respiratory tract infection, throat swab can be sent for culture. Antihistamines are the mainstay of treatment. A physician reference is warranted for further treatment.

Ans. 3

a. Single well defined, round plaque with a dusky, violaceous center and erythematous periphery on the back. Differential diagnosis can be fixed drug eruption (FDE), insect bite reaction, psoriasis, and erythema multiforme.
b. The drug history is relevant to the diagnosis as the most likely diagnosis in the case is FDE. Drugs commonly implicated include antibiotics (like cotrimoxazole, tetracyclines, penicillin, metronidazole, etc.), NSAIDs, dapsone, barbiturates, quinine, etc. The previous history of similar lesions is also significant as it points toward the classical history of FDE.

FDE occurs at the same site in every episode due to skin-resident memory T cells that get activated on exposure to the causative drug. FDE is a form of delayed hypersensitivity reaction.

c. Patient should be asked an exhaustive drug intake history—both allopathic and ayurvedic/homeopathic. Examination should be done for any mucosal involvement (oral and genital). Suspected offending drug should be stopped. Depending on the number and site of lesions, treatment may be topical corticosteroids or systemic corticosteroids. Patient should be given a drug reaction card documenting the potential drugs that he is susceptible to reacting and he should be advised to show it to the practitioner before using any drug.

Ans. 4

a. Stevens-Johnson syndrome/toxic epidermal necrolysis (SJS/TEN), pemphigus vulgaris, acute lupus erythematosus, generalized bullous FDE, and staphylococcal scalded skin syndrome
b. Purpuric, dusky macules coalescing into a rash, atypical target lesions, vesicles and large flaccid bulla over erythematous skin, painful oral mucosal erythema with ulcers, hemorrhagic crusting of lips, ocular involvement in the form of conjunctivitis, keratitis, pseudomembranes formation, urogenital tract can show mucosal erythema, blistering, and erosions with dysuria
c. The role of the emergency physician in SJS/TEN treatment involves early detection, withdrawal of offending medications/agents, early consultation with relevant specialists, supportive care, and/or ICU/burn unit referral. Maintenance of an ambient body temperature (31-32°C), proper fluid-electrolyte balance, nutritional support, and maintenance of a strict aseptic environment are crucial. Sterile Vaseline gauze dressing should be performed for the denuded skin. Disease-specific therapy should be initiated as soon as possible which includes corticosteroids/cyclosporine/intravenous immunoglobulin.
d. Acute complications are thermoregulatory dysfunction, fluid and electrolyte dysfunction (if >50% BSA involvement), anemia and leukopenia, hypoalbuminemia, hyperglycemia; Life-threatening complication: Septicemia; *Long-term complications* are postinflammatory dyspigmentation, onychomadesis (shedding of nails), abnormal photosensitivity, and sweating; Ocular: Corneal and conjunctival scarring, dry eye, trichiasis; Entropion; Oral mobility limitation due to gingival synechiae; Lung: Bronchiolitis obliterans; Gastrointestinal tract (GIT): Esophageal stricture; Urogenital: Vaginal and introital adhesions. Severity of the disease can be assessed by SCORTEN which provides a fair idea about the prognosis **Table 1**.

TABLE 1: SCORTEN score.

Total SCORTEN score	***Probability of death (%)***
0–1	3
2	12
3	35
4	58
≥5	90
Parameters	***Points***
Age >40 years	1
Presence of a malignancy	1
Epidermal detachment >30%	1
Heart rate >120 beats/minute	1
Bicarbonate <20 mmol/L	1
Urea >10 mmol/L (28 mg/dL)	1
Glycemia >14 mmol/L (252 mg/dL)	1

Ans. 5

a. Herpes zoster ophthalmicus. The unilateral presentation with a sharp midline demarcation is indicative of dermatomal involvement. The severe pain along with fluid-filled vesicles is also characteristic.

b. Since the infection has affected the trigeminal nerve's ophthalmic division (V1), the potential complications are related to the eyes, such as blepharitis, conjunctivitis, keratitis, uveitis, secondary glaucoma, neurotrophic keratopathy, and necrotizing retinitis. These can be severe leading to vision loss. Other complications include postherpetic neuralgia and secondary bacterial infections.

c. Patients should be started on antiviral treatment as soon as possible within 72 hours of disease onset. Acyclovir 800 mg five times a day/valacyclovir 1,000 mg thrice a day/famciclovir 500 mg thrice a day for at least 7 days is the recommended therapy. Role of corticosteroids is controversial. Ophthalmic assessment should be done in cases of involving the eye to facilitate appropriate ocular management.

Ans. 6

a. *Complete hemogram with a differential count*—to look for anemia and signs of infection; *Serum albumin*—to look for hypoalbuminemia; *Liver transaminases*—as baseline workup for immunosuppressive therapy; *Serum electrolytes, creatinine, and blood urea*—to evaluate kidney function; *Random blood glucose*—for baseline; *Chest X-ray*—to look for infection; *Urine examination*—to look for protein loss or infective focus;

Skin swabs for culture from raw areas—for bacterial overgrowth; *Urine/blood culture*—to look for septicemia; *Urine pregnancy test*—to rule out pregnancy; *Skin biopsy*—for diagnosis

b. Pemphigus vulgaris, other pemphigus variants, pemphigoid and its variants, erosive lichen planus, acute lupus erythematosus, erythema multiforme, and dermatitis herpetiformis

c. Patient should be monitored closely with strict temperature charting, input/output charting. Priority is to be given to maintaining fluid and electrolyte imbalances as skin barrier is damaged in these cases. Patient needs aseptic precautions and Vaseline gauze dressings to protect the raw areas. Antibiotics as per the sensitivity reports may be given to combat infection. Nutritional support, analgesics, and antihistamines are other supportive measures. The mainstay of treatment is corticosteroid therapy or biologic therapy (rituximab infusion). Other immunosuppressives, such as azathioprine, mycophenolate mofetil (MMF), methotrexate (MTX), and cyclophosphamide are adjuncts.

Ans. 7

a. Methotrexate toxicity is causing these symptoms. The early signs are ulcerative stomatitis, sore throat, and fever. Patients may present with tenderness or erythema of psoriasis lesions and skin ulcerations. Other manifestations can be nausea, diarrhea, and abdominal pain.

b. *Complete hemogram*—to look for pancytopenia as bone marrow suppression is expected and can be deadly in these patients. *Liver transaminases*—to look for liver function, MTX can cause hepatocellular injury, cirrhosis, and fibrosis. *Kidney function tests*—to ensure renal function as MTX is renotoxic and also because kidney is the major source of MTX excretion.

c. Patients of MTX toxicity are prone to infection/sepsis due to bone marrow suppression. So, they should ideally be managed in the intensive care unit (ICU) with reverse barrier nursing. Oral, skin and wound care. Intravenous hydration to maintain a urine output of 2 $L/m^2/day$ until MTX level has fallen to 0.2 μmol/L. Urine alkalization by sodium bicarbonate (urine pH >7 promotes MTX excretion and prevents MTX crystallization). Folinic acid/leucovorin rescue—20 mg 6 hourly IV for the first day followed by 10 mg 6 hourly till blood counts return to normal. Granulocyte colony-stimulating factor (G-CSF) 300 IU SC till leukocyte count returns to normal. Glucarpidase can be used if available which is extremely effective in lowering methotrexate level and prevent harmful effects of methotrexate in patient with kidney disease.

Ans. 8

a. Patient appears to have an autoimmune connective tissue disease, most likely systemic lupus erythematosus (SLE). Her skin lesions appear to be of acute LE type with crusted erosions on trunk and a crusted type of malar rash on face. This condition closely mimics TEN. For a patient to be diagnosed as having SLE, the SLICC (Systemic Lupus International Collaborating Clinics) or EULAR criteria need to be fulfilled. *SLICC criteria* have been described in the **Table 2**. At least four criteria with ≥1 clinical + ≥1 immunological criteria or biopsy proven lupus nephritis with presence of ANA/anti-dsDNA antibodies are required to confirm SLE.

b. Complete blood count with erythrocyte sedimentation rate (ESR) and C-reactive protein (CRP), liver function tests, renal function tests, urine routine examination and microscopy, 24-hour urinary protein levels, complement levels, ANA test, anti-dsDNA, anti-Sm, urine pregnancy test (in married female), echocardiogram of heart, ultrasonography (USG) of abdomen, X-rays/USG of affected joints, skin biopsy with direct immunofluorescence in patients with skin lesions

c. Treatment varies according to the disease severity. For this case, patient should be managed as an indoor patient until her skin lesions and general condition improve. She should be started on corticosteroids and immunomodulators such as MTX/azathioprine/MMF to control disease activity. She should also receive antimalarial like hydroxychloroquine along with supportive measures for nutrition and hydration. For her skin lesions, Vaseline gauze dressing is essential. She should practice strict photoprotection and use a broad-spectrum sunscreen. For those with specific organ involvements, additional therapeutic options are to be considered.

TABLE 2: SLICC criteria for diagnosis of SLE.

Clinical criteria	*Immunological criteria*
• *Acute cutaneous lupus:* Lupus malar rash (not malar discoid), bullous lupus, TEN variant of SLE, maculopapular lupus rash, and photosensitive lupus rash • *Subacute cutaneous lupus* (nonindurated psoriasiform and/or annular polycyclic lesions that resolve without scarring, although occasionally with postinflammatory dyspigmentation or telangiectasias)	ANA above laboratory reference range
Chronic cutaneous lupus: Localized (above the neck) and/or generalized (above and below the neck) classical discoid rash, hypertrophic (verrucous) lupus, lupus panniculitis (profundus), mucosal lupus, lupus erythematosus tumidus, chilblains lupus, discoid lupus/lichen planus overlap	Anti-dsDNA above laboratory reference range, except ELISA (2x above laboratory reference range)

Contd...

Contd...

Clinical criteria	*Immunological criteria*
Oral ulcers: Palate, buccal, tongue, or nasal ulcers; in absence of other causes	Anti-Sm
Nonscarring alopecia: In absence of other causes	*Antiphospholipid antibody:* Lupus anticoagulant, false-positive RPR, medium or high titer anticardiolipin (IgA, IgG, or IgM), anti-β_2-glycoprotein (IgA, IgG, or IgM)
Synovitis: Involving ≥2 joints, characterized by swelling or effusion or tenderness in ≥2 joints and 30 minutes or more of morning stiffness	*Low complement:* Low C3, low C4, and low CH50
Serositis: Typical pleurisy for >1 day, pleural effusions, or pleural rub, typical pericardial pain for >1 day, pericardial effusion, pericardial rub, or pericarditis by EKG (in absence of other causes)	*Positive direct Coombs test:* In the absence of hemolytic anemia
Renal: Urine protein/creatinine (or 24 hour urine protein) representing 500 mg of protein/24 hour, RBC casts	–
Neurologic: Seizures, psychosis, mononeuritis multiplex (in absence of other causes), myelitis, peripheral or cranial neuropathy (in absence of other causes), acute confusional state (in absence of other causes)	–
Hemolytic anemia: In absence of other causes	–
Leukopenia or lymphopenia: <4,000/mm^3 at least once (leukopenia) or <1,000/mm^3 at least once (lymphopenia); in absence of other causes	–
Thrombocytopenia: <100,000/mm^3 at least once; in absence of other causes	–

Ans. 9

a. *Differential diagnosis:* Generalized pustular psoriasis, AGEP, subcorneal pustular dermatosis, Reiter disease, and candidiasis. The most likely diagnosis in this case is generalized pustular psoriasis. The patient already has a history of psoriasis and psoriatic arthritis. The image shows nail involvement which is classical of psoriasis in the form of subungual pus, onychomadesis, and dystrophy of nails. His skin also shows "lakes of pus" appearance with few dried pus areas exfoliating.

b. Hypovolemia and oligemia leading to acute kidney injury, malabsorption, hypoalbuminemia, hyperthermia, hypocalcemia, septicemia, cholestatic jaundice, acute respiratory distress syndrome, telogen effluvium, amyloidosis, and loss of nails
c. Generalized pustular psoriasis patients require admission to hospital with prompt intensive care. Hydration with intravenous fluids, nutritional supplementation, and protection of skin with Vaseline gauze dressings are the first step. Investigations should be done to identify the general condition of the patient—complete hemogram, ESR, and liver and kidney function tests. Skin biopsy to confirm the diagnosis. The triggers for pustular psoriasis should be identified, these can be infection, irritating topical agents, stress, pregnancy, hypocalcemia or withdrawal of systemic agents like steroids, cyclosporine. Fever and joint pain can be treated with antipyretics and NSAIDs. Drug of choice is acitretin. Other options are cyclosporine, MTX, adalimumab, infliximab, and etanercept.

Ans. 10

a. Vesicle and bulla. *Vesicles* are small, clear, fluid-filled blisters of <1 cm in diameter. They are seen in herpes infections (herpes labialis, herpes genitalis, varicella, and herpes zoster), autoimmune blistering disorders (pemphigus vulgaris, dermatitis herpetiformis, etc.), contact dermatitis, etc. *Bullae* are clear, fluid-filled blisters of >1 cm in diameter. They are seen in burns, contact dermatitis, drug reactions, autoimmune blistering disorders (pemphigus vulgaris, bullous pemphigoid, etc.), inherited disorders of skin fragility (epidermolysis bullosa simplex, etc.).
b. Acute irritant contact dermatitis is the most likely diagnosis. It can present in the form of no skin lesions but only subjective sensations, such as stinging, burning, sensation of dryness, and tightness. Skin lesions can present as a spectrum ranging from a little dryness, redness to bulla, and eczematous lesions to even an acute burn.
c. The large bullae should be drained with aseptic precautions keeping the roof intact. The patient can be started on oral antihistamines, oral anti-inflammatory agents, and dressing with Vaseline gauze. Corticosteroids can be given topically or orally in severe cases. For prevention, patients should avoid the irritant. They can use personal protective equipment, such as gloves, boots, and masks as appropriate.

Ans. 11

a. The patient has erythroderma or exfoliative dermatitis which is defined as redness and scaling affecting ≥90% of the body surface area.
Causes in adults: Eczema—atopic dermatitis, contact dermatitis, airborne contact dermatitis, chronic actinic dermatitis, psoriasis, and lymphoma; Drugs—allopurinol, β-lactam antibiotics, anticonvulsants, NSAIDs,

antiretrovirals, and sulfonamides; Hereditary dermatoses—ichthyosiform erythroderma and pityriasis rubra pilaris; Bullous dermatoses—pemphigus foliaceus and bullous pemphigoid; Others—dermatophytosis and crusted scabies, subacute cutaneous lupus erythematosus, and idiopathic

b. *Complication:* Hemodynamic and metabolic disturbances (increased skin perfusion leads to fluid loss by transpiration), hypothermia, hypoalbuminemia (due to the protein lost in exfoliated scales), infection, and high output cardiac failure

c. The patient should be hospitalized and monitored closely for vitals. A warm and humid environment is required along with fluid and electrolyte correction and nutritional supplementation (high-protein diet). Secondary infection if any should be treated. Antihistamines can provide symptomatic relief. Topically, bland emollients with wet dressings are to be used. Low-to-medium potency topical corticosteroids can be applied as well. The specific treatment should be initiated only after delineating cause of erythroderma. For eczematous diseases, systemic corticosteroids/immunomodulators are suitable. For psoriatic erythroderma, steroid-sparing immunosuppressives are preferred.

Ans. 12

a. *Differential diagnosis:* Acute eczema, allergic contact dermatitis, irritant contact dermatitis, stasis dermatitis, cellulitis, and pellagra

b. Eczema can be classified as exogenous (occurring due to external agent) or endogenous (occurring due to constitutional reasons). *Examples of exogenous eczema* are irritant/allergic contact dermatitis, photodermatitis, and phytophotodermatitis. *Examples of endogenous eczema include* atopic eczema, seborrheic dermatitis, pityriasis alba, asteatosis eczema, stasis dermatitis, and prurigo nodularis.

   Another technique of classifying eczema can be through its morphology and stage.

   - Acute eczema—presents with vesicles, edema, oozing, and crusting and is the initial stage; intensely itchy
   - Subacute eczema—presents with erythema, scaling, fissuring; itchy, painful, and stinging sensation
   - Chronic eczema—thickened skin (lichenification), excoriations; itchy

c. Patient appears to have acute eczema. He should be asked to keep legs elevated. He should be treated with wet compresses, antihistamines, and topical/oral corticosteroids. Antibiotics can be added if secondary infection is suspected.

Ans. 13

a. Multiple pinpoint pustules on a background of erythema are visible on the upper limb and trunk. Differential diagnosis of a pustular rash is as follows:
   - Acute generalized exanthematous pustulosis—short duration, drug history present, lack of prior history of psoriasis, absence of psoriatic stigmata of joints or nails, and flexural predominance of pustules
   - Pustular psoriasis—longer duration of pustules, prior history of psoriasis, no relevant drug history, typical psoriatic lesions, nail, or joint involvement suggestive of psoriasis
   - Subcorneal pustular dermatosis—less acute course, flaccid pustules which may demonstrate hypopyon.
   - Drug rash with eosinophilia and systemic symptoms (DRESS)—a smaller number of pustules, internal organ involvement present more commonly than AGEP
   - Candida infection—pustules only in flexural areas, in immunocompromised patients, yeast can be detected in microbiological samples.

b. *Drugs:* Acetaminophen; antimicrobials—penicillin, macrolides, tetracyclines, quinolones, cephalosporins, cotrimoxazole, azoles, hydroxychloroquine, carbamazepine, NSAIDs, and calcium channel blockers.

c. AGEP is a self-limiting disease with a favorable prognosis. Management includes withdrawal of the offending drug, supportive care, and symptomatic treatment of pruritus and skin inflammation. Since reexposure to the causative agent can induce another episode of AGEP, patients should be counseled to avoid the offending drug and be provided with a written list of the generic and brand names of the offending drug. Patients with severe forms of AGEP usually are hospitalized for treatment. Older or compromised patients with fever and widespread eruption may require fluid, electrolyte, and nutritional support. Systemic corticosteroids for a short period of time are usually enough to treat the condition. The skin lesions require bland emollient applications.

Ans. 14

a. There are multiple erythematous macules and papules, few coalescing together with scaling over both palms and soles extending to the dorsal part of toes as well. Few vesicles containing a turbid fluid are visible on palms. Maculopapular rash may be seen in viral infections—measles, rubella, dengue, chikungunya, erythema infectiosum, and infectious mononucleosis; Bacterial infections—scarlet fever and enteric fever; Drug eruptions; Erythema multiforme; Urticaria; Rheumatic fever; Pityriasis rosea; Lupus erythematosus; Gianotti-Crosti syndrome

b. *Red-flag signs:* Child appears toxic/unwell and is lethargic, pallor, respiratory distress—tachypnea and grunting; Poor feeding; Dry mucous membranes; Persistent tachycardia; Reduced urine output; Nonblanching rash; Fever for ≥5 days; Seizure
c. The patient appears to have hand, foot, and mouth disease (HFMD). As the condition is self-limiting in nature, treatment is supportive. Adequate hydration, rest, soothing lotions, and symptomatic treatment for fever, and throat pain are suitable. Topical corticosteroids are given for a short duration by dermatologists for faster relief.

Ans. 15

a. *Differential diagnosis:* Hansen's disease/leprosy; Urticaria; Lupus erythematosus; Dermatophytosis; Psoriasis; Neurofibromatosis; Granuloma annulare; Mycosis fungoides
b. Patient is mentioned to be from Bihar (leprosy endemic state), has inability to feel sensations in lesions which are swollen/tender/erythematous (sensory loss on lesions is seen in leprosy), has annular "inverted saucer-shaped" lesions which are classically seen in leprosy (borderline tuberculoid type) and gives history of taking medicine from red colored strip (suggestive of multidrug therapy given as part of the government program for leprosy treatment). All these points are suggestive of Hansen's disease or leprosy. The patient should be further examined to determine the severity and type of leprosy.
   - Full skin examination to note various morphologies of skin lesions present—hypopigmented patch, skin-colored/erythematous plaques, nodules, and ulcer
   - Head-to-toe examination—loss of lateral one-third of eyebrows, ear infiltrates, deformities, and eye examination
   - Nerve examination—palpation of peripheral nerves to look for thickening, pain, and nodularity
   - Sensory examination—test on lesions and normal skin both for crude and fine touch, temperature, and pain. Motor examination—voluntary muscle tests to check for power of muscles
   - Slit-skin smear test—to look for acid-fast bacilli
   - Skin biopsy for histopathology
c. Patient requires to be managed under a dermatologist as leprosy patients require a long-term follow-up and must be closely monitored under the NLEP (National Leprosy Elimination Program). After diagnosis of patient's type of leprosy (tuberculoid leprosy or lepromatous leprosy), patient is started on appropriate multidrug therapy (MDT). Patients also need to be evaluated for presence of reactions; this patient appears to be in type 1 reaction for which NSAIDs and oral corticosteroids need to be administered.

Obstetrics and Gynecology Emergencies OSCE

Patibandla Sree Sowjanya

QUESTIONS

Q1. **A 24-year-old G_1P_1 with 32 weeks gestation presented to emergency department (ED) with vaginal bleeding for last few hours associated with abdominal pain. On examination, heart rate (HR): 110 beats/min, blood pressure (BP): 90/60 mm Hg, and respiratory rate (RR): 20 breaths/min. Uterus is tender and feels tense and woody on palpation.**

a. What is the most likely diagnosis?
b. Name four risk factors associated with this condition.
c. Give four steps how would you manage this patient in ED?

Q2. **A 22-year-old with 34 weeks gestation presents to ED with severe frontal headache and visual blurring. She is from a nearby village and has not attended antenatal clinics and her last scan was 18 weeks. This is her first pregnancy and fit otherwise. She has been experiencing headaches more and more frequently. Her vitals are HR: 90 beats/min, BP: 170/110 mm Hg, RR: 17 breaths/min, and temperature: 98.4°F.**

a. What critical condition to be considered for this patient?
b. Describe the features suggestive of the diagnosis.
c. Give the signs you might expect to see.

Q3. **A 28-year-old patient presents to ED after finding out she is pregnant for the first time. Her last menstrual period (LMP) was 7 weeks ago. She is concerned that her blood group is B negative and her husband's blood group is O positive and may need special treatment during pregnancy.**

a. Outline basic pathophysiology of rhesus diseases.
b. Name three potentially sensitizing events.
c. Enumerate complications of hemolytic disease of newborn.

Q4. **A 22-year-old lady is brought to ED after fainting at work. She complained of severe abdomen pain. Her LMP was 7 weeks ago. She denies vaginal discharge or bleeding. On examination,**

HR: 130 beats/min and BP: 80/50 mm Hg. Rebound tenderness noted in left iliac fossa (LIF).

a. What is the most likely diagnosis?
b. What are the risk factors for this diagnosis?
c. What are the signs and symptoms suggestive of this diagnosis?

Q5. A 29-year-old primi who was in labor for 14 hours presents to ED with profuse vaginal bleeding. Uterine atony was suspected to be the cause.

a. Give causes for primary postpartum hemorrhage (PPH).
b. What are the risk factors for uterine atony?
c. Name the technique performed to attempt to stop bleeding and drugs that could be given to stop bleeding.

Q6. A 21-year-old woman, 11 weeks pregnant, presents to ED with persistent and severe nausea and vomiting. She has been having morning sickness since 5 weeks but her symptoms are getting worse. She has tried oral medications cyclizine and promethazine but not able to retain medication or food. She is feeling weak and lightheaded. Her vitals are HR: 128 beats/min and BP: 90/60 mm Hg. She is afebrile and rest of the examinations is within normal limits.

a. What is the diagnosis of the condition?
b. What are the characteristics of this condition?
c. Name the complications associated with this condition.

Q7. A 46-year-old woman presents to ED with vaginal bleeding. Her LMP was 10 weeks ago and home pregnancy test was positive 2 weeks ago. The bleeding was heavy and has been ongoing for last 24 hours. She noticed larger clots and her serum β-human chorionic gonadotropin (β-hCG) shows levels of 150,000 IU/L.

a. What is your diagnosis?
b. What is the most useful investigation and characteristic finding you can expect?
c. What are the risk factors associated with this condition?
d. What is the definitive treatment of this condition?

Q8. For each of the following patients presenting with vaginal bleeding, give three different differential diagnoses:

a. A 20-year-old presenting with very heavy regular periods with clots and flooding
b. A 60-year-old postmenopausal with vaginal bleeding
c. A 25-year-old presenting with postcoital bleeding

Q9. You are asked to give a presentation on antepartum hemorrhage to your AED colleagues.

a. What is the definition of the antepartum hemorrhage?
b. What is the pathophysiology of placenta previa?
c. What are the risk factors for placenta previa?
d. How do you differentiate placenta previa and abruptio placenta?

Q10. A 28-year-old woman presents to ED with vaginal bleeding. She is 10 weeks pregnant and concerned that she is having miscarriage.

a. State four main categories of miscarriage and how they are differentiated from each other?
b. What investigation would help to classify the type of miscarriage?
c. What are the risk factors of miscarriage?

Q11. A 25-year-old lady presents to ED complaining of foul fishy smelling watery vaginal discharge. She denies itchy, pain, or urinary symptoms. On examination, you notice a thin white discharge coating the vagina.

a. What is the most likely diagnosis?
b. What are the most common risk factors?
c. What is the definitive treatment?

Q12. A 23-year-old anxious female presents to ED asking for emergency contraception after having unprotected sexual intercourse yesterday evening.

a. Name the methods of emergency contraception that are available.
b. Give four important factors that should be considered for providing emergency contraception.

Q13. For each of the following trimesters, give two possible causes for bleeding in pregnancy.

a. First trimester
b. Second trimester
c. Third trimester

Q14. A 23-year-old university student attends AED complaining of a foul-smelling frothy gray-green discharge. She is also complaining of vulval itch, irritation, and superficial dyspareunia. She has recently started a relationship with a new partner. On examination, you note vulvovaginal inflammation and a strawberry cervix.

a. What is the most likely diagnosis?
b. What is the quickest way to confirm your diagnosis?
c. What is the first-line treatment for this condition?

Q15. A 40-year-old woman presents to the ED or emergency department with vaginal discharge. She describes the discharge as thick and white, and also complains of vulval itching and irritation and some discomfort on passing urine. On examination, you note some vulval erythema and excoriations as well as a thick white cheese-like discharge.

a. What is the most likely diagnosis?
b. Give a risk factor for this condition.
c. What is the first-line treatment for this condition?

ANSWERS

Ans. 1

a. Abruptio placenta
b. *Risk factors:* Trauma, preeclampsia, smoking, previous cesarean section, multiple pregnancy, and previous placental abruption
c. Insert two large bore IV cannulae, start IV fluid bolus, and crossmatch 6 units blood
   Analgesia as required, cardiotocography to monitor fetus, and urgent OBG consultation

Ans. 2

a. Preeclampsia
b. Severe headaches—unrelieved by analgesia, visual problems—blurring of vision, flashing lights, double vision, floating spots, and persistent epigastric pain/right upper quadrant pain. Sudden swelling of face, hands, or feet
c. Hyperreflexia, clonus, papilledema, and fetal distress

Ans. 3

a. *Rhesus:* Negative mothers can become sensitized to and produce antibodies against fetal rhesus positive red blood cells causing destruction of these cells.
b. Amniocentesis, cordocentesis. Antepartum hemorrhage, fall/abdomen trauma
   Threatened miscarriage, ectopic pregnancy, intrauterine death
c. Neonatal anemia, neonatal jaundice, kernicterus, and hydrops fetalis

Ans. 4

a. Ectopic pregnancy
b. *Risk factors:* Previous ectopic pregnancy, history of (H/o) pelvic inflammatory disease (PID), H/o tubal or pelvic surgery, sterilization/reversal of sterilization, and assisted reproductive techniques
c. *Symptoms:* Abdominal or pelvic pain, vaginal bleeding, dizziness, fainting, syncope, shoulder tip pain, passage of tissue, pain on defecation;

Signs: Abdominal tenderness, left iliac fossa/right iliac fossa (LIF/RIF) mass, peritonism/rebound tenderness/guarding, adnexal tenderness/mass, cervical excitation, and shock

Ans. 5

a. Retained placenta, genital tract trauma, and clotting disorders
b. *Risk factors of uterine atony:* Past H/o PPH/retained placenta, halothane anesthesia, large placental site (large baby, multiple pregnancy, and severe rhesus disease), placenta previa, placenta abruption, preeclampsia/PIH, trauma to uterus/cervix, Older mothers/maternal obesity
c. *Technique:* Bimanual uterine compression; Drugs: Oxytocin 5 units slow IV infusion, ergotamine 0.5 mg slow IV or IM, and carboprost 0.25 IM (maximum eight doses)

Ans. 6

a. Hyperemesis gravidarum
b. *Characteristics:* Prolonged and severe nausea and vomiting, dehydration, electrolyte imbalance, ketosis, body weight loss > 5% of pregnancy weight
c. *Complications:* Acidosis, abnormal liver function tests (LFTs), hyponatremia leading to lethargy, seizures, and respiratory arrest; vitamin deficiencies—vitamin B_6 and B_{12} leading to peripheral neuropathy, vitamin B_1 deficiency leading to Wernicke's encephalopathy, retinal hemorrhage, splenic avulsion, Mallory-Weiss tear/esophageal rupture, and pneumothorax

Ans. 7

a. Molar pregnancy
b. Pelvic ultrasound—absent fetus, snowstorm appearance
c. Age <16 years and >45 years previous molar pregnancy
d. Surgical evacuation of the uterus

Ans. 8

a. *Menorrhagia:* Dysfunctional uterine bleeding, endometriosis/adenomyosis, uterine fibroids, PID/endometritis, hypothyroidism, copper intrauterine device (IUD), and clotting disorders
b. *Postmenopausal bleeding:* Atrophic vaginitis, endometrial hyperplasia, endometrial carcinoma, vaginal cancer, ovarian cancer, and hormone replacement therapy (HRT)
c. *Postcoital bleeding:* Pelvic inflammatory disease, cervical ectropion, cervical or endometrial polyps, vaginal cancer, cervical cancer, trauma, endometrial cancer, and atrophic vaginitis

Ans. 9

a. Vaginal bleeding after 24th weeks of pregnancy
b. *Placenta previa:* Placenta is inserted wholly or in part into lower segment of uterus

c. *Risk factors of placenta previa:* Previous H/o placenta previa, previous cesarean section, advancing maternal age, increasing parity, uterine abnormalities, smoking, and assisted reproductive techniques
d. Differentiation between placenta previa and abruptio placenta

Placenta previa	***Placenta abruption***
Painless	Painful
No tender uterus	Tender woody uterus on palpation
No signs of fetal distress	Fetal distress
Clinical shock in proportion to visible *per vaginal (PV)* bleed	Clinical shock out of proportion to visible PV bleed

Ans. 10

a. *Miscarriage:* Loss of pregnancy before 24 weeks gestation, usually occurring before 12 weeks gestation.
   Complete miscarriage: All the products of conception expelled from uterus, bleeding stopped, and OS closed.
   Threatened miscarriage: Mild PV bleeding ± pain, cervical OS closed
   Inevitable miscarriage: Heavy PV bleeding + pain, cervical OS open
   Missed (delayed) miscarriage: No visible PV bleeding, products of conception not expelled, and often recognized on ultrasound
b. Transvaginal ultrasound
c. *Risk factors:* Chromosomal abnormalities, placental abnormalities, uterine abnormalities, incompetent cervix, >200 mg caffeine in a day; comorbidities—DM, HTN, SLE, CKD, thyroid disease; infections—Rubella, CMV, HIV, and listeriosis
   Medicines: NSAID and methotrexate

Ans. 11

a. Bacterial vaginosis
b. Active sexual life, copper IUD
c. Metronidazole 400 mg

Ans. 12

a. Levonorgestrel, ulipristal acetate, and copper IUD
b. Consider time frame for unprotected sexual intercourse, exclude pregnancy
   Carry out risk assessment for sexually transmitted infection (STI)
   Consider risk for sexual abuse, rape, or nonconsensual sex
   Consider if patient is on regular medication which can interact with oral medication
   Provide adequate follow-up/aftercare advice
   Consider the age >18 years
   Offer advice regarding regular contraception or protection against STI

Ans. 13

a. Any two of spontaneous miscarriage—ectopic pregnancy and molar pregnancy

Any two of spontaneous miscarriage—molar pregnancy, placental abruption, and placenta previa

b. Ay two of placental abruption—placenta previa, vasa previa, and uterine rupture

Ans. 14

a. Trichomoniasis
b. High vaginal swab for wet film microscopy
c. Oral metronidazole

Ans. 15

a. Vulvovaginal candidiasis
b. Any one of—poorly controlled diabetes mellitus, immunocompromise, recent antibiotics
c. Intravaginal or oral antifungal (e.g., clotrimazole, pessary, or oral fluconazole)

Pediatric Emergencies OSCE: Part I

Nadeem Qureshi

QUESTIONS

Q1. **A 15-day-old neonate, born at full term gestation via normal vaginal delivery, was noted to have respiratory distress and bluishness by parents. The baby was referred to tertiary center for further management where at presentation, the baby was found to be lethargic, in distress, and had central cyanosis. On auscultation, no significant murmur could be appreciated. His arterial blood gas showed severe hypoxemia with metabolic acidosis. Chest X-ray is available for interpretation.**

a. Interpret the chest X-ray.

b. What are the most probable causes?

c. How to approach cyanosis in neonates?

d. What is the management?

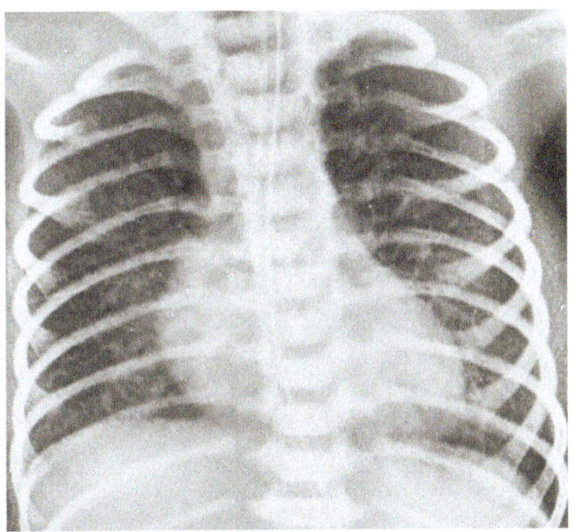

Q2. **A 6-day-old term neonate presented in medical emergency with complaints of lethargy, increased respiratory rates, and refusal to feed. The baby was mottled in color with poor peripheral perfusion. While the central pulses were palpable, the lower limb pulses were feeble.**

Chest X-ray and echocardiography was done. On echocardiography, severe left ventricular (LV) dysfunction with ejection fraction (EF) is 15–20%.

a. Interpret the chest X-ray.
b. What is the most probable diagnosis in neonates who presented with shock?
c. What is the management?

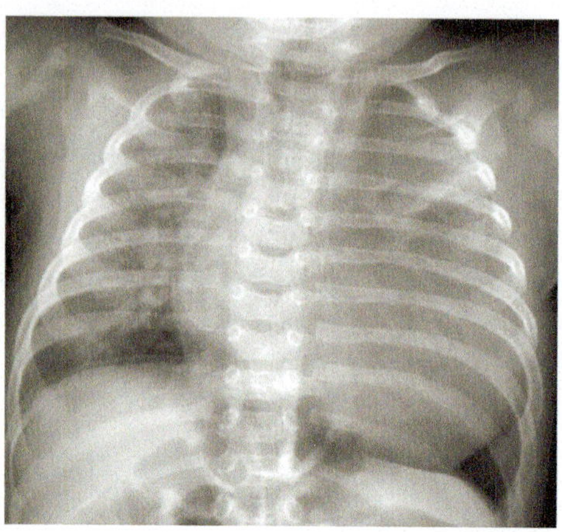

Q3. A 3-week-old neonate presented with tachypnea, tachycardia, and refusal to feed for 3 days. There was hepatomegaly and cardiomegaly on examination. Auscultation revealed gallop rhythm, no significant murmur. Chest X-ray frontal view showed cardiomegaly, no parenchymal lesion.

a. Interpret the ECG.
b. What is the further investigation modality for diagnosis?
c. What is the management of this condition?

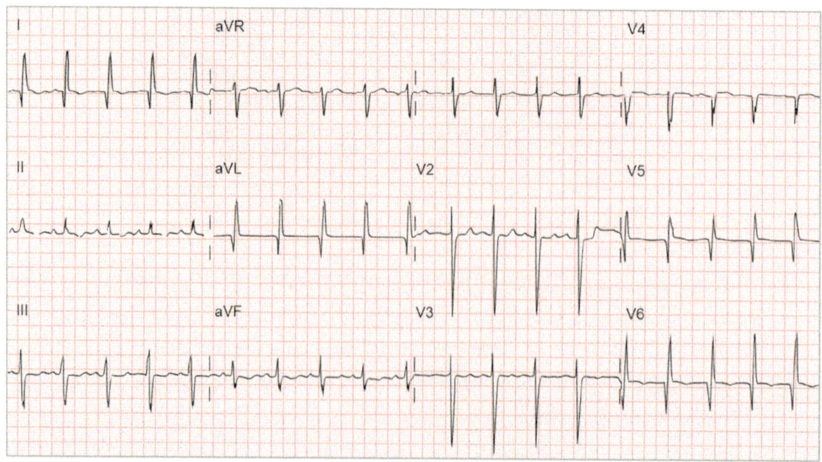

Q4. An 8-year-old boy presented to the medical emergency department with complaints of respiratory distress. Patient had history of breathlessness on exertion and orthopnea since months. Patient had past history of swelling in left knee followed by swelling of left ankle 2 months ago. He had tachycardia, cardiomegaly, and a loud apical pansystolic murmur with radiation to axilla. He also had hepatomegaly with liver 5 cm below costal margin.

a. Interpret the X-ray chest.
b. What are the congenital cardiac defects associated with congestive heart failure (CHF) in pediatric age group?
c. What is the management of this condition?

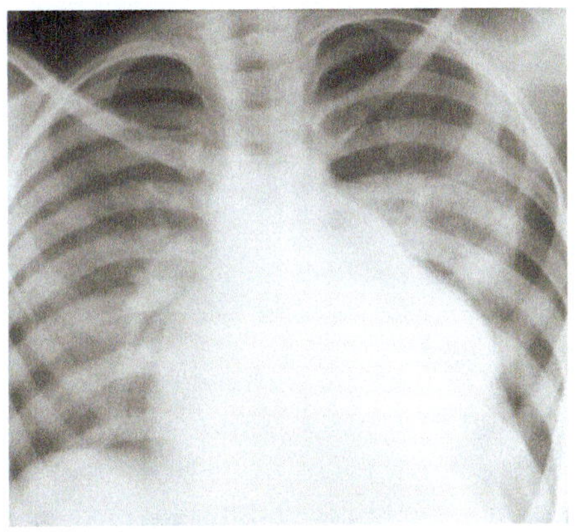

Q5. A 3-year-old child brought to emergency department who has accidentally ingested the cardiac medicine of his grandfather. Interpret the ECG.

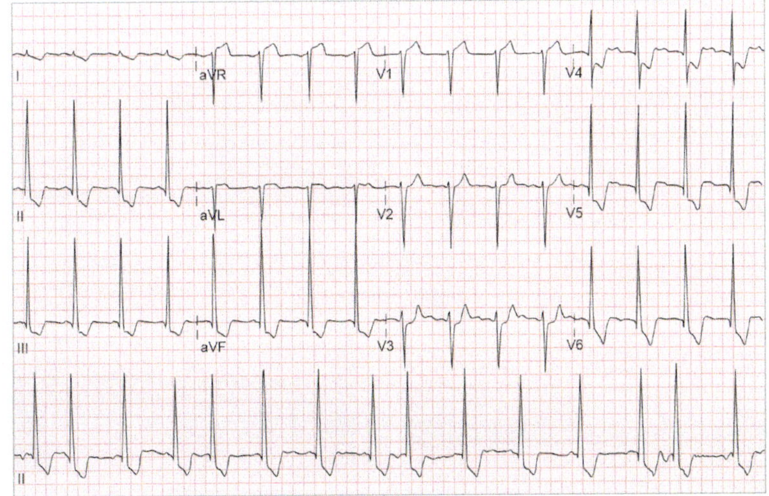

Q6. A child presenting with features of cardiac failure in emergency department.

a. Interpret the chest X-ray.
b. Interpret the echocardiography image shown below.
c. What is the Beck's triad?
d. What is the management of this condition?

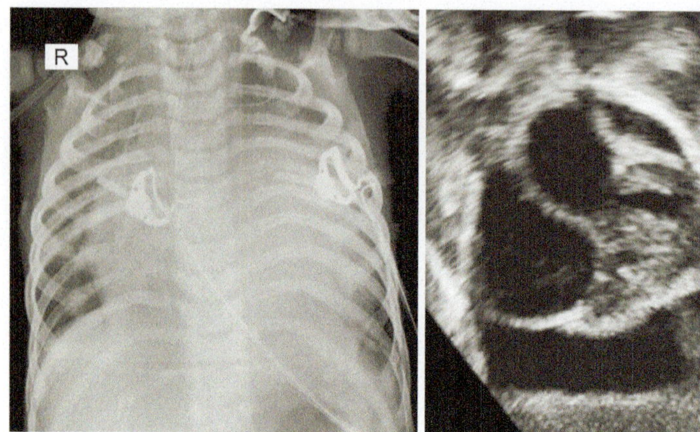

Q7. A neonate was brought to tertiary care emergency department with abdominal distension, bilious vomiting, and lethargy. A localized area of tenderness, discoloration of the abdominal wall, and sudden increase in the abdominal girth are found. There is a drop in the mean blood pressure. A plain X-ray may show multiple air fluid levels. A plain abdominal X-ray is available with the parents, which was done in primary health center.

a. Interpret the X-ray abdomen.
b. What is the significance of discoloration of the abdominal wall in this condition and most likely diagnosis?
c. What are the management steps in this condition?

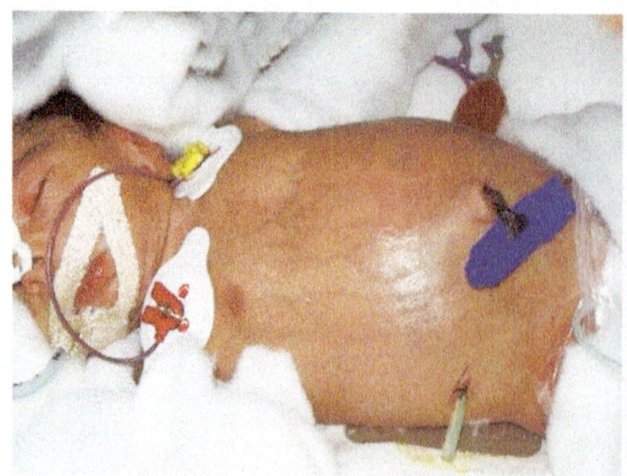

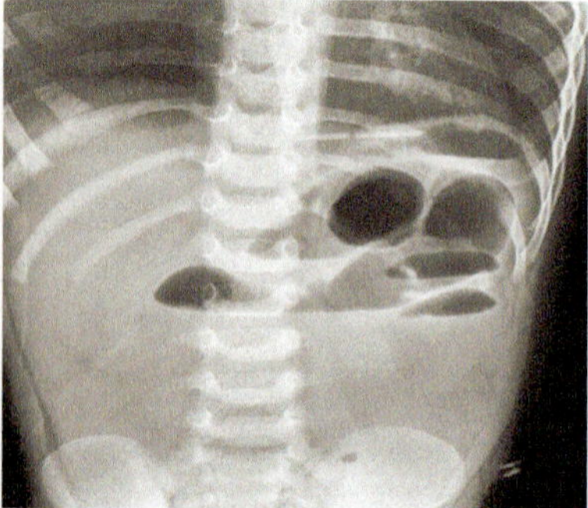

Q8. A neonate presents with vomiting and later dehydration in emergency department. The plain X-ray abdomen provided to emergency physician for interpretation.

a. Interpret the X-ray. What is this appearance called?
b. What are the steps in management of this condition?

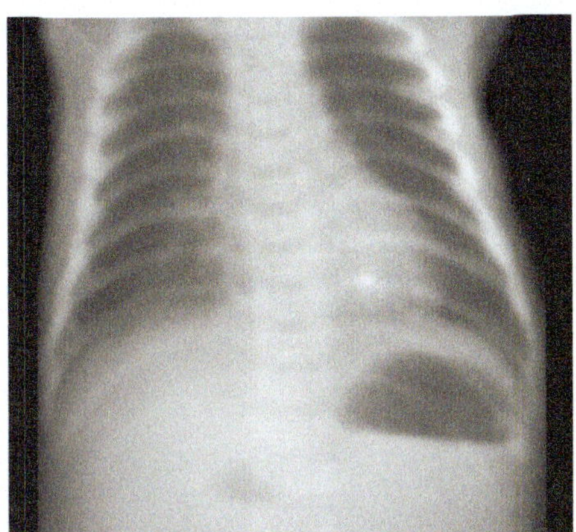

Q9. A baby of 3 weeks of age with projectile, forceful vomiting and an epigastric lump presented to emergency department. The baby is dehydrated and sick due to excessive vomiting. The baby has hypochloremic alkalosis. Clinical examination reveals a pyloric tumor. A plain X-ray abdomen provided to emergency physician.

a. Interpret the X-ray abdomen. What is the most likely diagnosis?
b. What is the definitive management of this condition?

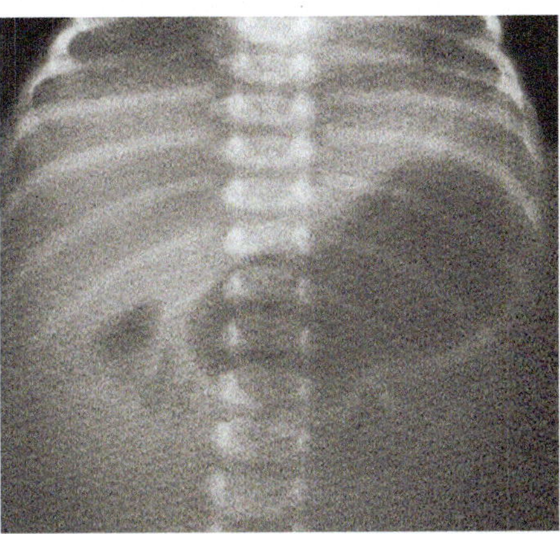

Q10. A child was brought to emergency department with complaints of abdominal pain. Initially, the child denied any history of trauma because of fear of parents. History of abdominal trauma while

playing football was revealed later on detailed history. A plain X-ray abdomen was provided to emergency physician.

a. What is the most probable diagnosis?

b. What are the steps in management?

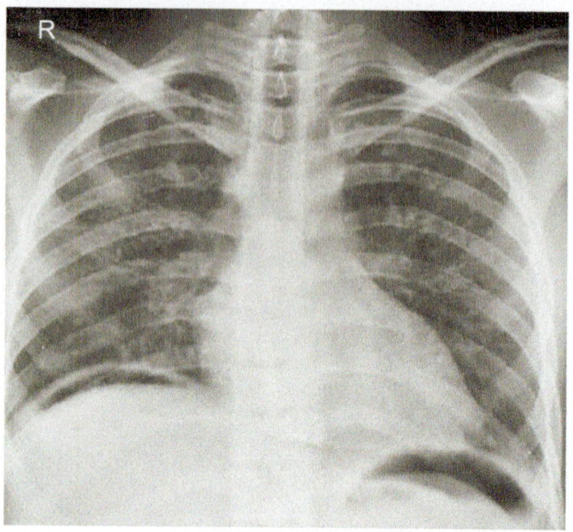

Q11. Identify the condition in newborn as baby passes delayed meconium after birth.

What is the management of the condition?

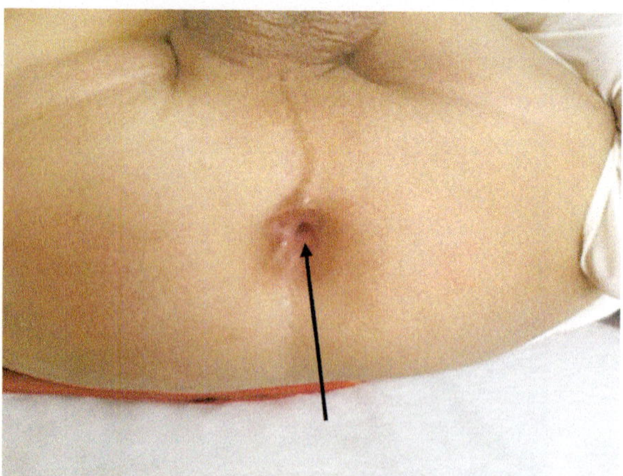

Q12. A newborn baby presented with delayed passage of meconium, abdominal distension, and vomiting. The baby is very sick and lethargic and has a tender abdomen.

a. Name the investigation as shown in image below.

b. Interpret the investigation and most probable clinical condition.

c. What is the management of the clinical presentation?

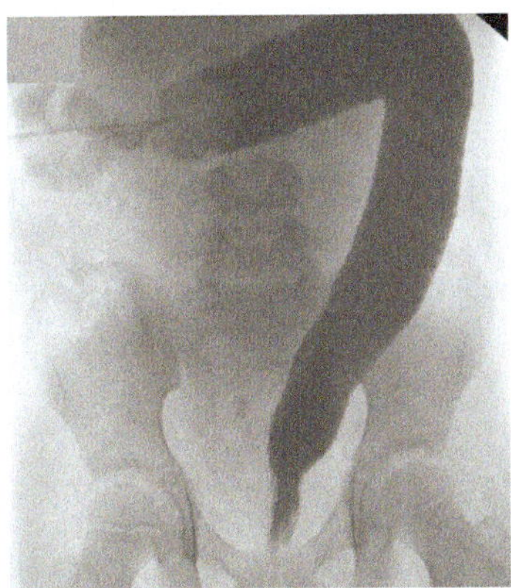

Q13. A child was brought to emergency with abdominal pain, vomiting, and distension of the abdomen. Emergency physician examined the child and found swelling in right inguinal area which is irreducible.

a. Identify the condition.
b. What is the differential diagnosis?
c. What is the complication if not managed timely?

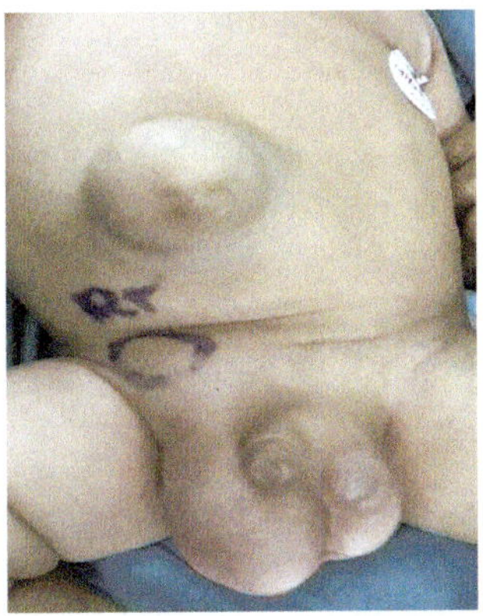

Q14. Describe the picture and name the condition.

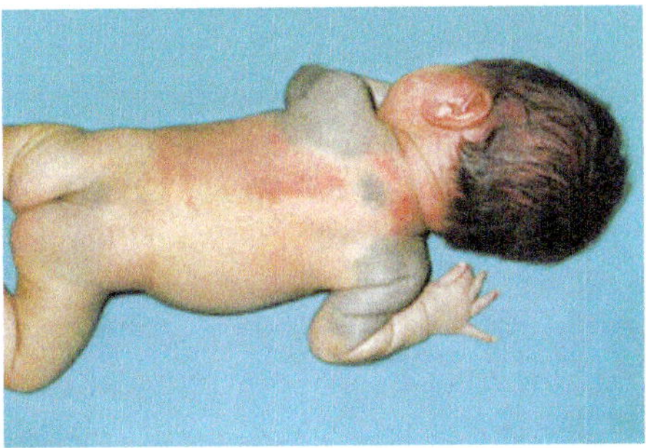

Q15. A 15 days old baby brought to emergency department and parents worried about skin lesion noticed over the trunk soon after the birth.

a. Identify the condition.
b. What is Darier sign?
c. What are the factors affecting these lesions?

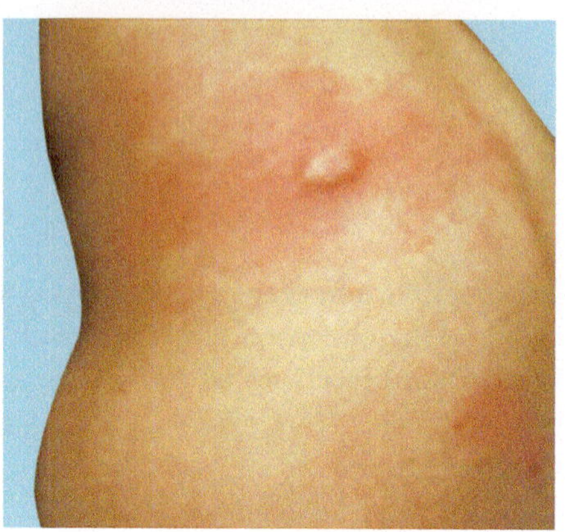

ANSWERS

Ans. 1

a. *Chest X-ray:* Mild cardiomegaly with increased pulmonary vascular markings
b. Most probably congenital heart disease, the most common congenital heart diseases that present with neonatal cyanosis include complete transposition of the great arteries, tetralogy of Fallot (with critical pulmonary stenosis or pulmonary atresia), obstructive total anomalous, pulmonary venous connection, single ventricle with critical pulmonary stenosis/pulmonary atresia, tricuspid atresia with critical pulmonary stenosis/pulmonary atresia, and critical pulmonary stenosis/pulmonary atresia with intact interventricular septum
c. *Approach to cyanosis:* Differentiate cardiac from pulmonary causes of cyanosis. Arterial oxygen tension is measured in the right radial artery (preductal) while the patient on 100% oxygen for 10 minutes. The definitive diagnosis is readily established by detailed echocardiography. Prostaglandin E1 (alprostadil) IV infusion to keep the patent ductus arteriosus (PDA) open (dose 10–60 ng/kg/min, if poor response saturations and acidosis not improving) the dose can be increased to maximum 300–400 ng/kg/min
d. *Definitive management includes management of the cause:* For transposition of the great vessels—Arterial switch operation, total

anomalous; Pulmonary venous connection—surgical rerouting of pulmonary veins; Severe valvular pulmonary stenosis—balloon valvotomy and ductal stenting/BT shunt for duct-dependent pulmonary circulation.

Ans. 2

a. Chest X-ray of a neonate presenting in emergency with shock. X-ray reveals cardiomegaly and prominent vascular markings with retrocardiac lung collapse
b. It is very important to have a high index of suspicion for congenital heart disease in neonates presenting with shock as most commonly it is mistakenly diagnosed and managed as neonatal sepsis. While babies with sepsis are medically managed those with duct-dependent systemic circulation need aggressive resuscitation and prompt intervention usually. These babies can present directly with cardiovascular collapse after ductal closure and are therefore often critically ill at presentation.
c. Management includes prostaglandin therapy, blood volume expansion, stabilization with inotrops, oxygen and mechanical ventilation in unresponsive cases. Confirmation of diagnosis by echocardiography followed by relief of obstruction by surgical correction.

Ans. 3

a. Deep Q waves in leads I, aVL, V5, and V6 and T wave inversion seen in lead I. 12-lead ECG of an infant with anomalous left coronary artery from the pulmonary artery (ALCAPA). Anomalous origin of coronary artery from pulmonary artery (ALCAPA), the babies usually present with features of CHF due to myocardial ischemia leading to LV dilatation and dysfunction.

   The presentation can be delayed up to 3–4 weeks of age till the pulmonary vascular pressures falls substantially. Babies with CHF usually present with feeding difficulties and excessive sweating. They are tachypneic and tachycardiac at rest and can have wheeze due to LV failure. Gallop rhythm, hepatomegaly, and cardiomegaly are other important signs.
b. Echocardiography revealed severe LV dysfunction with EF 15–20%. On echocardiography, left coronary was seen arising anomalously from pulmonary artery and baby was diagnosed to have ALCAPA.
c. *Management:* Oxygen therapy, general neonatal care which includes maintenance of temperature and glucose levels. Nasogastric feeding, diuretics, correction of coexistent metabolic derangements, such as anemia, hypoglycemia, electrolyte imbalance, and acidosis. Inotropes/vasodilators, such as low-dose dobutamine, dopamine, and milrinone to decrease systemic vascular resistance and improve cardiac contractility. Mechanical ventilation is usually required in heart failure with impending cardiogenic shock.

Ans. 4

a. Chest X-ray showed cardiomegaly with straightening of left heart border [left atrial (LA) enlargement], LV type of apex and signs of pulmonary venous hypertension; Chest X-ray frontal view of a 8-year-old child with rheumatic heart disease, severe mitral regurgitation. There is cardiomegaly with pulmonary venous hypertension. Features of left LA dilatation, i.e., straightening of left heart border and widening of carinal angle are seen.
b. Congenital cardiac defect associated with CHF in pediatric age group are large/multiple ventricular septal defect (VSD), complete atrioventricular (AV) canal defect with AV regurgitation, large PDA and AV malformation. Acquired causes of pediatric CHF are rheumatic heart disease, cardiomyopathy arrhythmia, and pericardial tamponade. Heart failure secondary to congenital heart disease is a gradual process while heart failure due to acquired causes is more commonly an acute process.
c. *Management:* Treatment of the precipitating factors, such as infective endocarditis, intercurrent infections, anemia, electrolyte imbalances, arrhythmia, pulmonary embolism, and drug toxicity.

Ans. 5

The 12-lead ECG suggestive of digitalis effect: Prolongation of PR interval with sagging of ST segment. History of accidental ingestion of high dose of digoxin. Digitalis is especially useful as it decreases heart rate and increases myocardial contractility; however its use has to be closely monitored in view of its narrow therapeutic index

Ans. 6

a. Chest X-ray showing cardiomegaly with globular heart shadow in a child with large pericardial effusion
b. *Echocardiography:* Subcostal coronal view showing large pericardial effusion. On pericardial tap, serous fluid was drained and was of tubercular etiology.
c. Beck's triad comprising hypotension, diminished heart sounds, and engorged neck veins venous hypertension in cardiac tamponade
d. *Management:* In hemodynamically stable patient with no features of cardiac tamponade, a definitive diagnosis by echocardiography and drainage via pericardiocentesis or surgical drainage is required. Urgent decompression of the pericardial space is mandatory and lifesaving if signs of cardiac tamponade are present. This is achieved by aspirating from a subxiphoid approach with a cannula aiming at left shoulder and at angle of 30–45 from skin and obtaining as much fluid as possible before removing cannula. Blood volume expansion with 20 mL/kg crystalloid IV bolus; repeated as necessary.

Ans. 7

a. A plain X-ray abdomen may show multiple air fluid levels. Signs of sudden deterioration drop in the mean blood pressure and sudden increase in the abdominal girth suggestive of intestinal obstruction or perforation.
b. A localized area of tenderness and a discoloration of the abdominal wall is a harbinger of intestinal gangrene, most likely *neonatal necrotizing enterocolitis* (NNEC), although *duodenal obstruction* constitutes half of the cases of neonatal intestinal obstruction.
c. Neonate was brought to emergency department with abdominal distension, bilious vomiting, and lethargy. Intestinal obstruction in neonates recovers uneventfully on conservative management. However, NNEC is very deceiving and babies can deteriorate suddenly. Surgical approach can vary from making a stoma with drainage of intraperitoneal collection to a resection and anastomosis.

Ans. 8

a. The plain X-ray shows a *double-bubble appearance* suggestive of duodenal obstruction. *Duodenal obstruction* constitutes half of the cases of neonatal intestinal obstruction. They include duodenal atresia/stenosis (intrinsic) or malrotation and annular pancreas (extrinsic) obstruction. One-third of babies with duodenal obstruction have trisomy 21 or Down's syndrome.
b. Resuscitation surgery is required and standard operation is a Kimura's diamond-shaped-duodenoduodenostomy.

Ans. 9

a. A plain X-ray abdomen is mostly nonspecific, but gastric dilatation with paucity of distal bowel gas is suggestive of infantile hypertrophic pyloric stenosis (IHPS)
b. *Management surgery:* Ramstedt's pyloromyotomy which is the gold standard for this condition.

Ans. 10

a. X-ray showing air under the diaphragm suggestive of intestinal perforation. Blunt trauma abdomen may give rise to mesenteric tear or omental torsion.
b. Management of lower and splenic trauma respond to conservative management along with blood transfusion and very few babies require surgery.

Ans. 11

Image and clinical presentation suggestive of anorectal malformation (ARM). Depending on the tightness of the anal opening in newborn, a stoma may be required for a high ARM or an anoplasty for a low anorectal malformation.

Ans. 12

a. Barium enema
b. Barium enema showing narrow segment most probably Hirschsprung's disease correlating with clinical condition
c. An acute obstruction which fails to respond to nasogastric aspiration requires early surgery and a stoma.

Ans. 13

a. Irreducible inguinal hernia
b. Obstructed hernia and torsion of testis
c. Bowel will become gangrenous if not managed timely

Ans. 14

Mongolian spots: Single or multiple slate and gray or bluish black irregular macules commonly seen over buttocks and lumbosacral area. These are more common in African American and Asian infants. These are due to accumulation of melanocytes deep within dermis and usually self-resolve over years. Special variants of Mongolian spots, nevus of Ota (involving face, periocular area) and nevus of Ito (involving shoulder) may persist. Mongolian spots should not be confused with bruising.

Ans. 15

a. *Urticaria pigmentosa:* It presents at birth or first few months of life. It is characterized by multiple small reddish-brown papules or plaques over the trunk. These lesions are caused by vascular effects of histamine released from infiltrating mast cells in the cutaneous tissue.
b. *Darier sign:* Development of a wheal and flare reaction after firm stroking of the lesion is a positive Darier sign. Lesions are usually self-limited and resolves by adolescence.
c. *Factors affecting these lesions:* In infancy, these lesions can sometimes blister and wide spread erosions can result in dehydration and sepsis. With temperature changes, metabolic insults, such as fever or viral illnesses, large numbers of degranulating lesions can produce flushing and systemic symptoms of histamine release. These patients should be counseled to avoid certain medications and iodinated contrast media.

16 CHAPTER

Pediatric Emergencies OSCE: Part II

Amritesh Ranjan, Preeti Dwivedi, Manish Agrawal

QUESTIONS

Q1. Calculate the size of (a) cuffed and (b) uncuffed endotracheal tube required for 6 years old girls who has need for ventilation. Also (c) calculate the depth of insertion.

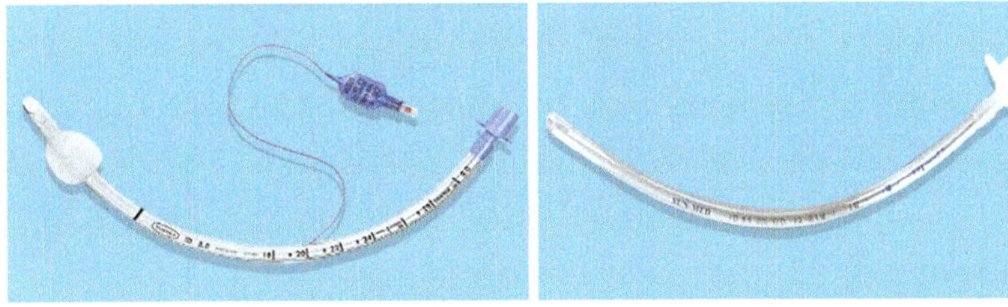

Q2. A child is admitted in intensive care unit and a nurse notify the ECG to pediatrician on duty.

a. Interpret the ECG.
b. What are the types?
c. What is the treatment for the condition?

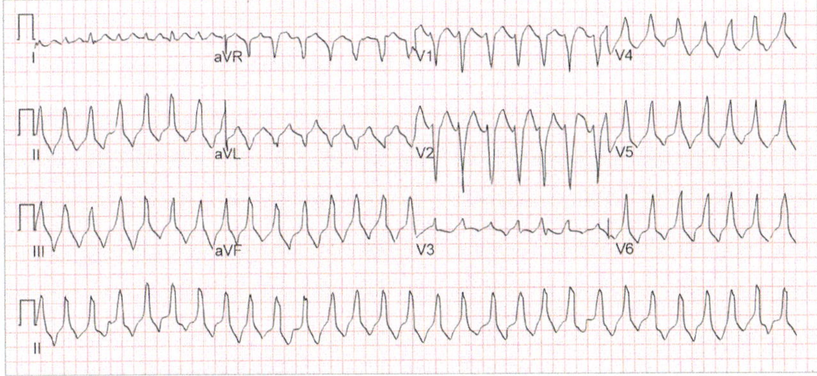

Q3. Interpret X-ray of neck.

a. Name the sign.
b. Name the condition in which this sign is found?
c. Name the causative organism.
d. What is the management of such condition?

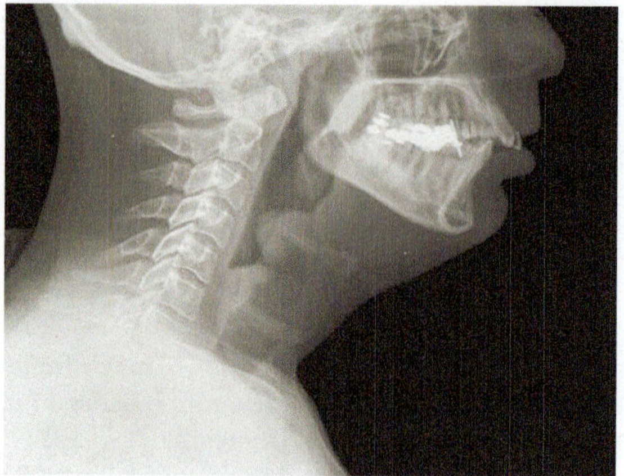

Q4. A child presents to emergency department (ED) with complaint of blood in urine. How will you establish whether it is glomerular or extraglomerular?

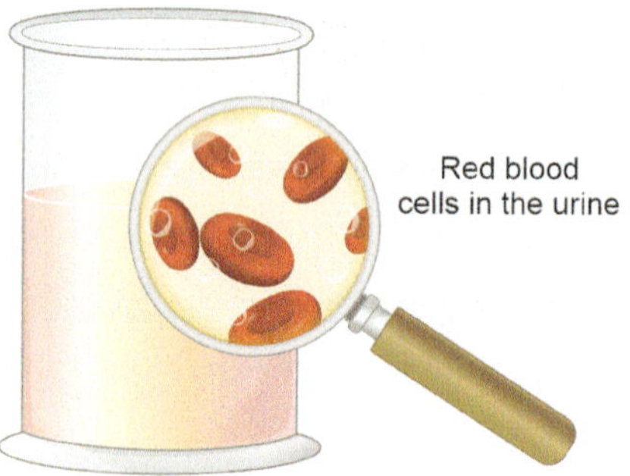

Q5. An 8-year-old girl presents to ED with complaints of staring look, frequent falls, and regaining posture within few minutes. There are multiple bruises on the body.

a. What do you suspect?
b. How will you confirm your suspicion?
c. How will you confirm your diagnosis?
d. What is the management?

Q6. Answer the following questions regarding hypertension in children.

a. Classify blood pressure (BP) in children.
b. Define hypertensive crisis/emergency and hypertensive urgency.
c. Mention four drugs—two oral and two IV along with dosage that can be used in hypertensive crisis.

Q7. Study the following image.

a. Name the investigations done. What is the typical appearance called?
b. Name the disease with which findings are consistent?
c. What does it suggest?
d. What is the clinical presentation of this disease?

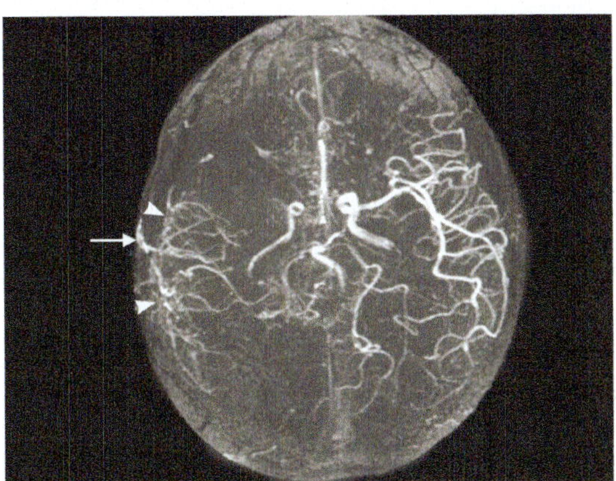

Q8. A 10-year-old boy known case of (k/c/o) Burkitt lymphoma who was started on chemotherapy 5 days back presents to ED with dysuria/oliguria/hematuria with flank pain. Patient also had vomiting, cramps, and now is in altered mental status.

a. What do you suspect?
b. What is the triad of this condition?
c. What is the management—mainstay/drug used?

Q9. A 6-year-old girl presents to ED with case of (c/o) increased respiratory rate/abnormal breathing, fruity odor from breath, nausea/vomiting (N/V) and pain abdomen, lethargy, and confused state.

a. What is your impression for this condition?
b. What are the diagnostic criteria?
c. How do you classify this condition?
d. How do you measure corrected sodium in this condition?

Q10. A child brought to the emergency with flat pink rashes on trunk arm and legs.

a. What are the Ravelli criteria for diagnosing macrophage activation syndrome (MAS) in patient with systemic onset juvenile idiopathic arthritis (SOJIA)?
b. What are the differentiating features of MAS and SOJIA flare?

Q11. A 16-year-old was brought to ED with c/o nausea, vomiting, pain in lower abdomen, and pain in testis. On examination, scrotum is red/edematous, tender to touch, and painful. He also gives a similar history 2 months back but that lasted for 2 minutes and resolved on its own.

a. What is the condition suspected?
b. What are the investigations?
c. What is the management?

Q12. A 40-day-old infant presents to ER with predominant nonbilious and projectile vomiting 15–20 minutes after feed over the period of time this complaint has increased. Child is looking dehydrated, has significant weight loss and lethargic. Mother c/o noticing an abdominal lump after feeding in right upper quadrant.

a. Name the condition.
b. Name the metabolic derangements in this child.
c. What is the management/treatment of choice for this condition?
d. What is paradoxical aciduria?

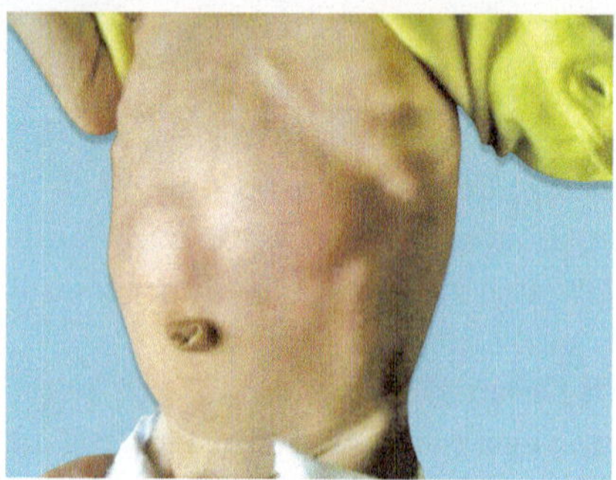

Q13. See the picture below and write answers of the below questions.

a. Identify the instrument.
b. What is the indication for the use of it?
c. Name the sites where it can be used?
d. What is the contraindication?

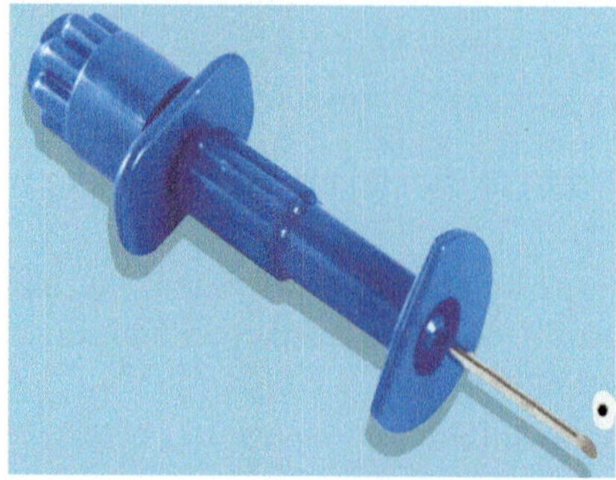

Q14. A 3-year-old child was brought to ER with history of (h/o) accidental ingestion of methanol.

a. What is the clinical presentation and write specific antidote?
b. What is the differential diagnosis (D/D) of miosis in a child with h/o poisoning?
c. Give specific antidote for poisoning/overdose:
   - Organophosphorus
   - Paracetamol
   - Digoxin
   - Lead

Q15. A 10-year-old child playing cricket became unconscious on the field.

a. Name three conditions associated with syncope.
b. What complications this child may develop?
c. What investigations to be done?
d. What is the ECG diagnosis?

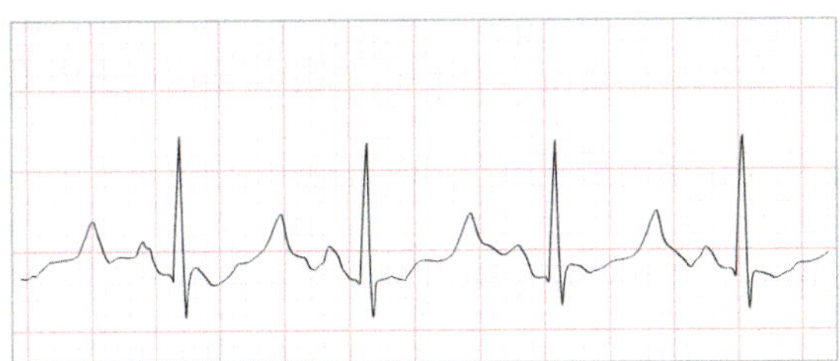

Q16. A 4-year-old child has sudden eruption on his back.

a. What is the most likely diagnosis?
b. What is the most appropriate management?
c. Which are in high-risk category?

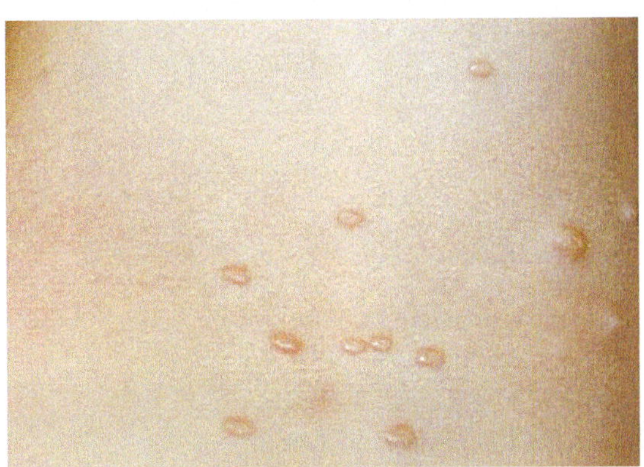

Q17. A newborn brought to an emergency, who stops feeding and their bodies become stiff and on examination sever muscle contraction and spasm.

a. Name of the condition the neonate is suffering from.
b. Name the facial appearance.
c. What test is being shown here?
d. How can it be prevented?

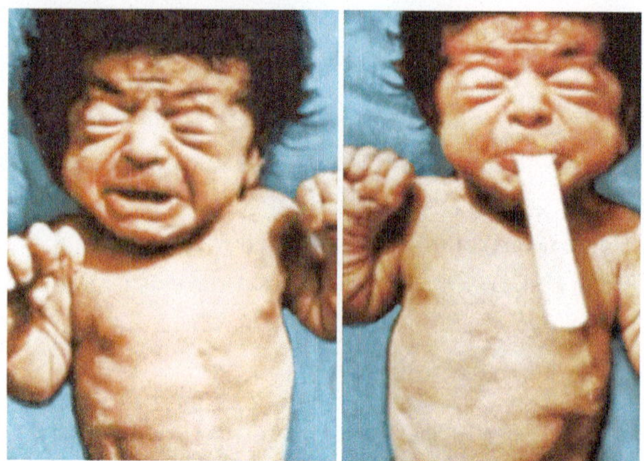

Q18. A 2.1 kg full term male baby came to ED with c/o abdominal distension, respiratory distress, and excessive salivation. Interpret the X-ray. Name the clinical condition.

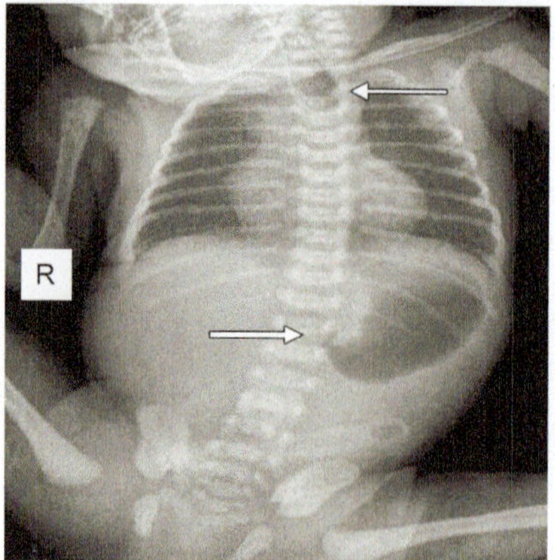

Q19. A below X-ray is provided to Emergency physician for interpretation.

a. Comment on the X-ray.
b. What would be the neurological sign?
c. What is the diagnosis and management?

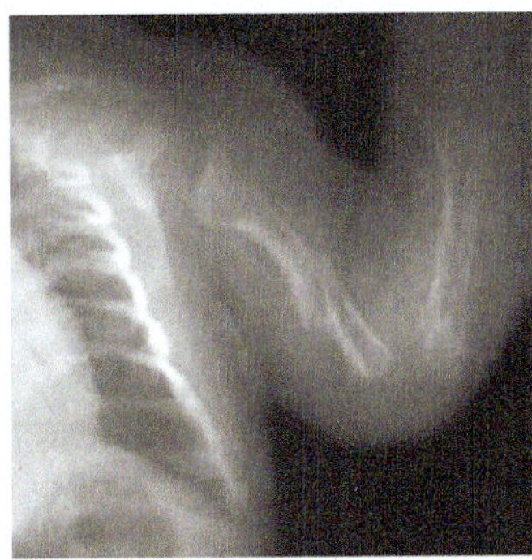

Q20. **A 3 kg full term baby came with complaints of vomiting (greenish in color) and not accepting feeding properly and abdominal distension. He has h/o cow milk given via bottle. X-ray is shown below. Name the condition.**

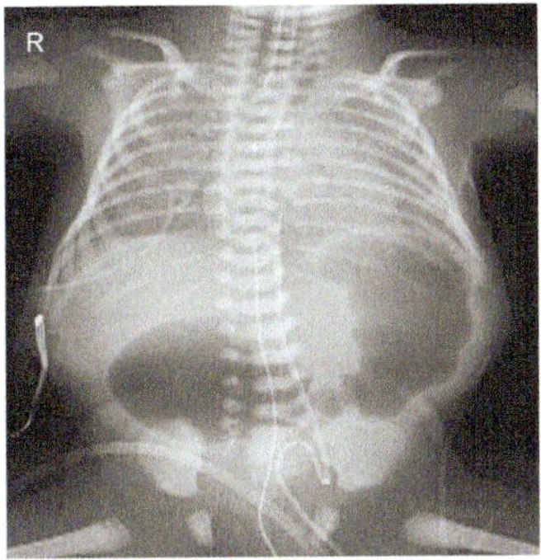

Q21. **A 3-month-old infant came with c/o abnormal movement of body and paleness of skin. Baby had h/o delayed cry with seizures with neonatal intensive care unit (NICU) admission. CT scan is given below.**

a. Confirm the diagnosis.
b. What is the common presentation of this disease?

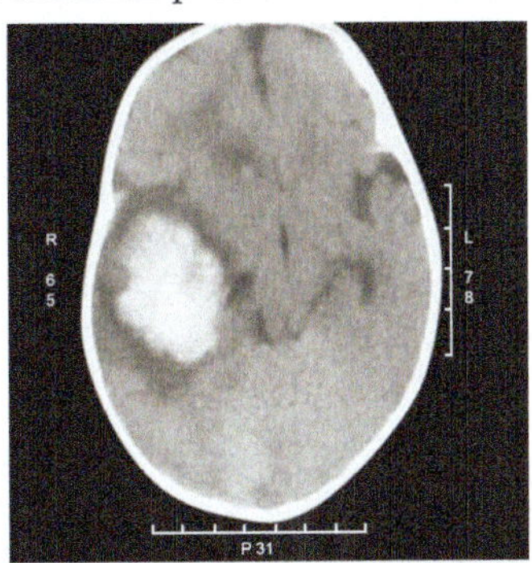

ANSWERS

Ans. 1

a. *Cuffed:* Age (years)/4 + 3.5
b. *Uncuffed:* Age (years)/4 + 4
c. *Depth of insertion:* Age (years)/2 + 12

Ans. 2

a. Supraventricular tachycardia (SVT)
b. *Types:*
   1. Atrioventricular nodal reentry tachycardia (AVNRT) (most common)
   2. Atrioventricular reciprocating tachycardia (AVRT) (second most common in younger people)
   3. Atrial tachycardia (AT) (with preexisting heart disease)
c. *Treatment:*
   - Carotid sinus massage
   - *Vagal maneuvers:* Coughing and holding your breath, ice pack on face
   - Medications adenosine
   - Cardioversion

Ans. 3

a. Thumb sign
b. Acute epiglottitis
c. Parainfluenza 1/2/3 and influenza A/B/RSV and *Mycoplasma*
d. Airway management and antibiotics

Ans. 4

	Glomerular	***Extraglomerular***
Color	Red/smoky brown/cola colored	Red/pink
Clots	Absent	Present
Proteinuria	+/–	Usually absent
RBC morphology	Dysmorphic	Normal
RBC cast	May be present	Absent

Ans. 5

a. Absence seizure
b. PPT by hyperventilation
c. 3 Hz spike and wave discharge on EEG
d. Ethosuximide and valproate

Ans. 6

Blood pressure classification in pediatric age

- *Normal:* SBP/DBP <90 percentile

- *Prehypertension:* SBP/DBP 90–95 or BP >120/80 mm Hg even if <90 centile
- *Stage 1:* SBP/DBP ≥95–99 + 5 mm Hg
- *Stage 2:* SBP/DBP >99 + 5 mm Hg

b. • Hypertension crisis is severe life-threatening elevation of BP with end-organ damage
   • Hypertensive urgency is severe life-threatening elevation of BP without end-organ damage

c. Drugs for BP control
   Oral:
   • Clonidine (central α-agonist) (0.05–0.1 mg)
   • Enalapril [angiotensin-converting enzyme (ACE) inhibitor] (0.05–0.1 mg/kg)
   • Nifedipine (calcium channel blocker) (0.1–0.2 mg/kg)
   Intravenous:
   • Esmolol (β-blocker): Loading dose—100–500 mg/kg; Maintenance dose—50–300 mg/kg/min
   • Labetalol (α- and β-blocker): Bolus—0.2–1 mg/kg

Ans. 7

a. MR angiogram suggestive of "puff of smoke" on cerebral angiogram
b. Moyamoya disease
c. Internal carotid vessels show stenosis of bilateral (B/L) internal carotid artery (ICA), B/L middle cerebral artery (MCA), and A1 segment of right anterior cerebral artery
d. Acute hemiparesis/acute ischemic stroke

Ans. 8

a. Tumor lysis syndrome
b. Hyperkalemia, hyperuricemia, and hyperphosphatemia (also with hypocalcemia)
c. *Treatment:*
   • *Hydration:* 3,000 mL/m^2/24 h (1/2 DNS)
   • Allopurinol (10 mg/kg/day) × 7 days followed by (5 mg/kg/day) × 7 days
   • *Rasburicase:* 0.15–0.2 mg/kg IV × 5–6 days

Ans. 9

a. Diabetic ketoacidosis
b. • *Hyperglycemia BSL:* >200 mg/dL
   • *Venous pH:* <7.3 or HCO_3^- <15 mmol/L
   • *Ketonemia (Blood:* β-hydroxybutyrate ≥3 mmol/L)

c. • *Mild:* pH <7.3 and HCO_3^- <15 mmol/L
   • *Moderate:* pH <7.2 and HCO_3^- <10 mmol/L
   • *Severe:* pH <7.1 and HCO_3^- <5 mmol/L

d. Actual sodium concentration = by adding 1.6 mEq/L for each 100 mg/dL rise in glucose above 100 mg/dL. $(\text{Sodium})_c$ = Measured Na^+ + (Glucose level – 100) × 0.016.

Ans. 10

a. A febrile patient with known or suspended SOJIA is classified as having MAS. If the following criteria are met:
   Ferritin >684 ng/mL and any two of the following:
   1. Platelet count <181 × 10^9/L
   2. AST >48 U/L
   3. TGs >156 mg/dL
   4. Fibrinogen ≤360 mg/dL

b. Differentiating feature of MAS and SOJIA are given in table below:

Feature	**SOJIA**	**MAS**
Fever	Quotidian	Persistent
HSM	+	+
ZN	+	+
Clinical feature	Arthritis, synovitis	Hemorrhages, altered mental status
Hb	N/↓	↓↓
TLC	↑↑	↓
PC	↑↑	↓
ESR	↑	↓
Fibrinogen	↑	↓
AST/ALT	N/↑	↑
Albumin	N	↓
PT/APTT	N	↑↑
Ferritin	↑	↑↑
LDH	N	↑
TGs	N	↑
Urine	N	↑

Ans. 11

a. Testicular torsion
b. (1) Color Doppler USG and (2) Radioisotope scan done to establish blood flow in testes.
c. Inguinal/scrotal exploration

Ans. 12

a. Infantile hypertrophic pyloric stenosis
b. Hypokalemia, hypochloremia, metabolic (acidosis), and alkalosis

c. Ramstedt's pyloromyotomy

d. *Vomiting:*
   - Loss of H^+ = Alkalosis
   - Loss of Cl^- = Hypochloremia
   - Loss of K^+ = Hypokalemia

     ↓
   - Blood → Metabolic acidosis
   - Renal compensation → Kidney → Loss of HCO_3^- → $NaHCO_3$ → Na conservation → Loss of H^+ → Paradoxical aciduria

     ↓
   - Na conservation → Loss of K^+ → Hypokalemia

Ans. 13

a. Intraosseous needle with stylet

b. Emergent vascular access in cardiac arrest/shock. Where IV is not possible.

c. (1) Proximal tibia—anteromedial flat surface 1–2 cm below and medial to tibial tuberosity; (2) Distal tibia—just above medial malleolus

d. *Contraindications:* (1) Osteogenesis imperfecta, (2) crush injury at the site, (3) osteomyelitis, and (4) injection of overlying tissue

Ans. 14

a.
   - Headache, inebriation, and Eye-Snow Field Lesion
   - Ethanol/fomepizole
   - Organophosphorus compound (OPC)/barbiturates/nicotine/opiates

b.
   - *Organophosphorus:* Atropine/PAM
   - *Paracetamol:* N-acetyl cysteine
   - *Digoxin:* DigiFab
   - *Lead:* EDTA/BAL

Ans. 15

a. Hypertrophic obstructive cardiomyopathy (HOCM), Wolff-Parkinson-White (WPW) syndrome, and complete AV block

b. Ventricular arrhythmia, tachycardia, and torsade de pointes

c. ECG

d. Long QT syndrome

Ans. 16

a. Molluscum contagiosum

b. Watchful

c. Immunocompromised state/HIV

Ans. 17

a. Neonate is suffering from tetanus neonatorum.

b. Risus sardonicus

c. Spatula test
d. Tetanus immunization of mother and aseptic umbilical cord cutting

Ans. 18

Pyloric atresia

Ans. 19

a. Humerus fracture
b. Asymmetrical Moro reflex
c. Diagnosis—osteogenesis imperfecta; Management—pamidronate infusion

Ans. 20

Duodenal atresia

Ans. 21

a. Leukomalacia
b. Most common presentation is spastic diplegia. It is a form of cerebral palsy that causes tight, contracted muscles, especially in legs.

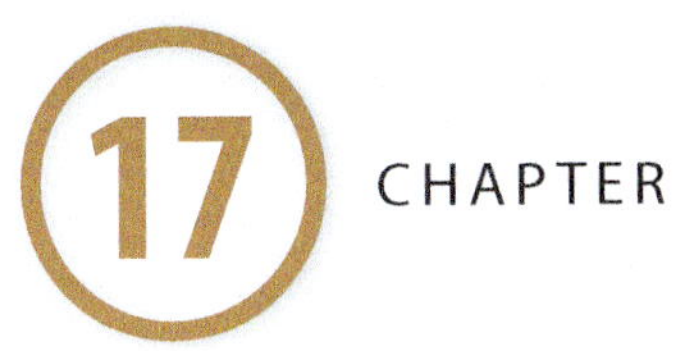

Geriatric Emergencies OSCE

M Sai Surendar

QUESTIONS

Q1. **A 75-year-old woman with history of hypertension and diabetes presents with sudden onset of severe left-sided pleuritic chest pain. She denies fever, cough, or shortness of breath. On examination, she is afebrile, tachycardia (110 beats/min) and has normal oxygen saturation on room air. Breath sounds are clear bilaterally.**

a. What is the most likely diagnosis?

b. What is the next step in management?

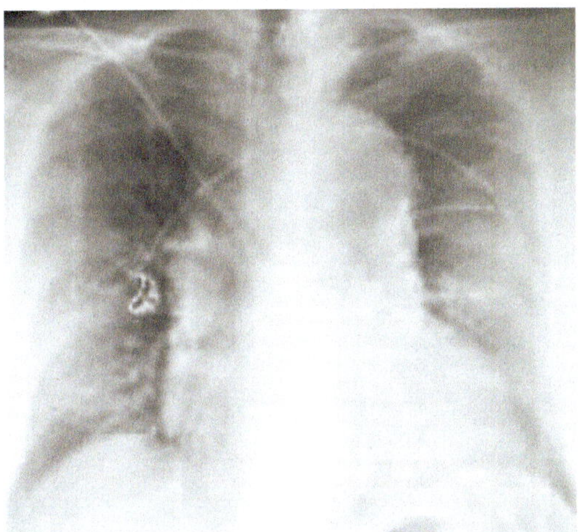

Q2. **An 82-year-old man with a history of dementia presents with *acute onset of confusion, agitation, and ataxia*. He is afebrile and has normal vital signs. His neurological examination shows bilateral asterixis.**

a. What is the most likely diagnosis?

b. What is the next step in management?

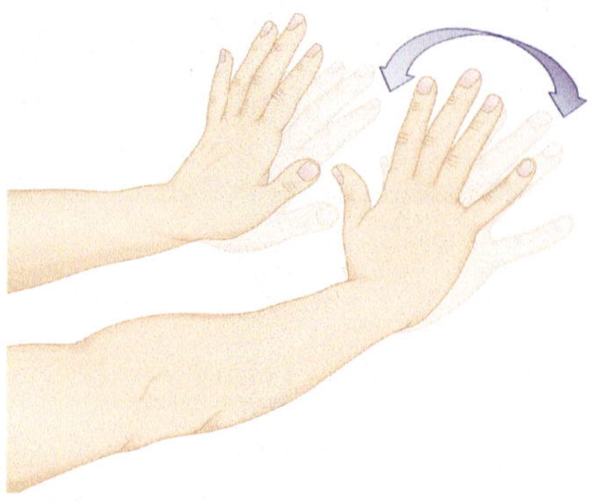

Q3. **An 88-year-old woman with a history of chronic obstructive pulmonary disease (COPD) presents with acute onset of respiratory distress and altered mental status. She is cyanotic and has shallow rapid breathing. Her oxygen saturation is 85% on room air.**

a. What is the most likely diagnosis?
b. What is the immediate management?

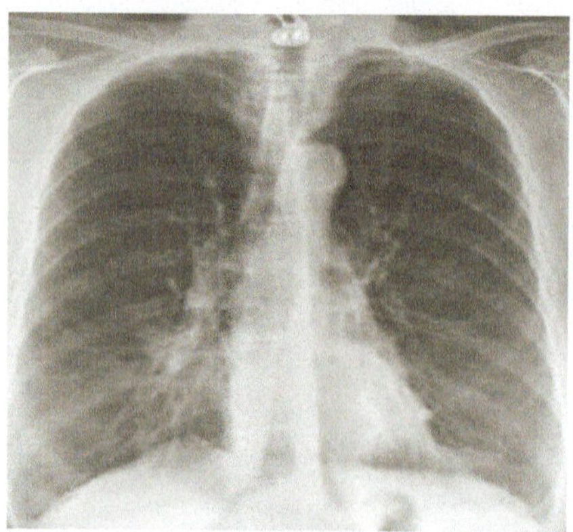

Q4. **A 72-year-old woman with a history of atrial fibrillation presents with sudden onset of dizziness and palpitations. She denies chest pain or shortness of breath. Her pulse is irregular at 140 beats/min.**

a. What is the most likely diagnosis?
b. What is the next step in management?

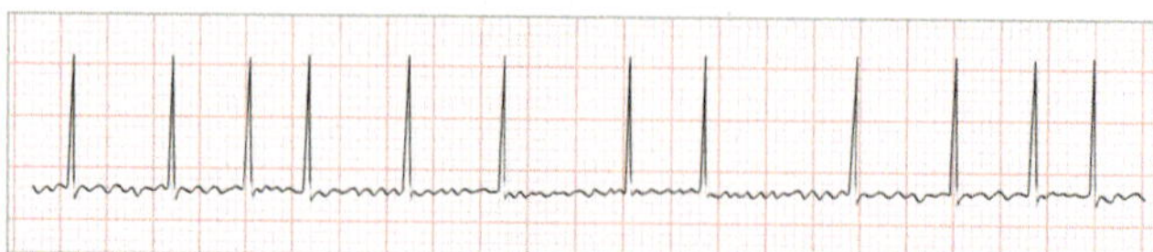

Q5. An 80-year-old man with a history of heart failure presents with progressive shortness of breath and swelling of his legs. He is afebrile and normal vital signs. His lung auscultation reveals bilateral crackles.

a. What is the most likely diagnosis?
b. What is the initial management?

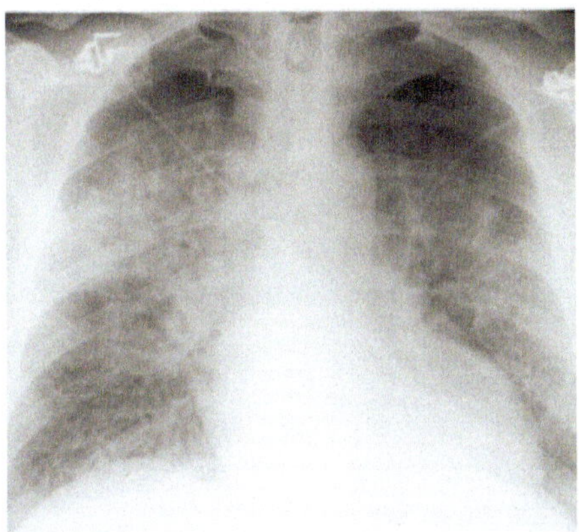

Q6. A 78-year-old woman is unable to bear weight on her injured hip. On examination, the affected leg is shortened and externally rotated.

a. What is the most likely diagnosis?
b. What is the initial management?

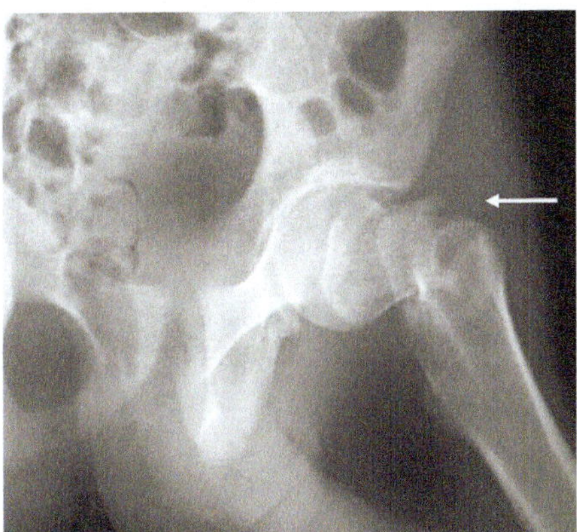

Q7. A 70-year-old woman presents with a history of sudden onset of severe right-sided weakness and facial droop. She is awake and alert but unable to speak.

a. What is the most likely diagnosis?
b. What will be immediate action?

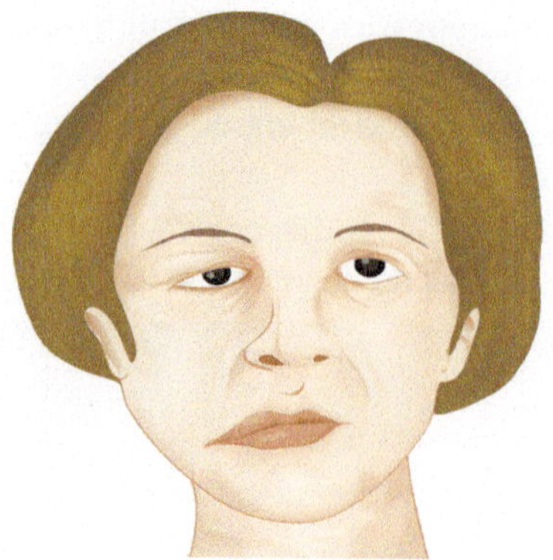

Q8. **An 82-year-old man with a history of Parkinson's disease presents with acute onset of abdominal pain and constipation. He denies fever or vomiting.**

a. What is the most likely diagnosis?
b. What is the initial management?

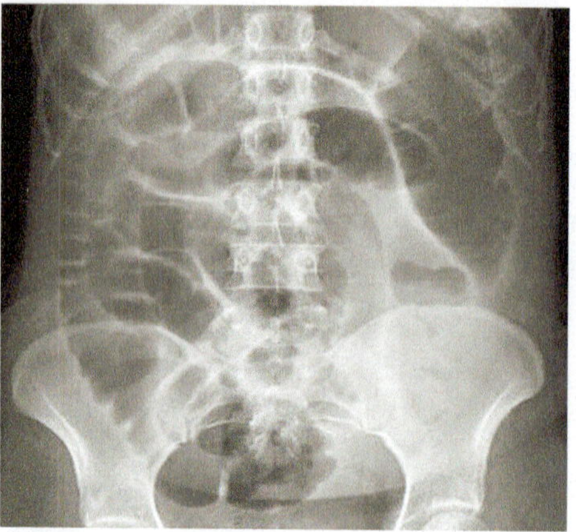

Q9. **A 75-year-old woman with a history of polypharmacy presents with dizziness, light headedness, and near syncope. She denies fever or chest pain. Her blood pressure is 90/60 mm Hg.**

a. What is the most likely diagnosis?
b. Write management.
c. Define polypharmacy.

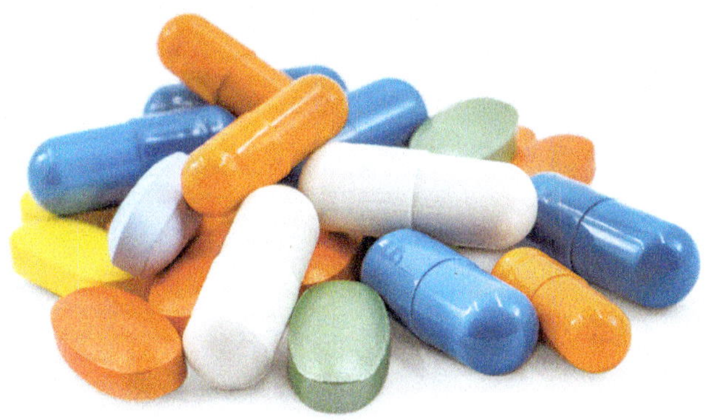

Q10. **An 80-year-old woman with a history of hypertension and atrial fibrillation presents to the emergency department with sudden onset of chest pain radiating to her left arm. ECG performed in emergency department.**

a. Interpret the ECG.

b. What is the initial management?

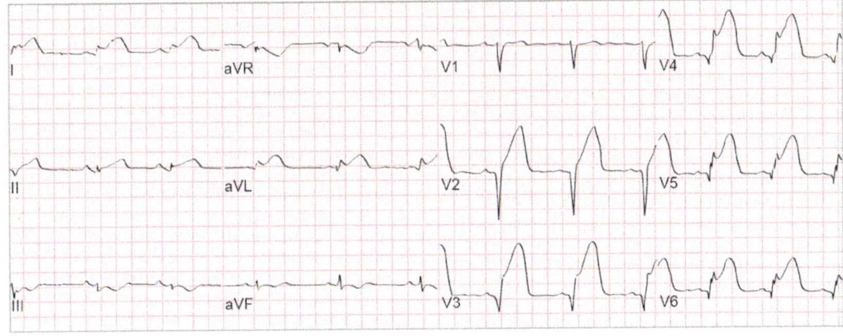

Q11. **A 70-year-old male came with complaints of right-sided chest pain and shortness of breath for 2 days. No history of trauma and auscultation chest bilateral air entry, clear, and heart sound present. His vitals are stable. Echocardiogram and chest X-ray are normal.**

a. What is the differential diagnosis?

b. What will be next line management?

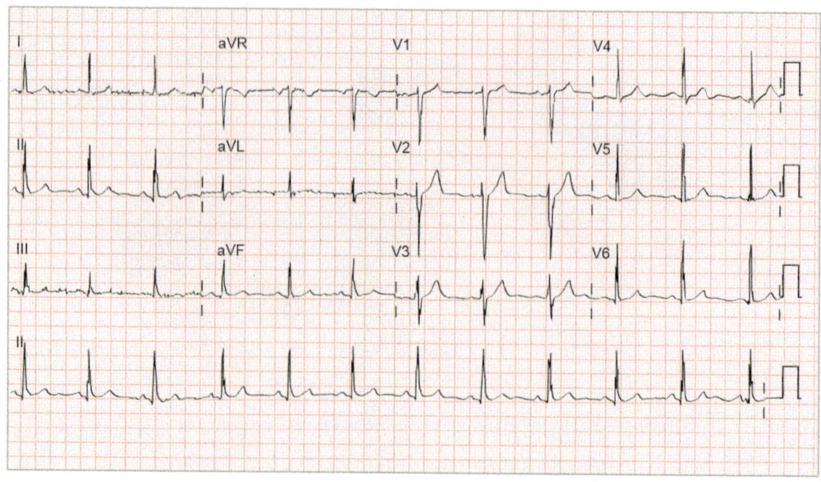

Q12. An 85-year-old woman presents with a history of dementia and complains of sudden onset of severe chest pain, shortness of breath, and confusion.

a. What are the most likely causes?

b. What is the immediate management to stabilize the patient?

Q13. A 90-year-old woman living alone complains of dehydration, and is weak and confused. She has not been seen by anyone for several days. Her vitals are blood pressure (BP): 90/60 mm Hg, pulse: 110 beats/min, blood glucose: 90 mg/dL, SpO_2: 96%, chest: B/L air entry +, clear.

a. What are the potential causes of patient dehydration and confusion?

b. What are measures for older patients' safety at home and ethical consideration in making decision about a patient living situation?

Q14. An 82-year-old woman presents with a history of hypertension and atrial fibrillation, lives alone with mild cognitive decline but independent in activities of living, complains of sudden onset of severe headache described as "*the worst headache of my life*" right-sided facial droop and slurred speech, left arm weakness, and difficulty of gripping objects. She is alert and oriented to person and place but appears confused and anxious.

a. What is the most likely diagnosis?

b. What are the immediate priorities in managing this patient and complications?

Q15. **A 78-year-old man with a history of *dementia* and chronic kidney disease lives with his wife taking multiple medications for his conditions including a diuretic. He found confused, disoriented, appears weak, dry mouth, and thirst. He speaks incoherently and exhibits erratic behavior, wandering around the house. His vital signs show elevated heart rate and low blood pressure.**

a. What are the potential causes of the patients' dehydration and delirium?
b. How can the severity of the dehydration and delirium to be assessed?

ANSWERS

Ans. 1

a. *Most likely diagnosis:* Acute aortic dissection; ECG show ST segment elevation or depression; X-ray may be normal or showing widening mediastinum.
b. *Gold standard investigation:* Aortic CT scan

Ans. 2

a. *Most likely diagnosis:* Metabolic encephalopathy; Other possibilities: Toxicity, cerebrovascular accident (CVA), sepsis, and electrolyte imbalance.
b. *Next step in management:* Admission in intensive care, appropriate investigations and treatment of cause.

Ans. 3

a. *Most likely diagnosis:* Acute exacerbation of COPD
b. *Management:* One or more bronchodilators, inhaled corticosteroids; High-flow O_2/ventilation support (noninvasive ventilation/mechanical ventilation)

Ans. 4

a. *Most likely diagnosis:* Paroxysmal supraventricular tachycardia
b. *Management:* Consider vagal maneuver, adenosine, or synchronized cardioversion

Ans. 5

a. *Most likely diagnosis:* Acute on chronic heart failure possibly due to nonadherence of medication and dietary indiscretion or intercurrent Illness.
b. *Initial management:* Oxygen inhalation, nitrates, diuretics, angiotensin-converting enzyme (ACE) inhibitors, and fluid restriction

Ans. 6

a. *Most likely diagnosis:* Neck or intertrochanteric (IT) fracture femur.
b. *Management:* The goals of treatment are different for the elderly versus the young adults. In the elderly patient, the goals are mobility with weight-bearing as tolerated and minimizing complications seen with prolonged bed rest. Multiple surgical options are considered: reduction and internal fixation, hemiarthroplasty, or total hip arthroplasty. Considerations include the patient's physiological age, level of activity, medical comorbidities, and the degree of bone density.

Ans. 7

a. *Most likely diagnosis:* Cerebrovascular accident
b. *Initial management:* Support airway, breathing, and circulation (ABC); prehospital stroke assessment; estimate time of onset of symptoms; triage to stroke center, perform blood glucose, ECG, obtain IV access; activate stroke team and do CT brain; if hemorrhage refer to neurosurgeon, if no hemorrhage (probable ischemic stroke)—thrombolytic therapy

Ans. 8

a. *Most likely diagnosis:* Acute abdomen secondary to fecal impaction
b. A common complication in Parkinson's disease due to slowed intestinal motility. Consider laxatives/enema

Ans. 9

a. *Most likely diagnosis:* Orthostatic hypotension
b. *Management:* Review medications for potential offending agents and consider adjusting doses or discontinuing them.
c. Based on a review of current data, using five or more medications is termed as "polypharmacy". Polypharmacy is common in older adult due to multiple comorbidities.

Ans. 10

a. *ECG interpretation:* ST segment elevation in anteroseptal and lateral wall suggestive of STEMI acute coronary syndrome.
b. *Management:* Patient should be kept under continuous monitoring, control of blood pressure, antiplatelets, and low-molecular-weight heparin (LMWH) cardiologist opinion.

Ans. 11

a. *Differential diagnosis:* To rule out acute coronary syndrome/anxiety/functional symptoms
b. *Management:* Consider reassurance and counseling

Ans. 12

a. *Most likely causes:* Acute coronary syndrome, pulmonary embolism, aortic dissection, and pneumonia. Consider ECG X-ray, echocardiography cardiac enzyme, and D-dimer.

b. *Management:* Oxygen supplementation, cardiac monitoring, arterial blood gas analysis, triple rule-out CT coronary angiography, and VQ scan

Ans. 13

a. Potential causes are urinary tract infection, sepsis, and polymedication. Older adults are more susceptible to accidents and injuries than are younger adults because of internal and external factors.

b. Measures to be taken for elder population safety such as illumination of living area, use of assistive devices; *behaviors monitoring tools by which* sensors and warning systems that alert caregivers whenever the care recipient changes location or behavior. Use of telemedicine tools. Use of assistive technologies can monitor bed movements, medication use, ambient environmental conditions, and emergency communication. All modern technologies improve the quality of care and safety of older patients with Alzheimer's disease.

Ans. 14

a. *Most likely diagnosis:* Intracerebral hemorrhage and subarachnoid hemorrhage.

b. *Immediate priorities:* Maintaining airway, breathing, and circulation, quick neurological assessment maintaining intracranial pressure, CT head, and neurosurgeon opinion.

Ans. 15

a. Potential causes of dehydration in this case are diuretics, sepsis, CVA, or delirium.

b. There are several tools available for assessment of confusion in emergency department. *Richmond agitation sedation scale* (RASS), *Glasgow Coma Scale* described 40 years ago and most familiar among physicians. *Confusion assessment method (CAM):* It is helpful for nonpsychiatric trained physician to diagnose delirium quickly and accurately. CAM consists of four components: (1) Acute onset mental status changes fluctuating course, (2) inattention, (3) disorganized thinking, and (4) altered level of consciousness. First two components are mandatory and either of two from rest of two necessary for diagnosis of delirium.

Infectious Diseases Emergencies OSCE

M Rajadurai, J Joshua Vijay

QUESTIONS

Q1. **A 35-year-old patient arrives at the emergency department complaining of acute onset of bloody diarrhea. The patient reports that the symptoms began suddenly earlier in the day and have been associated with abdominal cramping. The patient denies any recent travel, but mentions eating at a local restaurant yesterday. There is no known history of chronic gastrointestinal issues.**

Patient's presentation:

- ***Chief complaints:*** **Acute onset of bloody diarrhea and abdominal cramping.**
- ***Vital signs:*** **Blood pressure 120/80 mm Hg, heart rate 100 bpm, respiratory rate 18 bpm, and temperature 38.5°C (101.3°F).**
- ***Physical examination:*** **Mild abdominal tenderness in the lower quadrants, no signs of peritonitis, and no palpable masses.**

a. What are the key differential diagnoses that you would consider for this patient presenting with acute bloody diarrhea?

b. What initial diagnostic investigations would you order for this patient to further assess the cause of the acute bloody diarrhea?

c. Based on the patient's presentation and initial investigations, what would be your initial management plan for this patient with acute bloody diarrhea?

Q2. **A 28-year-old patient arrives at the emergency department presenting with a fever persisting for the past 5 days. The patient reports associated symptoms such as malaise, headache, and muscle aches. There is no clear history of recent travel, but the patient works in a daycare center. The patient denies any known sick contacts or exposure to unusual environments.**

Patient's presentation:

- ***Chief complaints:*** **Fever persisting for 5 days, malaise, headache, and muscle aches.**
- ***Vital signs:*** **Blood pressure 120/80 mm Hg, heart rate 100 bpm, respiratory rate 18 bpm, and temperature 39.2°C (102.6°F).**

- ***Physical examination:*** **No significant findings on general inspection. Mild pharyngeal erythema, no lymphadenopathy, and no respiratory distress.**

a. What are the key differential diagnoses that you would consider for this patient presenting with a fever persisting for 5 days?
b. What initial diagnostic investigations would you order for this patient to further assess the cause of the prolonged fever?
c. Based on the patient's presentation and initial investigations, what would be your initial management plan for this patient with a prolonged fever?

Q3. A 45-year-old male patient arrives at the emergency department with symptoms suggestive of urosepsis. The patient reports a 2-day history of dysuria, frequency, and urgency of urination. He also mentions lower abdominal pain and fever. There is no known history of kidney stones or recent urinary tract infections (UTIs).

Patient's presentation:

- ***Chief complaints:*** **Lower abdominal pain, dysuria, frequency, urgency of urination, and fever.**
- ***Vital signs:*** **Blood pressure 110/70 mm Hg, heart rate 120 bpm, respiratory rate 22 bpm, and temperature 38.9°C (102°F).**
- ***Physical examination:*** **Lower abdominal tenderness, costovertebral angle (CVA) tenderness, and suprapubic tenderness. The patient appears unwell.**

a. What are the key clinical features and signs that raise suspicion for urosepsis in this male patient?
b. What initial diagnostic investigations would you order for this male patient to confirm the diagnosis of urosepsis and guide further management?
c. Based on the patient's presentation and initial investigations, what would be your initial management plan for this male patient with urosepsis?

Q4. A 25-year-old patient arrives at the emergency department with a chief complaint of severe headache, photophobia, neck stiffness, and fever for the past 24 hours. The patient denies any recent upper respiratory tract infections or known exposure to individuals with similar symptoms. The patient appears unwell and is accompanied by a family member who reports concern about the sudden onset of symptoms.

Patient's presentation:

- ***Chief complaints:*** **Severe headache, photophobia, neck stiffness, and fever.**

- ***Vital signs:*** **Blood pressure 130/80 mm Hg, heart rate 110 bpm, respiratory rate 20 bpm, and temperature 39.5°C (103.1°F).**
- ***Physical examination:*** **Neck stiffness, positive Brudzinski's sign, and positive Kernig's sign. Photophobia is noted, and the patient is lethargic.**

a. What clinical features and signs raise suspicion for meningitis in this patient?

b. What initial diagnostic investigations would you order for this patient to confirm the diagnosis of meningitis and guide further management?

c. Based on the patient's presentation and initial investigations, what would be your initial management plan for this patient with suspected meningitis?

Q5. **A 60-year-old patient is brought to the emergency department with a chief complaint of fever, altered mental status, and hypotension. The patient has a history of diabetes mellitus and recently underwent surgery for a perforated appendix. The family reports that the patient has been unwell and febrile for the past few days, with a sudden deterioration in mental status and a decrease in urine output.**

Patient's presentation:

- ***Chief complaints:*** **Fever, altered mental status, and hypotension.**
- ***Vital signs:*** **Blood pressure 80/50 mm Hg, heart rate 120 bpm, respiratory rate 28 bpm, and temperature 39.8°C (103.6°F).**
- ***Physical examination:*** **Altered mental status, hypotension, tachycardia, tachypnea, cool, and mottled skin. No focal neurological deficits are noted.**

a. What clinical features and signs raise suspicion for septic shock in this patient?

b. What initial diagnostic investigations would you order for this patient to confirm the diagnosis of septic shock and guide further management?

c. Based on the patient's presentation and initial investigations, what would be your initial management plan for this patient with septic shock?

Q6. **A 65-year-old patient is brought to the emergency department with a chief complaint of severe diarrhea, abdominal cramps, and fever for the past 3 days. The patient reports recent antibiotic use for a respiratory infection. The stool is described as loose and foul-smelling. The patient appears dehydrated and is visibly uncomfortable.**

Patient's presentation:

- ***Chief complaints:*** **Severe diarrhea, abdominal cramps, and fever.**
- ***Vital signs:*** **Blood pressure 110/70 mm Hg, heart rate 120 bpm, respiratory rate 24 bpm, and temperature 38.5°C (101.3°F).**
- ***Physical examination:*** **Abdominal tenderness, hyperactive bowel sounds, and signs of dehydration (e.g., dry mucous membranes, decreased skin turgor).**

a. What clinical features and signs raise suspicion for pseudomembranous colitis in this patient?
b. What initial diagnostic investigations would you order for this patient to confirm the diagnosis of pseudomembranous colitis and guide further management?
c. What would be your initial management plan for this patient with pseudomembranous colitis?

Q7. A 65-year-old patient with a known history of chronic obstructive pulmonary disease (COPD) presents to the emergency department with increased dyspnea, cough, and sputum production over the past 24 hours. The patient reports worsening of symptoms despite using their rescue inhaler. There is no recent history of respiratory infections or changes in medication. The patient is visibly distressed and exhibits increased work of breathing.

Patient's presentation:

- ***Chief complaints:*** **Increased dyspnea, cough, and sputum production.**
- ***Vital signs:*** **Blood pressure 140/90 mm Hg, heart rate 110 bpm, respiratory rate 28 bpm, temperature 37.8°C (100°F), and oxygen saturation 88% on room air.**
- ***Physical examination:*** **Use of accessory muscles, prolonged expiratory phase, wheezing on auscultation, and increased tactile fremitus.**

a. What clinical features and signs raise suspicion for a COPD exacerbation in this patient?
b. What initial diagnostic investigations would you order for this patient to confirm the diagnosis of a COPD exacerbation and guide further management?
c. Based on the patient's presentation and initial investigations, what would be your initial management plan for this patient with a COPD exacerbation?

Q8. A 50-year-old patient presents to the emergency department with a chief complaint of severe pain, swelling, and erythema in the

left leg. The patient reports a recent injury while gardening and noticed the development of blisters and increasing discomfort over the past 24 hours. The patient is febrile and appears systemically unwell.

Patient's presentation:

- ***Chief complaints:*** **Severe pain, swelling, and erythema in the left leg.**
- ***Vital signs:*** **Blood pressure 130/80 mm Hg, heart rate 120 bpm, respiratory rate 24 bpm, and temperature 39.5°C (103.1°F).**
- ***Physical examination:*** **Left leg shows marked swelling, erythema, and tenderness. Blisters are present, and there are areas of skin discoloration. The patient is in significant pain, with localized signs of cellulitis.**

a. What clinical features and signs raise suspicion for necrotizing soft tissue infection of the leg in this patient?

b. What initial diagnostic investigations would you order for this patient to confirm the diagnosis of necrotizing soft tissue infection and guide further management?

c. Based on the patient's presentation and initial investigations, what would be your initial management plan for this patient with necrotizing soft tissue infection of the leg?

Q9. **A 45-year-old patient presents to the emergency department with a chief complaint of persistent cough, shortness of breath, and fever for the past 3 days. The patient reports productive cough with yellow-green sputum. The patient denies recent travel or known exposures to individuals with respiratory infections.**

Patient's presentation:

- ***Chief complaints:*** **Persistent cough, shortness of breath, and fever.**
- ***Vital signs:*** **Blood pressure 130/80 mm Hg, heart rate 100 bpm, respiratory rate 22 bpm, and temperature 38.9°C (102°F).**
- ***Physical examination:*** **Decreased breath sounds on auscultation, increased tactile fremitus, and dullness to percussion over the right lower lung field.**

a. What clinical features and signs raise suspicion for community-acquired pneumonia in this patient?

b. What initial diagnostic investigations would you order for this patient to confirm the diagnosis of community-acquired pneumonia and guide further management?

c. Based on the patient's presentation and initial investigations, what would be your initial management plan for this patient with community-acquired pneumonia?

Q10. A 25-year-old patient who presents with a chief complaint of a sore throat. The patient reports a gradual onset of throat pain, difficulty swallowing, and a mild fever over the past 2 days. There is no known exposure to individuals with similar symptoms. The patient denies cough, shortness of breath, or recent travel.

Patient's presentation:

- ***Chief complaints:*** **Sore throat, difficulty swallowing, and mild fever.**
- ***Vital signs:*** **Blood pressure 120/80 mm Hg, heart rate 80 bpm, respiratory rate 16 bpm, and temperature 37.8°C (100°F).**
- ***Physical examination:*** **Red and inflamed pharynx with visible exudate on the tonsils. There is no cervical lymphadenopathy.**

a. What clinical features raise suspicion for a viral etiology in this patient's sore throat?
b. What common viral pathogens could be causing this patient's sore throat?
c. What would be your initial management plan for this patient with a viral sore throat?
d. When would you consider a bacterial cause for this patient's sore throat and order a throat culture or rapid strep test?

Q11. A 55-year-old patient undergoing chemotherapy for leukemia presents to the emergency room with a chief complaint of fever. The patient completed a recent cycle of chemotherapy and is now experiencing a temperature of 38.5°C (101.3°F). The patient reports feeling weak but denies any specific respiratory or gastrointestinal symptoms.

Patient's presentation:

- ***Chief complaint:*** **Fever.**
- ***Vital signs:*** **Blood pressure 120/80 mm Hg, heart rate 110 bpm, respiratory rate 20 bpm, and temperature 38.5°C (101.3°F).**
- ***Medical history:*** **Undergoing chemotherapy for leukemia.**

a. What is the significance of febrile neutropenia in a patient undergoing chemotherapy?
b. What are the common causative organisms in febrile neutropenia, and why is empirical antibiotic therapy initiated?
c. What initial diagnostic tests would you order for a patient with febrile neutropenia?
d. What would be your initial management approach for this patient with febrile neutropenia?

Q12. A 28-year-old patient presents to the emergency department with a chief complaint of abdominal pain that started around the umbilicus and has migrated to the right lower quadrant over the past 24 hours. The patient describes the pain as constant and increasing in intensity. There is associated nausea, but no vomiting. The patient reports a lack of appetite and low-grade fever. On examination, there is tenderness in the right lower quadrant, and rebound tenderness is noted.

Patient's presentation:

- ***Chief complaint:*** **Abdominal pain in the right lower quadrant.**
- ***Vital signs:*** **Blood pressure 120/80 mm Hg, heart rate 90 bpm, respiratory rate 18 bpm, and temperature 38.2°C (100.8°F).**
- ***Physical examination:*** **Tenderness in the right lower quadrant with rebound tenderness. Rovsing's sign is positive.**

a. What clinical features and signs raise suspicion for acute appendicitis in this patient?

b. What additional physical examination findings and maneuver may be helpful in the assessment of acute appendicitis?

c. What diagnostic tests would you order to confirm the diagnosis of acute appendicitis?

d. What would be your initial management plan for this patient with suspected acute appendicitis?

Q13. A 60-year-old patient with a history of cirrhosis secondary to alcoholic liver disease presents to the emergency department with complaints of abdominal pain, fever, and increasing abdominal distension over the past 48 hours. On examination, the patient has tense ascites, and there is tenderness to palpation in the lower abdomen.

Patient's presentation:

- ***Chief complaints:*** **Abdominal pain and increasing abdominal distension.**
- ***Vital signs:*** **Blood pressure 110/70 mm Hg, heart rate 100 bpm, respiratory rate 20 bpm, and temperature 38.9°C (102°F).**
- ***Medical history:*** **Cirrhosis secondary to alcoholic liver disease.**

a. What clinical features and signs suggest the possibility of spontaneous bacterial peritonitis (SBP) in this patient?

b. What is the pathophysiology of SBP, and why are patients with cirrhosis at increased risk?

c. What diagnostic tests would you order to confirm the diagnosis of SBP?

d. What would be your initial management plan for this patient with suspected SBP?

Q14. A 45-year-old patient with a history of mitral valve prolapse presents to the emergency room with complaints of fever, fatigue, and new-onset murmur. The patient reports recent dental work. On examination, there is a new regurgitant murmur heard at the apex.

Patient's presentation:

- ***Chief complaints:*** **Fever, fatigue, and new-onset murmur.**
- ***Vital signs:*** **Blood pressure 130/80 mm Hg, heart rate 100 bpm, respiratory rate 18 bpm, and temperature 38.5°C (101.3°F).**
- ***Medical history:*** **Mitral valve prolapse.**

a. What clinical features and signs raise suspicion for infective endocarditis in this patient?

b. What are the common causative organisms of infective endocarditis, and why is recent dental work significant in this context?

c. What diagnostic tests would you order to confirm the diagnosis of infective endocarditis?

d. What would be your initial management plan for this patient with suspected infective endocarditis?

Q15. A 35-year-old patient presents to emergency room consultation with a chief complaint of persistent cough, weight loss, and evening fevers for the past 2 months. The patient reports a history of close contact with an individual diagnosed with active tuberculosis. On examination, there are crackles heard over the right upper lung field.

Patient's presentation:

- ***Chief complaints:*** **Persistent cough, weight loss, and evening fevers.**
- ***Vital signs:*** **Blood pressure 120/80 mm Hg, heart rate 90 bpm, respiratory rate 18 bpm, and temperature 38.2°C (100.8°F).**
- ***Medical history:*** **Close contact with an individual diagnosed with active tuberculosis.**

a. What clinical features and signs raise suspicion for pulmonary tuberculosis in this patient?

b. What diagnostic tests would you order to confirm the diagnosis of pulmonary tuberculosis?

c. What are the potential complications or challenges in the management of pulmonary tuberculosis?

Q16. A 45-year-old patient presents with a chief complaint of progressive shortness of breath, pleuritic chest pain, and fever for the past week. The patient has a history of pneumonia treated with oral antibiotics 2 weeks ago. On examination, decreased breath sounds and dullness to percussion are noted on the right side.

Patient's presentation:

- ***Chief complaints:*** **Progressive shortness of breath, pleuritic chest pain, and fever.**
- ***Vital signs:*** **Blood pressure 130/80 mm Hg, heart rate 100 bpm, respiratory rate 24 bpm, and temperature 38.9°C (102°F).**
- ***Medical history:*** **Recent pneumonia treated with oral antibiotics.**

a. What clinical features and signs raise suspicion for empyema in this patient?
b. What diagnostic tests would you order to confirm the diagnosis of empyema?
c. What is the initial management approach for a patient with empyema in the emergency department?

ANSWERS

Ans. 1

a. The key differential diagnoses for acute bloody diarrhea include:
   - *Infectious causes:* Bacterial infections (e.g., *Salmonella, Shigella,* and *Campylobacter*); Viral infections (e.g., norovirus and rotavirus); Parasitic infections (e.g., amebiasis and giardiasis).
   - *Inflammatory bowel disease (IBD):* Crohn's disease and ulcerative colitis.
   - *Ischemic colitis:* Reduced blood flow to the colon.
   - *Gastroenteritis:* Inflammation of the stomach and intestines.
   - *Diverticulitis:* Inflammation or infection of diverticula in the colon.

b. The initial diagnostic investigations for a patient with acute bloody diarrhea may include:
   - *Stool studies:* Stool culture to identify bacterial pathogens. Stool examination for ova and parasites.
   - *Clostridium difficile* toxin assay
   - *Complete blood count (CBC):* Assess for signs of infection or anemia.
   - *Basic metabolic panel (BMP):* Evaluate electrolyte imbalances.
   - *C-reactive protein (CRP) and erythrocyte sedimentation rate (ESR):* Indicators of inflammation.

- *Abdominal imaging:* Depending on clinical suspicion, consider imaging studies such as abdominal ultrasound or computed tomography (CT) scan.

c. The initial management plan for a patient with acute bloody diarrhea includes:
   - *Fluid resuscitation:* Administer intravenous fluids to address dehydration, especially if there are signs of hypovolemia.
   - *Empirical antibiotics:* If the suspicion for bacterial infection is high, start empirical antibiotics while awaiting stool culture results.
   - *Isolation precautions:* Implement appropriate isolation precautions to prevent potential transmission of infectious agents.
   - *Symptomatic treatment:* Provide symptomatic relief for abdominal cramping and discomfort.

Ans. 2

a. The key differential diagnoses for a patient with a fever persisting for 5 days include:
   - *Viral infections:* Influenza, Epstein–Barr virus (EBV) infection (infectious mononucleosis), and *Cytomegalovirus* (CMV) infection.
   - *Bacterial infections:* Streptococcal pharyngitis, UTI, respiratory tract infections (e.g., pneumonia).
   - *Systemic inflammatory conditions:* Systemic lupus erythematosus (SLE) and rheumatoid arthritis.
   - *Vector-borne infections:* Lyme disease and tick-borne diseases.
   - *Drug reactions:* Some medications can cause fever as a side effect.
   - *Hematological disorders:* Hematologic malignancies (e.g., leukemia).

b. The initial diagnostic investigations for a patient with prolonged fever may include:
   - *CBC:* To assess for leukocytosis, anemia, and thrombocytopenia.
   - *Blood cultures:* To identify possible bacterial bloodstream infections.
   - *Urinalysis and urine culture:* To rule out UTI.
   - *Chest X-ray:* If there are respiratory symptoms, to evaluate for pneumonia.
   - *Infectious disease screen:* Testing for common viral infections (e.g., influenza, EBV, CMV).
   - *Throat swab for culture:* If there is suspicion of streptococcal pharyngitis.

c. The initial management plan for a patient with a prolonged fever includes:
   - *Empirical antibiotics:* If there is clinical suspicion of a bacterial infection, start empirical antibiotics pending further test results.
   - *Antipyretics:* Administer antipyretic medications (e.g., acetaminophen) to alleviate symptoms and reduce fever.

- *Hydration:* Ensure adequate hydration, especially if there are signs of dehydration.
- *Disposition:* Based on the patient clinical condition and investigations, admission to be planned.

Ans. 3

a. The key clinical features and signs suggestive of urosepsis in this male patient include:
   - *Dysuria, frequency, and urgency:* Symptoms of a UTI.
   - *Lower abdominal pain:* Pain or discomfort in the lower abdomen, often indicative of a UTI involving the bladder.
   - *Fever:* Elevated body temperature is a common sign of systemic infection.
   - *Hemodynamic instability:* Signs such as tachycardia and hypotension may indicate sepsis.
   - *CVA tenderness:* Tenderness over the CVA may suggest involvement of the kidneys.
   - *Suprapubic tenderness:* Tenderness over the suprapubic area may indicate bladder involvement.

b. The initial diagnostic investigations for a male patient with suspected urosepsis may include:
   - *Urinalysis:* To identify signs of infection (e.g., pyuria and hematuria) and assess for the presence of nitrites.
   - *Blood cultures:* To identify the causative organism and guide antibiotic selection.
   - *CBC:* To assess for leukocytosis, a common finding in systemic infections.
   - *Blood urea nitrogen (BUN) and creatinine:* To assess renal function and identify potential kidney involvement.
   - *Urinary culture:* To confirm the specific bacterial pathogen and guide antibiotic therapy.
   - *Imaging studies:* Renal ultrasound or CT scan may be considered to evaluate for obstructive uropathy or other structural abnormalities.

c. The initial management plan for a male patient with urosepsis includes:
   - *Empirical antibiotics:* Administer broad-spectrum antibiotics promptly, considering the local antimicrobial resistance patterns and adjusting based on culture results.
   - *Intravenous fluids:* Administer intravenous fluids to address hypotension and maintain adequate hydration.
   - *Analgesics:* Provide pain management
   - *Monitoring:* Regularly monitor vital signs, fluid balance, and response to treatment.

d. *Urology consultation:* Consider consulting urology for further evaluation and management, especially if there is concern about obstruction or structural abnormalities or complicated UTI.

Ans. 4

a. The clinical features and signs that raise suspicion for meningitis in this patient include:
   - *Severe headache:* Persistent and severe headache is a common symptom of meningitis.
   - *Photophobia:* Light sensitivity is a classic symptom of meningitis.
   - *Neck stiffness:* Stiffness and resistance to neck flexion (Brudzinski's sign) are indicative of meningeal irritation.
   - *Fever:* Elevated body temperature is often present in cases of infectious meningitis.
   - *Positive Kernig's sign:* Resistance to knee extension when the hip is flexed at a 90° angle.
   - *Lethargy:* Generalized weakness and lethargy are common in patients with meningitis.

b. The initial diagnostic investigations for a patient with suspected meningitis may include:
   - *Lumbar puncture:* To obtain cerebrospinal fluid (CSF) for analysis including cell count, glucose, and protein levels.
   - *Blood cultures:* To identify the causative organism and guide antibiotic therapy.
   - *CBC:* To assess for leukocytosis, anemia, and thrombocytopenia.
   - *Chest X-ray:* To rule out pneumonia or other respiratory infections.
   - *CT brain imaging:* In some cases, particularly before lumbar puncture, to assess for any contraindications for features of raised intracranial pressure

c. The initial management plan for a patient with suspected meningitis includes:
   - *Empirical antibiotics:* Administer broad-spectrum antibiotics promptly to cover likely pathogens, adjusting based on culture results.
   - *Antiviral medications:* If viral etiology is suspected, antiviral medications may be considered.
   - *Analgesics and antipyretics:* Provide pain management and antipyretic medications to alleviate symptoms.
   - *Intravenous fluids:* Administer intravenous fluids to address dehydration.
   - *Isolation precautions:* Implement appropriate isolation precautions to prevent potential transmission of infectious agents.
   - *Admission to ICU:* Consider admission to the ICU for close monitoring, especially if signs of increased intracranial pressure are present.

Ans. 5

a. The clinical features and signs that raise suspicion for septic shock in this patient include:
   - *Hypotension:* Systolic blood pressure <90 mm Hg or a mean arterial pressure (MAP) <65 mm Hg.
   - *Tachycardia:* Heart rate >90 bpm.
   - *Tachypnea:* Respiratory rate >20 bpm.
   - *Altered mental status:* Confusion, lethargy, or decreased level of consciousness.
   - *Fever:* Elevated body temperature, although hypothermia can also be observed.
   - *Cool and mottled skin:* Peripheral vasoconstriction leading to cool and mottled skin.
   - *Decreased urine output:* Oliguria or anuria, indicating impaired renal perfusion.

b. The initial diagnostic investigations for a patient with suspected septic shock may include:
   - *Blood cultures:* To identify the causative organism and guide antibiotic therapy.
   - *CBC:* To assess for leukocytosis or leukopenia.
   - *Lactate level:* To assess for tissue hypoperfusion.
   - *Blood gas analysis:* To evaluate acid-base status and assess for respiratory alkalosis or acidosis.
   - *Coagulation profile:* Prothrombin time (PT), activated partial thromboplastin time (aPTT), and platelet count.
   - *BMP:* To assess electrolyte imbalances and renal function.
   - *Urinalysis:* To assess for signs of UTI or sepsis-related kidney injury.
   - *Chest X-ray:* To evaluate for potential sources of infection (e.g., pneumonia).
   - *Echocardiography:* To assess cardiac function and identify potential sources of infection (e.g., endocarditis).

c. The initial management plan for a patient with septic shock includes:
   - *Empirical broad-spectrum antibiotics:* Administer antibiotics promptly to cover likely pathogens, adjusting based on culture results.
   - *Intravenous fluid resuscitation:* Administer crystalloid fluids rapidly to address hypovolemia and improve tissue perfusion.
   - *Vasopressor therapy:* Initiate vasopressor therapy (e.g., norepinephrine) to support blood pressure and perfusion.
   - *Monitoring:* Regularly monitor vital signs, urine output, and laboratory parameters.
   - *Oxygen therapy:* Provide supplemental oxygen to maintain adequate oxygenation.

- *Admission to ICU:* Transfer the patient to the ICU for close monitoring and advanced hemodynamic support.
- *Source control:* Identify and address the source of infection (e.g., surgical intervention for an intra-abdominal source).

Ans. 6

a. The clinical features and signs that raise suspicion for pseudomembranous colitis in this patient include:
   - *Recent antibiotic use:* Recent use of antibiotics, especially broad-spectrum antibiotics, is a major risk factor for *C. difficile* infection.
   - *Severe diarrhea:* Frequent, watery diarrhea that may be foul-smelling.
   - *Abdominal cramps:* Abdominal pain or cramps are common symptoms.
   - *Fever:* Elevated body temperature may be present.
   - *Dehydration:* Signs of dehydration, such as decreased skin turgor and dry mucous membranes.
   - *Abdominal tenderness:* Tenderness on abdominal examination, usually diffuse.

b. The initial diagnostic investigations for a patient with suspected pseudomembranous colitis may include:
   - *Stool testing for C. difficile toxin:* To detect the presence of *C. difficile* toxins in the stool.
   - *CBC:* To assess for leukocytosis, which may be elevated in severe cases.
   - *BMP:* To assess electrolyte imbalances and renal function.
   - *Imaging studies:* In some cases, abdominal imaging (e.g., CT scan) may be performed to assess for complications or extent of colitis.

c. The initial management plan for a patient with pseudomembranous colitis includes:
   - *Discontinuation of causative antibiotic:* If possible, discontinue the antibiotic responsible for triggering the infection.
   - *Initiation of specific antibiotic therapy:* Start specific antibiotics targeting *C. difficile*, such as oral metronidazole or oral vancomycin.
   - *Supportive care:* Provide supportive care including intravenous fluids to address dehydration and electrolyte imbalances.
   - *Isolation precautions:* Implement appropriate isolation precautions to prevent the spread of *C. difficile.*
   - *Monitoring:* Regularly monitor vital signs, fluid balance, and response to treatment.

Ans. 7

a. The clinical features that raise suspicion for a COPD exacerbation in this patient include:
   - *Increased dyspnea:* Worsening shortness of breath is a hallmark of a COPD exacerbation.

- *Cough and sputum production:* Increased cough and sputum production may indicate an exacerbation.
- *Limited response to rescue inhaler:* Poor response to the patient's rescue inhaler suggests a more severe exacerbation.
- *Use of accessory muscles:* Increased work of breathing with the use of accessory muscles.
- *Prolonged expiratory phase:* Prolonged expiration, characteristic of obstructive lung diseases.
- *Wheezing on auscultation:* Wheezing or decreased breath sounds on lung examination.
- *Decreased oxygen saturation:* Hypoxemia, as evidenced by decreased oxygen saturation.

b. The initial diagnostic investigations for suspected COPD exacerbation may include:
   - *Arterial blood gas (ABG) analysis:* To assess oxygen and carbon dioxide levels, especially if the patient is hypoxic or has signs of respiratory distress.
   - *Chest X-ray:* To rule out other potential causes of respiratory distress.
   - *CBC:* To assess for signs of infection or other abnormalities.
   - *Electrocardiogram (ECG):* To evaluate for cardiac comorbidities contributing to symptoms.
   - *Peak expiratory flow (PEF) or spirometry:* To assess lung function and severity of airflow obstruction.

c. The initial management plan for a patient with a COPD exacerbation includes:
   - *Bronchodilator therapy:* Administer short-acting bronchodilators (e.g., salbutamol) via nebulizer or metered-dose inhaler to relieve bronchospasm.
   - *Corticosteroids:* Administer systemic corticosteroids (e.g., prednisone) to reduce airway inflammation.
   - *Supplemental oxygen:* Administer supplemental oxygen to maintain oxygen saturation above 90%.
   - *Monitoring:* Continuously monitor vital signs including oxygen saturation.
   - *Intravenous fluids:* Consider intravenous fluids if there is evidence of dehydration.
   - *Consider antibiotics:* If there are signs of bacterial infection (e.g., increased sputum purulence), consider antibiotics.
   - *Consider noninvasive ventilation:* In cases of respiratory distress and persistent hypoxemia, consider noninvasive ventilation [e.g., bilevel positive airway pressure (BiPAP)].

Ans. 8

a. The clinical features and signs that raise suspicion for necrotizing soft tissue infection of the leg in this patient include:
   - *Severe pain and swelling:* Disproportionate pain and swelling compared to the apparent injury or infection.
   - *Erythema and tenderness:* Marked erythema and tenderness over the affected area.
   - *Rapid progression:* Rapid progression of symptoms within a short time frame.
   - *Systemic signs of infection:* Fever, tachycardia, and other systemic signs of infection.
   - *Blisters and skin discoloration:* Presence of blisters, bullae, or areas of skin discoloration.
   - *Crepitus:* Crepitus on palpation may indicate gas production by bacteria.
   - *Compartment syndrome:* Signs of compartment syndrome, such as pain out of proportion, may be present.

b. The initial diagnostic investigations for a patient with suspected necrotizing soft tissue infection may include:
   - *Blood cultures:* To identify the causative organism and guide antibiotic therapy.
   - *CBC:* To assess for leukocytosis, which may be elevated in severe infections.
   - *Blood gas analysis:* To assess for acid-base imbalances and tissue hypoperfusion.
   - *Serum lactate level:* Elevated lactate levels may indicate tissue hypoxia and necrosis.
   - *Imaging studies:* X-ray to rule out any bony involvement and Doppler study of venous system to rule out deep vein thrombosis
   - *Surgical consultation:* Prompt consultation with a surgeon for evaluation and potential surgical intervention.

c. The initial management plan for a patient with necrotizing soft tissue infection of the leg includes:
   - *Empirical broad-spectrum antibiotics:* Administer intravenous antibiotics promptly to cover likely pathogens, adjusting based on culture results.
   - *Surgical exploration and debridement:* Urgent surgical consultation for exploration and debridement of necrotic tissue.
   - *Intravenous fluid resuscitation:* Administer intravenous fluids to address hypotension and maintain adequate perfusion.
   - *Pain management:* Provide analgesics to alleviate pain and discomfort.
   - *Monitoring:* Continuous monitoring of vital signs, fluid balance, and laboratory parameters.

- *ICU admission:* Consider admission to the ICU for close monitoring and advanced support. Serial clinical assessments to monitor the response to treatment and identify any signs of worsening infection.

Ans. 9

a. The clinical features and signs that raise suspicion for community-acquired pneumonia in this patient include:
   - *Persistent cough:* Persistent cough, often productive, is a common symptom.
   - *Shortness of breath:* Dyspnea or shortness of breath, particularly with exertion.
   - *Fever:* Elevated body temperature is a common sign of infection.
   - *Productive cough:* Presence of yellow-green sputum may indicate a bacterial infection.
   - *Decreased breath sounds:* Abnormal lung auscultation findings, such as decreased breath sounds.
   - *Increased tactile fremitus:* Increased vibration felt on palpation, suggesting consolidation.
   - *Dullness to percussion:* Dullness on percussion over a lung field, indicating possible consolidation.

b. The initial diagnostic investigations for a patient with suspected community-acquired pneumonia may include:
   - *Chest X-ray:* To assess for infiltrates or consolidation in the lungs.
   - *CBC:* To assess for leukocytosis, which may indicate infection.
   - *BMP:* To assess electrolyte imbalances and renal function.
   - *ABG:* To assess oxygenation status, especially in cases of respiratory distress.
   - *Sputum culture:* To identify the causative organism, although results may take time.
   - *Blood cultures:* To identify the causative organism and guide antibiotic therapy.

c. The initial management plan for a patient with community-acquired pneumonia includes:
   - *Empirical antibiotic therapy:* Administer empirical antibiotics based on the likely pathogen and local resistance patterns.
   - *Oxygen therapy:* Provide supplemental oxygen to maintain adequate oxygenation.
   - *Intravenous fluids:* Administer intravenous fluids if there are signs of dehydration or if the patient is unable to tolerate oral intake.
   - *Analgesics and antipyretics:* Provide pain management and antipyretic medications to alleviate symptoms.
   - *Monitoring:* Regularly monitor vital signs, oxygen saturation, and laboratory parameters.

- *Follow-up chest X-ray:* Arrange for follow-up chest X-ray to assess for resolution of infiltrates

Ans. 10

a. The clinical features that raise suspicion for a viral etiology in this patient's sore throat include:
   - *Gradual onset:* Sore throats caused by viruses often have a gradual onset.
   - *Fever:* A mild fever may be present in viral infections.
   - *Red and inflamed pharynx:* Viral infections can cause redness and inflammation of the pharynx.
   - *Exudate on tonsils:* While exudate can be seen in bacterial infections, it is also observed in some viral infections.
   - *Absence of cough and shortness of breath:* Viral pharyngitis may not be associated with cough or respiratory symptoms.

b. Common viral pathogens that could be causing this patient's sore throat include:
   - *Rhinovirus:* A common cause of upper respiratory infections.
   - *Coronavirus:* Various strains including those causing the common cold.
   - *Adenovirus:* Can cause respiratory and throat infections.
   - *Influenza virus:* Influenza viruses can cause sore throat along with systemic symptoms.
   - *EBV:* Causes infectious mononucleosis and can present with severe sore throat.

c. The initial management plan for a patient with a viral sore throat includes:
   - *Symptomatic treatment:* Advise the patient to get plenty of rest and stay hydrated.
   - *Pain relief:* Recommend pain relievers (e.g., acetaminophen or ibuprofen) for pain and fever.
   - *Warm saltwater gargle:* Suggest warm saltwater gargle to soothe the throat.
   - *Monitor for complications:* Instruct the patient to monitor for worsening symptoms or signs of complications.
   - *Follow-up:* Schedule a follow-up appointment if symptoms persist or worsen.

d. Consider a bacterial cause and order a throat culture or rapid strep test in the following circumstances:
   - *Severe symptoms:* If the patient presents with severe symptoms, persistent fever, or significant difficulty swallowing.
   - *Exudate and tonsillar swelling:* If there is marked exudate on the tonsils and significant tonsillar swelling.

- *Close contact with confirmed strep throat:* If there is a known exposure to individuals with confirmed streptococcal pharyngitis.
- *Persistent symptoms:* If symptoms persist beyond the usual duration of a viral infection.

Ans. 11

a. *Significance of febrile neutropenia in a patient undergoing chemotherapy:* Febrile neutropenia is a serious and potentially life-threatening condition commonly encountered in patients undergoing chemotherapy. Neutropenia refers to a low absolute neutrophil count (ANC), which increases the risk of severe infections. Fever in a neutropenic patient is considered a medical emergency, as it may be the only sign of a potentially serious infection. Prompt evaluation and initiation of empirical broad-spectrum antibiotics are crucial in this population to prevent complications and reduce mortality.

b. Common causative organisms in febrile neutropenia include bacteria such as:
   - *Gram-positive bacteria: Staphylococcus aureus*, coagulase-negative staphylococci, and *Streptococcus* species.
   - *Gram-negative bacteria: Escherichia coli, Klebsiella pneumoniae, Pseudomonas aeruginosa*, and *Enterobacter* species.
   - *Fungal infections: Candida* species and *Aspergillus* species in certain situations.
   - *Empirical antibiotic therapy is initiated promptly because:*
     - Neutropenic patients may not exhibit typical signs of infection, making early diagnosis challenging.
     - The risk of rapid progression to sepsis is high in this population.
     - Broad-spectrum antibiotics are chosen to cover a range of potential pathogens until specific causative organisms are identified through cultures.

c. Initial diagnostic tests for a patient with febrile neutropenia may include:
   - *Blood cultures:* To identify the causative organism and guide antibiotic therapy.
   - *CBC:* To assess the ANC and overall blood cell counts.
   - *Peripheral blood smear:* To assess for morphologic abnormalities in blood cells.
   - *BMP:* To assess electrolyte imbalances and renal function.
   - *Chest X-ray:* To evaluate for pulmonary infiltrates or other signs of infection.

d. The initial management approach for a patient with febrile neutropenia includes:
   - *Empirical antibiotics:* Prompt initiation of empirical broad-spectrum antibiotics to cover potential bacterial and fungal pathogens.

- *Intravenous fluids:* Administer intravenous fluids for hydration.
- *Hospital admission:* Consider hospital admission for close monitoring and further management.
- *Hematopoietic growth factors:* Depending on the clinical situation, hematopoietic growth factors [e.g., granulocyte-colony stimulating factor (G-CSF)] may be considered to accelerate neutrophil recovery after oncologist/hematologist opinion.

Ans. 12

a. The clinical features and signs that raise suspicion for acute appendicitis in this patient include:
    - *Migration of pain:* Pain starting around the umbilicus and migrating to the right lower quadrant is characteristic.
    - *Constant pain:* Constant, increasing pain that is not relieved by changes in position.
    - *Nausea and anorexia:* Nausea, with or without vomiting, and a lack of appetite.
    - *Low-grade fever:* Low-grade fever may be present.
    - *Localized tenderness:* Localized tenderness in the right lower quadrant, particularly on deep palpation.
    - *Rebound tenderness:* Rebound tenderness (pain upon release of pressure) in the right lower quadrant.
    - *Positive Rovsing's sign:* Positive Rovsing's sign, where palpation of the left lower quadrant elicits pain in the right lower quadrant.

b. Additional physical examination findings and maneuver helpful in the assessment of acute appendicitis include:
    - *McBurney's point tenderness:* Tenderness at McBurney's point, located one-third of the way from the anterior superior iliac spine to the umbilicus.
    - *Psoas sign:* Pain elicited by extending the patient's right leg against resistance (positive psoas sign) may indicate irritation of the psoas muscle due to inflamed appendix.
    - *Obturator sign:* Pain elicited by internal rotation of the right hip (positive obturator sign) may indicate irritation of the obturator muscle.
    - *Alvarado score:* Use of the Alvarado score, which includes clinical features and laboratory findings, to assess the likelihood of appendicitis.

c. Diagnostic tests to confirm the diagnosis of acute appendicitis may include:
    - *CBC:* To assess for leukocytosis, which may be present in inflammatory conditions.

- *Urinalysis:* To rule out UTI or other genitourinary pathology.
- *Abdominal imaging:* Abdominal ultrasound or CT scan to visualize the appendix and assess for signs of inflammation or perforation.
- *Pregnancy test:* In females of reproductive age, a pregnancy test may be performed to rule out ectopic pregnancy.

d. The initial management plan for a patient with suspected acute appendicitis includes:
   - *NPO status:* Advise the patient to remain nil per os (NPO) to prepare for potential surgical intervention.
   - *Intravenous fluids and analgesia:* Administer intravenous fluids for hydration and analgesia for pain relief.
   - *Surgical consultation:* Consult a general surgeon for further evaluation and plan of appendectomy.

Ans. 13

a. The clinical features and signs that suggest the possibility of SBP in this patient include:
   - *Cirrhosis history:* Patients with cirrhosis, particularly those with tense ascites, are at risk for SBP.
   - *Abdominal pain:* Abdominal pain, often localized in the lower abdomen, is a common symptom.
   - *Fever:* Fever is a typical sign of infection, and its presence raises suspicion for SBP.
   - *Increasing abdominal distension:* Increasing abdominal distension may indicate worsening ascites.
   - *Tense ascites:* Tense or new-onset ascites may suggest SBP.
   - *Tenderness to palpation:* Tenderness to palpation, particularly in the lower abdomen, is a concerning finding.
   - *Altered mental status:* Some patients may exhibit altered mental status, reflecting systemic involvement.

b. The pathophysiology of spontaneous bacterial peritonitis involves bacterial infection of ascitic fluid without an obvious intra-abdominal source. The increased risk in patients with cirrhosis is attributed to:
   - *Portal hypertension:* Cirrhosis leads to portal hypertension, causing splanchnic vasodilation and increased permeability of the intestinal mucosa.
   - *Intestinal bacterial overgrowth:* Bacterial overgrowth in the intestines due to impaired gut motility and mucosal defense mechanisms.
   - *Translocation of bacteria:* Translocation of bacteria from the intestinal lumen to the mesenteric lymph nodes and eventually to the ascitic fluid.
   - *Reduced immune function:* Cirrhosis is associated with immune dysfunction, reducing the ability to clear bacteria.

c. Diagnostic tests to confirm the diagnosis of spontaneous bacterial peritonitis may include:
   - *Ascitic fluid analysis:* Cell count, differential, and culture of ascitic fluid to identify the presence of infection.
   - *Blood cultures:* Blood cultures to identify the causative organism.
   - *CBC:* To assess for leukocytosis, which may indicate systemic infection.
   - *Liver function tests:* To assess liver function and severity of cirrhosis.
   - *Imaging studies:* Abdominal imaging (ultrasound or CT scan) to assess for other intra-abdominal pathology.
   - *Serum albumin level:* Serum albumin level to calculate the serum-ascites albumin gradient (SAAG) if not a known chronic liver disease (CLD).

d. The initial management plan for a patient with suspected spontaneous bacterial peritonitis includes:
   - *Empirical antibiotics:* Prompt initiation of empirical antibiotic therapy covering common pathogens, such as third-generation cephalosporins or other antibiotics based on local resistance patterns.
   - *Intravenous fluids:* Intravenous fluids for resuscitation and management of potential hemodynamic instability.
   - *Albumin infusion:* Infusion of intravenous albumin in certain situations, especially in patients with a high risk of renal impairment.
   - *Paracentesis:* Diagnostic and therapeutic paracentesis to assess ascitic fluid characteristics and reduce intra-abdominal pressure.

Ans. 14

a. The clinical features and signs that raise suspicion for infective endocarditis in this patient include:
   - *Fever:* Persistent fever is a common symptom in infective endocarditis.
   - *Fatigue:* Generalized fatigue and malaise are frequently reported.
   - *New-onset murmur:* The presence of a new regurgitant murmur, especially in a patient with a predisposing heart condition (such as mitral valve prolapse), raises concern for infective endocarditis.
   - *Recent dental work:* A history of recent dental work is a potential risk factor for infective endocarditis, particularly if there is concurrent mitral valve prolapse.
   - *Systemic signs:* Other systemic signs may include weight loss, night sweats, and arthralgia.

b. Common causative organisms of infective endocarditis include:
   - *Streptococcus viridans:* Often associated with dental procedures.
   - *Staphylococcus aureus:* Commonly seen in intravenous drug users and may also result from skin and soft tissue infections.
   - *Enterococci:* Often associated with underlying gastrointestinal or genitourinary tract pathology.

- Recent dental work is significant because dental procedures, particularly those involving manipulation of the gingival tissues or periapical region of teeth, can introduce bacteria into the bloodstream. In patients with underlying valvular abnormalities or prosthetic valves, these bacteria may adhere to the damaged valve, leading to infective endocarditis.

c. Diagnostic tests to confirm the diagnosis of infective endocarditis may include:
  - *Blood cultures:* Multiple sets of blood cultures to identify the causative organism.
  - *Echocardiography:* Transthoracic echocardiography (TTE) or trans-esophageal echocardiography (TEE) to assess for valvular vegetations and structural abnormalities.
  - *CBC:* To assess for leukocytosis, which may indicate systemic infection.
  - *ESR and CRP:* Elevated inflammatory markers.

d. The initial management plan for a patient with suspected infective endocarditis includes:
  - *Empirical antibiotics:* Prompt initiation of empirical broad-spectrum antibiotics based on the likely causative organism and local resistance patterns.
  - *Blood cultures:* Obtain blood cultures before initiating antibiotics to identify the specific pathogen.
  - *Echocardiography:* Urgent echocardiography (TTE or TEE) to assess for valvular involvement.
  - *Cardiac surgery consultation:* Consultation with a cardiac surgeon for consideration of valve replacement or repair in certain cases.
  - *Antipyretics and supportive care:* Antipyretic medications for fever control and supportive care as needed.

Ans. 15

a. The clinical features and signs that raise suspicion for pulmonary tuberculosis in this patient include:
  - *Persistent cough:* Cough lasting for >2 weeks is a common symptom.
  - *Weight loss:* Unexplained weight loss is a significant indicator.
  - *Evening fevers:* Low-grade evening fevers are characteristic of tuberculosis.
  - *History of close contact:* Close contact with an individual diagnosed with active tuberculosis increases the risk of exposure.
  - *Crackles on examination:* Crackles heard over the lung fields, especially in the upper lobes, may suggest tuberculosis-associated parenchymal involvement.

b. Diagnostic tests to confirm the diagnosis of pulmonary tuberculosis may include:
   - *Sputum smear microscopy:* Acid-fast bacilli (AFB) smear microscopy to detect mycobacteria in the sputum.
   - *Sputum culture:* Mycobacterial culture to confirm the presence of *Mycobacterium tuberculosis.*
   - *Chest X-ray:* Chest X-ray to assess for characteristic findings, such as upper lobe infiltrates, cavitation, or pleural effusion.
   - *Tuberculin skin test (TST) or interferon-γ release assay (IGRA):* To assess for exposure to *Mycobacterium tuberculosis.*
   - *CBC:* To assess for leukocytosis or anemia.
   - *ESR and CRP:* Elevated inflammatory markers may be present.

c. Potential complications or challenges in the management of pulmonary tuberculosis include:
   - *Drug resistance:* Development of drug-resistant strains, requiring alternative treatment regimens.
   - *Adherence issues:* Patient nonadherence to the prescribed treatment, leading to treatment failure or relapse.
   - *Hepatotoxicity:* Hepatotoxicity associated with certain antituberculosis medications, requiring close monitoring of liver function.
   - *Immune reconstitution inflammatory syndrome (IRIS):* Paradoxical worsening of symptoms or the emergence of new symptoms as the immune system recovers during treatment.
   - *Concurrent conditions:* Management challenges in patients with comorbidities such as human immunodeficiency virus (HIV) infection or diabetes.

Ans. 16

a. The clinical features and signs that raise suspicion for empyema in this patient include:
   - *Progressive shortness of breath:* Progressive dyspnea may suggest a worsening respiratory condition.
   - *Pleuritic chest pain:* Pleuritic chest pain, especially in the setting of recent pneumonia, is concerning for pleural involvement.
   - *Fever:* Persistent or worsening fever may indicate an ongoing infectious process.
   - *Decreased breath sounds:* Decreased or absent breath sounds on auscultation of the affected side.
   - *Dullness to percussion:* Dullness to percussion over the affected lung area, indicating the presence of fluid in the pleural space.
   - *Pleuritic rub:* Pleuritic rub may be present on auscultation in some cases.

b. Diagnostic tests to confirm the diagnosis of empyema may include:
    - *Chest X-ray:* Chest X-ray to assess for the presence of fluid collection, consolidation, or pleural effusion.
    - *Thoracic ultrasound:* Thoracic ultrasound for a more detailed evaluation of pleural fluid characteristics and to guide interventions.
    - *CT scan of the chest:* CT scan may be ordered for a comprehensive assessment of the extent of pleural involvement.
    - *Pleural fluid analysis:* Thoracentesis for pleural fluid analysis including cell count, differential, cultures, and biochemical studies.
    - *Blood cultures:* Blood cultures to identify the causative organism.

c. The initial management approach for a patient with empyema in the emergency department includes:
    - *Stabilization:* Ensure adequate oxygenation and respiratory support. Consider supplemental oxygen if needed.
    - *Empirical antibiotics:* Initiate empirical broad-spectrum antibiotics to cover common causative organisms including *Streptococcus pneumoniae* and *S. aureus*.
    - *Analgesia:* Provide analgesia for pain relief, especially pleuritic chest pain.
    - *Thoracentesis:* Consider therapeutic thoracentesis for drainage of infected pleural fluid and relief of respiratory distress.
    - *Consultation:* Consult a pulmonologist or thoracic surgeon for further management, especially if there is a need for more advanced interventions such as chest tube placement or video-assisted thoracoscopic surgery (VATS).

19 CHAPTER Toxicology Emergencies OSCE

S Senthilkumaran

QUESTIONS

Q1. A 35-year-old male was brought to the emergency department after a polypharmacy overdose (unknown medication toxicity) with altered mental state.

a. Enumerate five risk factors for suicide.

b. Enumerate three investigations with justification in this patient with unknown medication toxicity with altered mental status.

c. Assesses disposition decision criteria.

Q2. A 27-year-old, 50 kg female, presented to the emergency department after ingesting 80 tablets of 325 mg of aspirin.

a. What features stratify her as high risk?

b. What are important investigations would you request?

c. What particular factors need to be taken into account if she needs to be intubated?

Q3. A 50-year-old male has been brought to the emergency department after being found unresponsive at home by his wife. He was found next to an empty bottle of amitriptyline. He is currently receiving treatment for postherpetic neuralgia. His ECG shows a broad complex tachycardia with a rate of 120 bpm.

a. How tricyclic antidepressant (TCA) overdose leads to toxic effect?

b. Write typical ECG findings of TCA overdose.

c. Write antidote for TCA overdose.

Q4. A 32-year-old lady with a past medical history of hypothyroidism was brought to the emergency department claims to have taken 100 tablets of 150 µg of thyroxin, taken 4 hours ago. She is currently having "normal" vital signs and well oriented and is feeling tired but is otherwise asymptomatic.

a. What is your risk assessment?

b. Write justification of thyroid function tests in this patient.

c. What are the steps in management of symptomatic thyroxin overdose?

Q5. A 29-year-old lady with weight of 61 kg presents to the emergency department after taking 45 unknown antihypertensive tablets. On presentation, her Glasgow Coma Scale (GCS) score is 13, heart rate (HR) is 46 bpm, and blood pressure (BP) is 80/40 mm Hg. Her ECG is provided to emergency physician for interpretation.

a. What does the ECG show and how can this help guide care?
b. How does β-blocker overdose differ from calcium channel blocker overdose?
c. What do you do if the patient arrests?

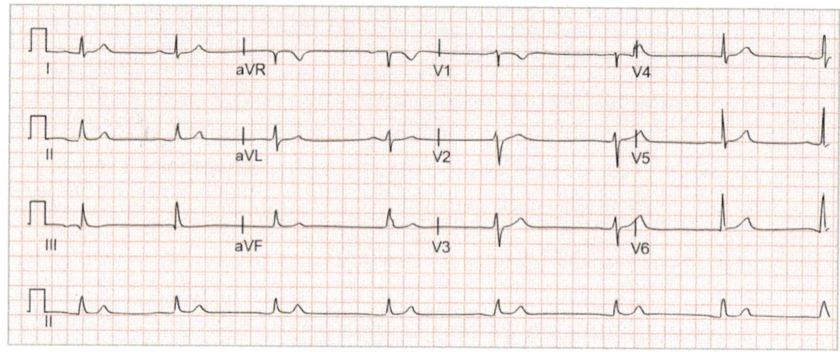

Q6. A 2.5-year-old male child presents to the emergency department with an accidental ingestion of antifreeze liquid. Subsequently, the child became drowsy. In emergency department, the child was stuporous and delirious with a diminished gag reflex and he is tachycardic and hypotensive.

a. Write few products which contain ethylene glycol.
b. Write clinical feature of severe ethylene glycol toxicity.
c. In suspected ethylene glycol toxicity write useful investigations.

Q7. A 29-year-old female consumed wild mushrooms harvested from mountains, developed pain abdomen, vomiting, and bloody diarrhea 4–6 hours after consumption.

a. What is the presentation of a patient with mushroom toxicity?
b. Summarize the treatment options for mushroom toxicity.
c. What are the potentially life-threatening complications?

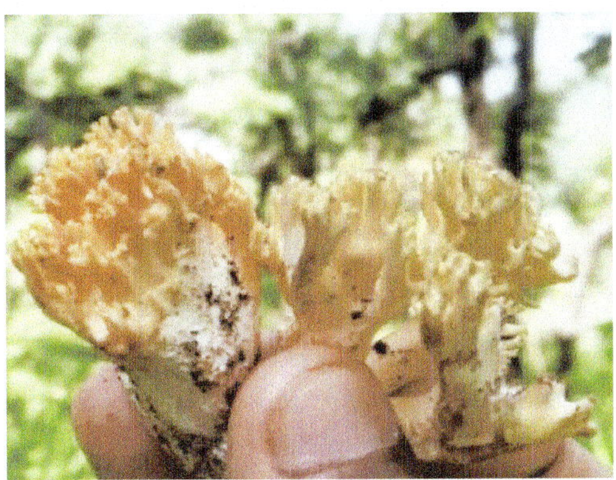

Q8. A 2-year-old male child presents to the emergency department after accidental ingestion of watch battery. After ingestion of battery baby is drooling saliva and not taking feed.

a. How do you approach to this patient?
b. Enumerate complications associated with accidental batteries ingestion.
c. What are the steps in managing this patient if X-ray showing the battery is located in the esophagus at the level of the aortic arch?

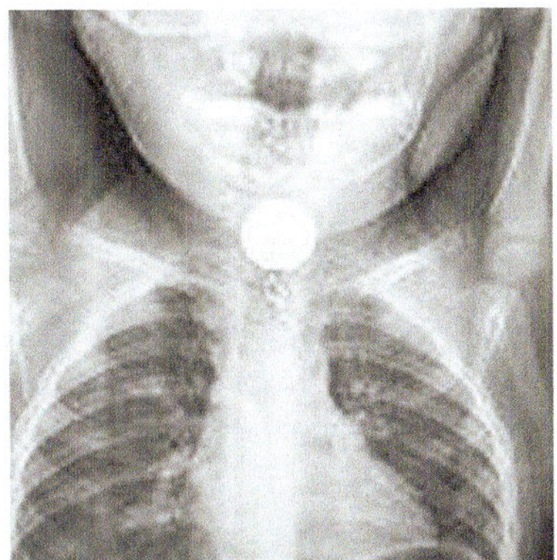

Q9. A 28-year-old female presents with a history of ingestion of 30 enalapril approximately 30 minutes ago.

a. Write clinical feature of angiotensin-converting enzyme (ACE) inhibitor overdose.
b. What are the steps in managing hypotension in ACE inhibitor overdose patient?
c. Is there any antidote available?

Q10. A 28-year-old lady ingested a large amount of rheumatoid arthritis medicine methotrexate and brought to the emergency medicine after 90 minutes for further management.

a. Write associated clinical feature associated with methotrexate use.
b. What are the steps in managing this patient?
c. What is the antidote?

Q11. A 49-year-old man was brought to the emergency department after 3 hours of consuming 30 usual diabetic medications (glipizide). He is now ataxic, confused, and slurred speech. Patient blood glucose is 30 mg/dL.

a. What is Whipple's triad?
b. What is the role of thiamine in the treatment of hypoglycemia?
c. How does octreotide treat it?

Q12. A 25-year-old lady was brought to the emergency department after ingestion of 50 olanzapine tablets 4 hours ago. She has a history of borderline personality disorder. In emergency room (ER), she was somnolent, actively seizing, and lost pulses. Immediately cardiopulmonary resuscitation (CPR) was initiated.

a. What types of interventions are indicated?
b. How to administer Intralipid?
c. What are adverse effects of Intralipid?

Q13. A 45-year-old male presented to the emergency department with shortness of breath, chest pain, and giddiness. He has a past medical history of systemic lupus erythematosus (SLE) and he is on methotrexate, dapsone, and hydroxychloroquine. His vitals are HR 98 beats/min, BP 140/90 mm Hg, respiratory rate (RR) 23 breaths/min, SpO_2 80% on 15 L via nonrebreather mask (NRBM). His ECG was normal sinus rhythm and chest X-ray (CXR) was unremarkable. His ABG given below:

a. What is the likely cause in this patient?
b. What is called oxygen saturation gap?
c. What is the treatment?

----*XXXX Diagnostics*----		
Blood	***Gas***	***Report***
248	20.36	Jan 05 2024
Patient ID	4318/024	
Measured		*37.0°C*
pH	7.208	
pCO_2	20.4	mm Hg
pO_2	348.2	mm Hg
Na	137	
K	3.9	
Cl	107	
Corrected		*38.6°C*
pH	7.439	
pCO_2	47.6	mm Hg
pO_2	123.5	mm Hg
Calculated data		
HCO_3 (act)	22.1	mmol/L
HCO_3 (std)	20.5	mmol/L
BE	8.6	mmol/L
O_2 CT	14.7	mL/dL
O_2 (sat)	98.3	%
CO_2 (ct)	32.4	mmol/L
pO_2 (A - a)	32.2	mm Hg
pO_2 (a/A)	0.79	
Entered data		
Temperature	38.6	°C
Hb (ct)	10.5	g/dL
FiO_2	100.0	%

Q14. A 30-year-old lady with mechanical mitral valve is brought to the emergency department after 30 minutes of ingestion of 50 tablets and 1 mg of warfarin. The patient is alert and well.

a. What is warfarin's mechanism of action?

b. What are the factors determine risk of bleeding apart from international normalized ratio (INR)?

c. Describe management plan in this patient who requires therapeutic anticoagulation.

Q15. A 23-year-old woman who is 35 weeks pregnant arrives at the emergency department after attempting suicide 2 hours prior by swallowing 50 prenatal iron tablets, which contain 325 mg of ferrous sulfate.

a. Is there any risk of iron toxicity to fetus?
b. Do you recommend chelation in this patient?
c. What are the surrogate markers of severe iron toxicity when serum levels are not available?

ANSWERS

Ans. 1

a. List five of the strongest risk factors for suicide. *SAD PERSONS* (mnemonic):
   - S—Male *S*ex (gender—more females attempt, more males succeed)
   - A—*A*ge <20 or >45
   - D—*D*epression in past history
   - P—*P*revious attempt
   - E—*E*thanol and drug abuse
   - R—*R*ational thinking loss (psychiatric illness)
   - S—*S*ocial supports lacking
   - O—*O*rganized plan
   - N—*N*o spouse, e.g., divorced, widowed, separated, or single
   - S—*S*ickness, chronic medical disease

b. Enumerate three investigations assess for medication toxicity:
   1. *Glucometer/blood glucose:* Altered mental state which may occur if the patient has taken an overdose (OD) of antidiabetic medications
   2. *ECG:* It may show features of sodium channel blockade, TCA ingestion, β-blocker/calcium channel blocker (CCB) ingestion, K high or low
   3. *Serum paracetamol:* Silent toxicity

c. Assesses disposition decision criteria:
   - Understanding by the patient and their social support
   - No longer intoxicated
   - Normal laboratory tests
   - Symptoms of toxicity controlled
   - Follow up confirmed for psychiatrist and/or internist

Ans. 2

a. Features to stratify her as high risk:
   - Dose >300 mg/kg
   - Tachypnea

b. Important investigations:
   - Arterial blood gas (ABG)
   - Salicylate level

c. To avoid intubation factors, need to be taken into account:
   - Avoid acidosis—give sodium bicarbonate prior to intubation
   - Hyperventilate once intubated
   - Avoid long-acting muscle relaxants to monitor for seizure activity

Ans. 3

a. Tricyclic antidepressants are weak bases that function as γ-aminobutyric acid type A (GABA-A) receptor blockers, noradrenaline, and serotonin reuptake inhibitors, and blocks the inactivated fast sodium channels. Blockage of these channels causes cardiotoxic effects and life-threatening dysrhythmias.
b. The important ECG findings suggestive of TCA toxicity are:
   QRS widening (>100 ms) and right axis deviation of the terminal QRS. In combination, these findings are almost pathognomonic of sodium channel blockade:
   - Right axis deviation of the terminal QRS is defined by terminal R wave >3 mm in aVR or R/S ratio >0.7 in aVR
   - QRS widening >100 ms is associated with seizures and >160 ms is associated with cardiac dysrhythmias
c. Sodium bicarbonate is the specific antidote for TCA overdose.

Ans. 4

a. Risk assessment in thyroxine overdose:
   - Mostly patients remain asymptomatic, may be symptomatic if >10 mg thyroxine is ingested, and may remain symptomatic up to 3 weeks. Thyroxine overdose symptoms are largely sympathomimetic and due to adrenergic stimulation.
b. *Utility of thyroid function tests in this patient:* Thyroid function tests are not routinely indicated following thyroxine overdose. Although elevated thyroxine levels are expected, they have little clinical correlation and do not alter management.
c. Symptomatic patient of thyroxin overdose (sympathomimetic features) may be treated with propranolol 10–40 mg q6h PO for symptomatic relief. If β-blockers are contraindicated, an alternative is diltiazem 60–180 mg q8h PO.

Ans. 5

a. *ECG findings:* Sinus bradycardia with a rate of about 45 beats/min, prolonged PR interval of 240 ms indicative of first-degree atrioventricular (AV) block
b. Difference between β-blocker overdose and calcium channel blocker overdose:
   - There are two key features that may help differentiate a calcium channel blocker overdose from a β-blocker overdose: (1) blood glucose and (2) level of consciousness.

- Calcium channel blocker overdoses tend to cause hyperglycemia, compared to a normal-to-low blood glucose in β-blocker overdoses.
- Beta-blocker overdoses tend to cause a depressed level of consciousness, and calcium channel blocker overdoses, a normal level of consciousness.

c. Management of cardiac arrest in this patient:
   - Cardiac arrest due to drug overdose and toxicity should be approached differently from cardiac arrest of other causes.
   - Sudden ventricular arrhythmias (i.e., pulseless VT) or progressive cardiogenic shock presenting as bradycardic pulseless electrical activity (PEA) are the main cause of cardiac arrest.
   - Cardiac arrest may occur in propranolol overdose
   - Good quality CPR is an important lifesaving measure. In the poisoned heart, cardioversion/defibrillation is unlikely to be successful. Avoid amiodarone.
   - Give boluses of IV sodium bicarbonate 1–2 mEq/kg every 1–2 minutes until return of perfusing rhythm.
   - Intubate and hyperventilate
   - Give adrenaline 1 mg every 3–5 minutes as per standard cardiac arrest algorithms
   - *Avoid amiodarone:* It will only make things worse.
   - Consider Intralipid

Ans. 6

a. Ethylene glycol is found in radiator coolants and antifreeze in concentrations 20–98%, deicing solutions, solvents, and brake fluids
b. *Clinical course of severe ethylene glycol toxicity:* This state of alcohol intoxication occurs within 1–2 hours and is characterized by euphoria, nystagmus, drowsiness, nausea, and vomiting. The patient has a high osmolar gap. Over the next 12 hours, the alcohol is metabolized into its toxic metabolites. As the high osmolar gap resolves, HAGMA (high anion gap metabolic acidosis) and hypocalcemia occur, with clinical manifestations that include dyspnea, tachypnea, tachycardia, hypertension, shock, coma, tetany, seizures, and death. Renal failure is heralded by flank pain and oliguria. Late-occurring cranial neuropathies may also occur about 5–20 days postingestion in survivors.
c. Investigations may be useful in suspected ethylene glycol toxicity.
   - Blood gas
   - Serum osmolarity
   - Hypocalcemia and evidence of renal impairment is highly suggestive of ethylene glycol toxicity.
   - Ethanol levels
   - Serum ethylene glycol levels

- *Urinalysis:* Oxalic acid crystals are pathognomonic for ethylene glycol poisoning, and para-amino hippuric crystals may also be seen. Urine fluorescence under a Wood's lamp may also be detected if the radiator coolant contained fluorescein.

Ans. 7

a. Clinical presentation of a patient with mushroom toxicity:
   - Severe gastroenteritis causing hypovolemic shock
   - Seizures or coma
   - Cholinergic crisis
   - Complications of organ failure (e.g., hepatic toxicity and renal toxicity)

b. Treatment options for mushroom toxicity:
   - *Decontamination:* Activated charcoal 50 g (1 g/kg in children) if onset of gastrointestinal (GI) symptoms occurs >6 hours postingestion. Consider multidose activated charcoal if suspected cyclopeptide hepatotoxicity as α-amanitin undergoes enterohepatic circulation
   - *Antidotes:*
     - *Cyclopeptide hepatotoxicity (e.g., GI symptoms onset >6 hours or increasing transaminases):* N-acetylcysteine Penicillin 1 MU/kg/day
     - *Cholinergic syndrome:* Atropine
     - *Seizures due to Gyromitra mushrooms:* Pyridoxine (similar management to isoniazid toxicity)

c. Potentially life-threatening complications of mushroom poisoning:
   - Hepatic encephalopathy
   - Acute kidney injury
   - Respiratory failure
   - Status epilepticus
   - Coma

Ans. 8

a. Initial approach to after accidental ingestion of watch battery:
   - Respiratory status and airway assessment in any suspected foreign body ingestion including pulse oximetry readings when indicated. Baby should remain in the upright position and NPO.
   - To locate the foreign body, radiographs from the nasopharynx to the anus, both anteroposterior and lateral, should be taken.

b. Complications of batteries ingestion may occur including electrical discharge, tissue damage, pressure necrosis, obstruction, and leakage of battery contents. Esophageal obstruction, esophageal perforation, and aspiration. Mercury batteries may pose a particular hazard if they break.

c. *Therapy indicated:* This battery requires emergent removal because of its location in the esophagus. Endoscopy is the removal method of choice.

Ans. 9

a. Clinical features of an ACE inhibitor overdose are hypotension, diarrhea, glomerulopathy, hyperkalemia, cough, rash, angioedema, and drug fever.
b. The hypotension should be managed with intravenous (IV) fluids and vasopressors.
c. Antidote:
   - In the presence of profound vasoplegic shock secondary to ACE inhibitor overdose, naloxone may be used to overcome the excess vasodepressor activity of endogenous opioids.
   - Long-acting vasopressin analog terlipressin is effective in treating refractory hypotension.

Ans. 10

a. Toxic side effects of methotrexate medication use include GI (nausea, vomiting, intestinal bleeding, stomatitis, mucositis, esophagitis), hematologic (leukopenia, anemia, and thrombocytopenia), hepatic (transaminitis, cirrhosis, and hyperbilirubinemia), pulmonary (acute lung injury), neurologic (hemiparesis, seizures, dysreflexia, encephalopathy, and coma), and renal (acute tubular necrosis).
b. Interventions in methotrexate toxicity therapy have three main goals: (1) clearance of methotrexate from the bloodstream, (2) folinic acid therapy, and (3) organ treatment.
c. Antidote for methotrexate toxicity:
   - Leucovorin is a metabolically functional folic acid and can bypass the antifolate effects of methotrexate. It should be used IV within 1 hour and the dose should equal or be greater than the dose of methotrexate. If methotrexate dose is unknown then can give 75 mg or 10 mg/m^2/dose in children. Then 12 mg is repeated every 6 hours for 4 doses.
   - To guide therapy, methotrexate levels can be obtained.
   - Use sodium bicarbonate and fluids to prevent nephrotoxicity.
   - Activated charcoal can be used within 1 hour of ingestion if patient is protecting their airway.

Ans. 11

a. *Whipple's triad:* Whipple triad is defined as (1) hypoglycemia symptoms, (2) hypoglycemia (blood glucose levels <55 mg/dL), and (3) relief of symptoms after ingesting glucose.
b. Role of thiamine in the treatment of hypoglycemia:
   - It is customary to deliver thiamine IV at a dose of 100 mg before giving the patient with altered mental status a glucose bolus. This is due to the concern that, in the absence of thiamine treatment, the glucose load could trigger or aggravate Wernicke's encephalopathy.

- Nevertheless, Wernicke's encephalopathy does not seem to be brought on by a single glucose bolus, though it can be brought on by prolonged carbohydrate administration (e.g., from total parenteral nutrition) without thiamine supplementation.

c. *Mechanism of octreotide:* Octreotide is a long-acting somatostatin analog works by inhibiting insulin secretion from the pancreas thus preventing persistent hypoglycemia.

Ans. 12

a. Interventions are indicated for olanzapine overdose:
   - Limit drug exposure
   - Prolonged normal resuscitation
   - Consider lipid emulsion administration
   - Prevention of acidosis

b. Method to administer Intralipid:
   - Lipid emulsion (20% Intralipid)—
   - 1 mL/kg bolus (over 1 minute) and start infusion 0.25 mL/kg/min. Continue CPR to distribute and repeat bolus every 3 minutes up to 3 mL/kg total dose until circulation restored. If hemodynamically unstable increase the infusion rate to 0.5 mL/kg/min. Maximum total dose—8 mL/kg

c. Adverse effects of Intralipid:
   - Interference with laboratory assays (e.g., Intralipid may cause spurious biochemistry results)
   - Interference with other therapies (e.g., Intralipid may decrease the effectiveness of lipid-soluble therapeutic agents)
   - It can theoretically result in hyperlipidemia, pulmonary injury, hepatosplenomegaly, thrombocytopenia, hyperlipidemia-induced pancreatitis, and fat embolism.
   - It lowers blood oxygen content, increases shunting, and causes pulmonary vasoconstriction
   - It can cause clogging of lipid molecules in the dialysis filters.

Ans. 13

a. *Likely cause of clinical presentation in this patient:* Acquired methemoglobinemia secondary to dapsone.

b. *Oxygen saturation gap:* The "oxygen saturation gap" is the difference between the calculated oxygen saturation from a standard blood gas machine and the reading from a pulse oximeter. If it is >5%, the patient's hemoglobin may be abnormal, representing carbon monoxide poisoning, methemoglobinemia, or sulfhemoglobinemia.

c. Management of this condition:
   - Stop causative agent—activated charcoal

- High-flow oxygen
- Methylene blue 1–2 mg/kg IV slow push over 5 minutes, expect significant clinical improvement within 10–60 minutes. Repeat dose of methylene blue between 30 and 60 minutes if still symptomatic.
- Methylene blue is itself an oxidant at doses >7 mg/kg and thus may cause methemoglobinemia in susceptible patients; hence, careful administration is essential.
- IV ascorbic acid has been used for methemoglobinemia when methylene blue is unavailable or contraindicated, such as in pregnant patients or those with G6PD deficiency.
- Exchange transfusion
- Hyperbaric oxygen treatment
- Cimetidine can be used in dapsone-induced methemoglobinemia to prevent further formation of its metabolite.
- IV hydration with dextrose 5% in water (D5W) is often effective.
- The nicotinamide adenine dinucleotide phosphate oxidase (NADPH)-dependent methemoglobin reductase enzyme system requires glucose for the clearance of methemoglobin.

Ans. 14

a. *Mechanism of action of warfarin:* Warfarin results in anticoagulation by inhibiting vitamin K metabolism, which depletes the reduced form of vitamin K needed for the synthesis of clotting factors (factors II, VII, IX, X, as well as proteins C and S).
b. Determining risk of bleeding (apart from INR):
   - In patients with warfarin poisoning or therapeutic overanticoagulation, the management is not solely dependent on the INR. If the patient is not actively bleeding but has an INR >5, we need to determine if the patient has low or high bleeding risk to decide on appropriate therapy.
   - *High risk of bleeding is considered in the presence of any of these factors:* Major surgery within the previous 2 weeks. Thrombocytopenia, antiplatelet drugs (e.g., aspirin and clopidogrel), and active GI disease (e.g., inflammatory bowel disease and peptic ulcer disease)
c. Management plan in the patient who requires therapeutic anticoagulation:
   - Vitamin K should only be given if the INR is sufficiently elevated and the bleeding risk is sufficiently high.
   - If INR 5–9 and bleeding risk is low, monitor INR, no vitamin K required; if bleeding risk is high, monitor INR, administer 0.5—1 mg vitamin K IV.
   - If INR >9 and bleeding risk is low, monitor INR, administer 1 mg vitamin K IV; if bleeding risk is high, monitor INR, administer 1 mg vitamin K IV, consider the administration of fresh frozen plasma (FFP).

Ans. 15

a. No, because the placenta has an active mechanism for iron to cross. It occurs by active endocytosis. So, if the mother has high iron levels, it is rare for the fetus to develop elevated iron levels.

b. Deferoxamine chelation therapy is an option for severe iron toxicity. The indications, duration, and end-points of therapy are controversial.
   - Indicated if serum level >90 µmol/L at 4–6 hours postingestion, presence of systemic toxicity and shock—metabolic acidosis and altered mental status
   - *Administers as infusion under cardiac monitoring:* Initial infusion rate of 15 mg/kg/hour, reduced if hypotension occurs, may be titrated up to 40 mg/kg/hour in severe toxicity
   - The infusion can be stopped when the patient is clinically stable and the serum iron level is <60 µmol/L. Ferrioxamine is excreted unchanged in the urine, which classically turns in rose color.
   - If the patient remains symptomatic with elevated iron levels, treatment should continue even if there is no urine color change after the first dose.

c. Serum glucose >150, WBC >15,000, and acidosis all suggest a serum iron concentration >300 µg/dL and used as surrogate markers of severe iron toxicity when serum levels are not available.

20 CHAPTER Trauma: Part I OSCE

Sanjay Shah

QUESTIONS

Q1. **A 21-year-old male presents to the emergency department having sustained a human bite injury to his hand from a punch, while involved in a brawl outside the pub 2 hours ago. On examination, he has superficial bite marks over the index and middle fingers on metacarpophalangeal joints. A hand X-ray shows no associated fractures. There is no associated tendon injury.**

a. Which are the indications to prescribe oral antibiotics for wound?
b. Which bite wounds are allowed to be healed without formal closure?
c. What is recommended choice of antibiotic for this patient?

Q2. **A 26-year-old gymnast is brought to the emergency department after falling awkwardly during practice and injuring her left knee. She is unable to bear weight and having pain. She is holding the left knee in flexed position. An X-ray is shown below:**

a. What is the diagnosis?
b. Which injuries are most dangerous due to this?
c. Explain the Ottawa knee rule.

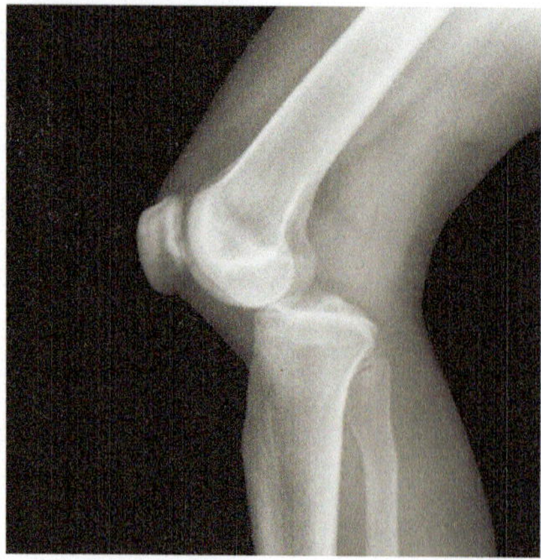

Q3. A 24-year-old racing driver is brought to the emergency department following a high-speed crash. A trauma computed tomography (CT) from head to pelvis shows a fractured cervical vertebra. On examination, he has weakness of the right side of his body with upgoing plantars, loss of pain, and temperature sensation in his left limbs, with normal fine-touch sensation over all four limbs.

a. This clinical picture is most likely seen in a lesion of which tract and of which side?
b. Narrate down incomplete lesions of spinal cord.

Q4. A 76-year-old man coming to the emergency department complained of knee pain after falling forward while in church.

a. What is diagnosis of this patient?
b. Write down mechanism of injury.
c. Write the management of this patient.
d. Give the definitions of *patella alta* and *patella baja*.

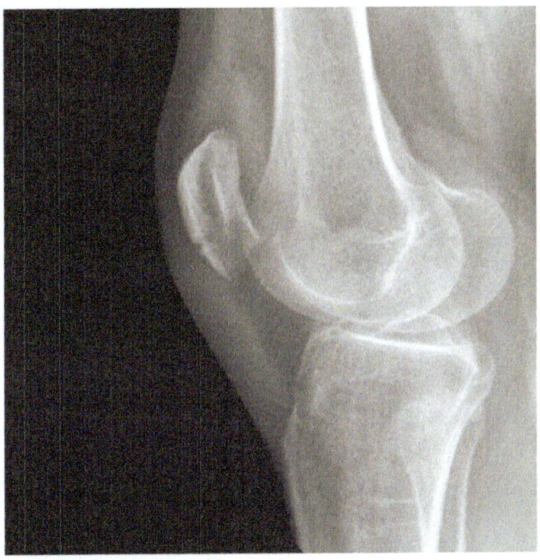

Q5. A 31-year-old man complaining of a severe pain in the lower right calf came to emergency department. He tells you that the pain started suddenly while playing badminton game. On examination, there is swelling and tenderness over the lower leg and plantar flexion is weaker on the right compared to the left.

a. Write down the diagnosis and diagnostic test for this patient.
b. Mentioned high-risk condition for this injury.
c. What is the mortise of the ankle and normal value for it?

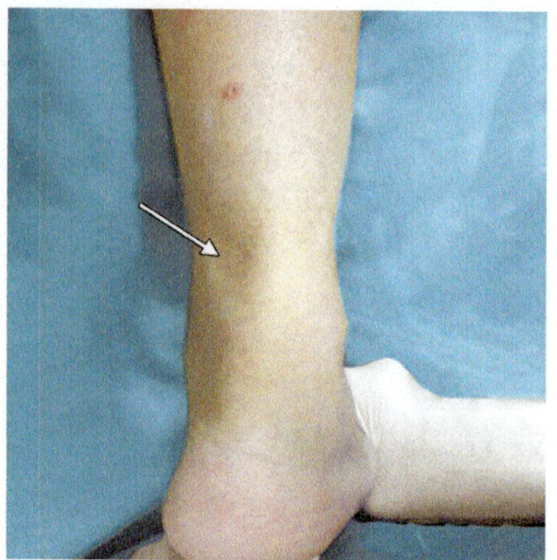

Q6. **A 13-year-old boy is brought to the emergency department by his father after developing left ankle pain following a tackle in a football match. An X-ray is done showing:**

a. Using the Salter-Harris classification, how would you classify this injury?
b. Write down Salter-Harris classification.
c. What is the complication of type V Salter-Harris?

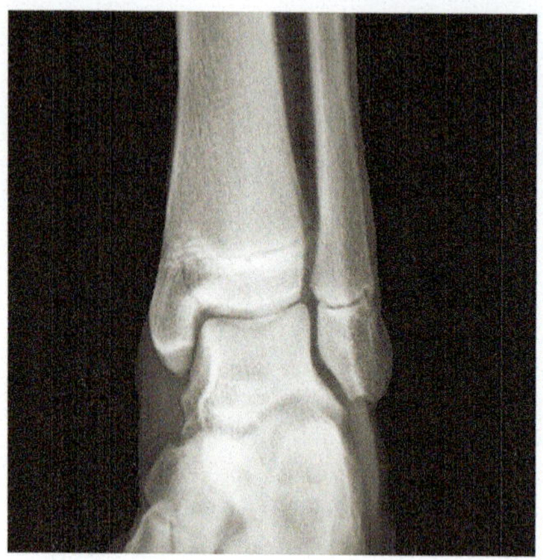

Q7. **A 36-year-old man presented to emergency department after being assaulted in a nearby park. He tells the triage nurse that he was kicked in the chest multiple times. He is complaining of chest pain and shortness of breath. His observations are recorded as follows:**

- ***Heart rate:*** **121 beats/min**
- ***Blood pressure:*** **132/89 mm Hg**

- ***Respiratory rate*: 25 breaths/min; a portable chest X-ray is arranged**

a. What is the single best diagnosis?
b. What does the chest X-ray show?
c. Enumerate pathophysiology for this injury.
d. Write the clinical features and management of this injury.

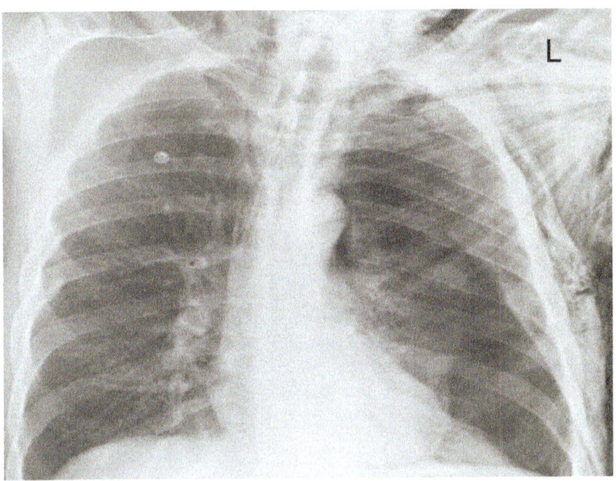

Q8. You are assessing a 36-year-old man came to emergency department who has been assaulted. Image is shown below.

a. What is the diagnosis?
b. Enumerate other clinical signs of it.
c. What are the contributors to secondary brain injury?
d. Write four suggested targets of goal-directed therapy for brain injury.

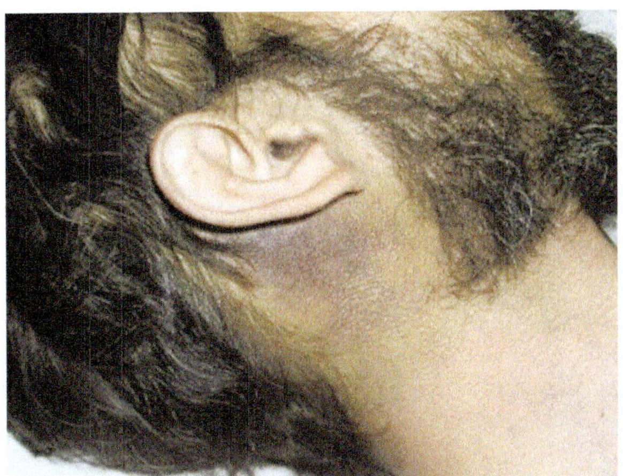

Q9. A 23-year-old man presents to the emergency department after fall down from his bicycle. He is complaining of pain in the right shoulder and is holding his right arm flexed at the elbow and close to his body. On examination, you notice a severe restriction in range of movement in all planes due to pain and a loss of the deltoid curve. X-ray shows below:

a. What is the diagnosis?
b. Write the clinical features of it.
c. Write the complications of it.
d. Write various methods for reduction.

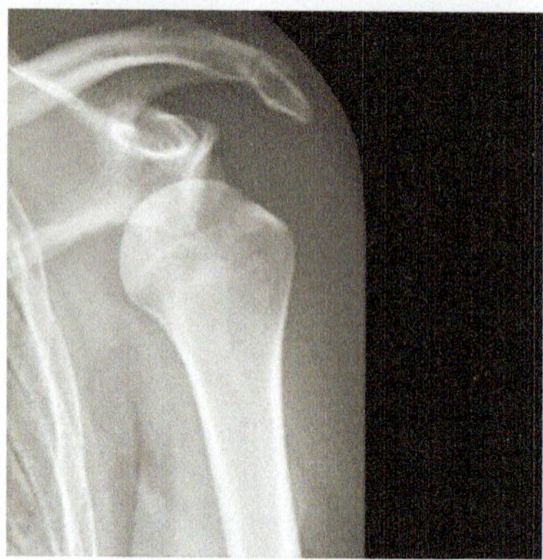

Q10. A 45-year-old female presents to the emergency department complaining of a painful right middle finger. She sustained a puncture wound to the palmar surface of the finger 5 days ago while gardening.

a. What is the diagnosis and mechanism of injury?
b. What is Kanavel's sign?
c. What is the management for this?

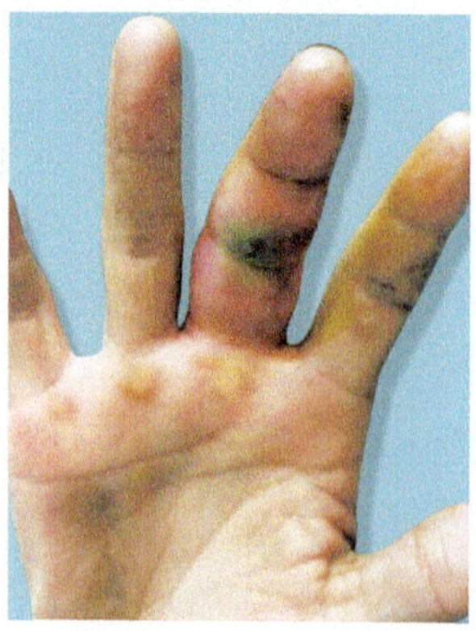

Q11. A 25-year-old rock climber presents to the emergency department complaining of pain in the right wrist following a fall. An X-ray is arranged.

a. What is the diagnosis and mechanism of action of this injury?
b. Mention about the examination and complication of this injury.
c. Enumerate borders and contents of anatomical snuffbox.

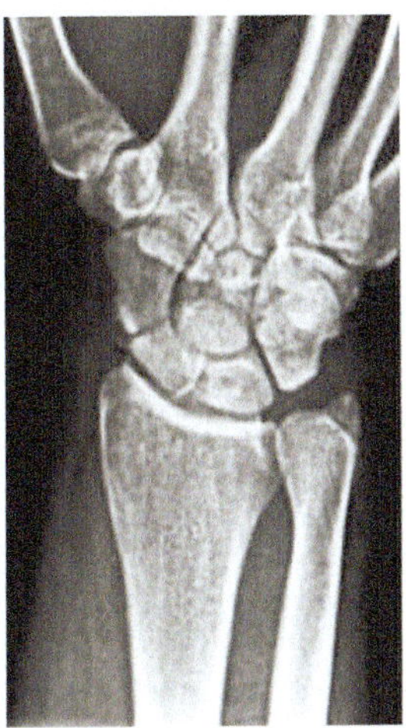

Q12. An 18-year-old boy presents to the emergency department with a burn injury on his left upper limb and chest. He was trying to light a bonfire using petrol when it flashed back over his hand and arm. The triage nurse thinks he has a deep partial-thickness burn.

a. What is the rule of 9?
b. What is the percentage of burns in this patient?
c. Write down the formula which is useful for the fluid resuscitation.
d. Enumerate the possible clinical findings of burn surface in this patient.
e. Enumerate complications of burn.

Q13. In a case of fall on an outstretched hand with injury over right elbow:

a. Which sign is seen in X-ray of elbow?
b. By this X-ray, which fracture would you suspect in case of adult and pediatric patient?
c. What is the most dangerous complication of this injury?
d. Narrate the appearance of elbow ossification center as per the age.

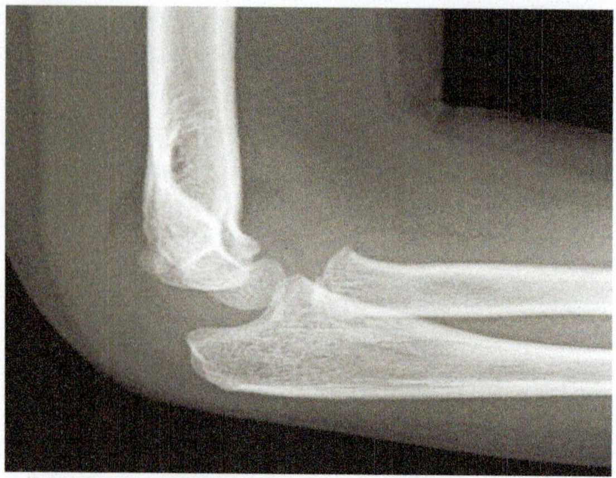

Q14. A 69-year-old woman presents to the emergency department after she had fall in a supermarket. She is able to give a clear history of tripping on a "wet floor sign". She is complaining of pain in the left wrist.

a. What is the diagnosis and what is the name of this deformity?
b. Enumerate complications of this injury.
c. Difference between Smith fracture and Colles' fracture.
d. Which nerve is involved in carpal tunnel syndrome?

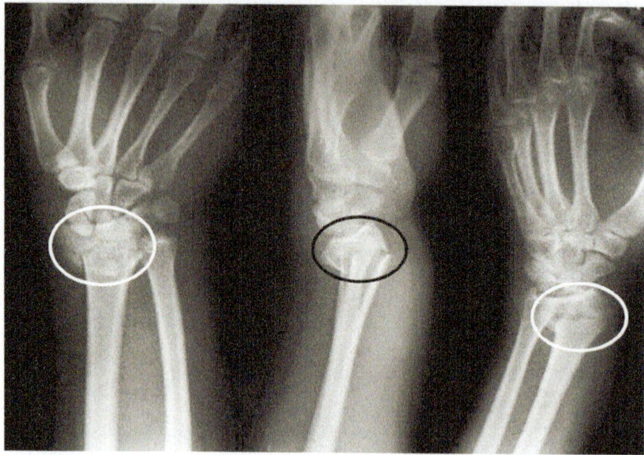

Q15. A 24-year-old female presented with history of road traffic accident. She is anxious with sustained injury over lower abdomen and her chest X-ray is normal. Pelvis X-ray is shown below. Her FAST (focused assessment with sonography in trauma) is positive for suprapubic (Douglas pouch).

a. Which injury is seen in this case?

b. Which procedure can be useful to control excessive hemorrhage in emergency department (even after external pelvic binder) before definitive management can be available?
c. Describe anatomic zones of that device placement.
d. Which zone can be avoided for this device placement and why?

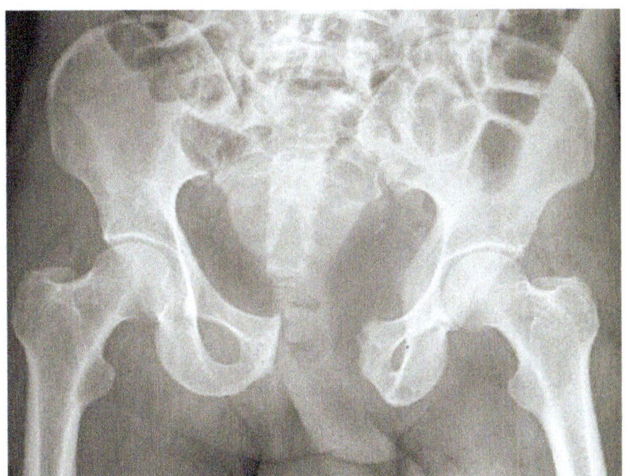

Q16. A 45-year-old woman is brought to the emergency department after slipping on an icy path. She has no significant past medical history. She complains of pain in her left ankle.

a. What is the diagnosis?
b. What are the examination clues in this patient?
c. How will you manage this patient?

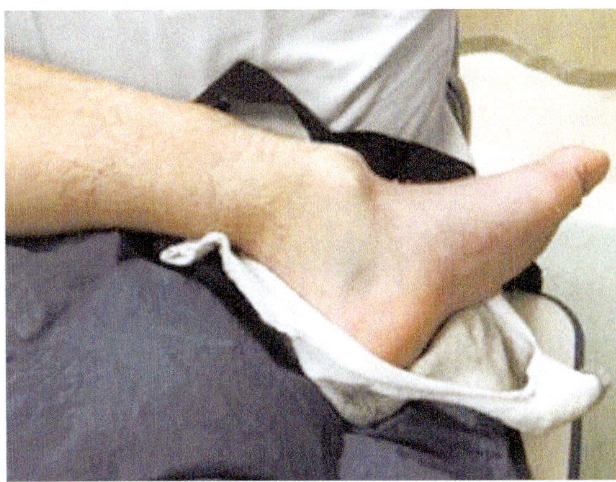

Q17. A 79-year-old man, taking aspirin for vascular disease, is brought to the emergency department with decreased consciousness after falling at home. He opens his eyes when you ask, localizes to pain,

and is using inappropriate words. His daughter accompanies him and tells you that he has fallen over a few times recently but is refusing more help or support at home. He drinks alcohol daily.

a. Which injury is shown here and describe cause of it?
b. Define Cushing reflex.
c. Formula to calculate cerebral perfusion pressure (CPP) and normal range of CPP and intracranial pressure (ICP).
d. How will you manage this patient?

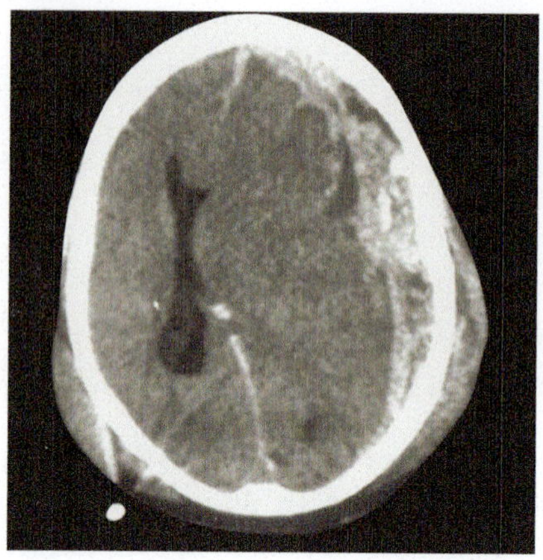

Q18. A 38-year-old female suffered from domestic violence. She has multiple bruises over face and both upper limb. Her X-ray paranasal sinuses (PNS) are shown below:

a. What is your diagnosis and what is the name of this sign?
b. Enumerate X-ray findings.
c. Which muscle is most likely to be involved?

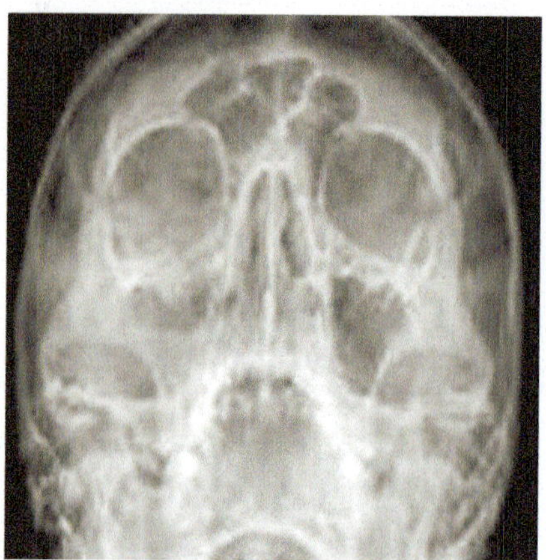

Q19. **A 24-year-old female presented with suicidal attempt of hanging, she is in drowsy state and her CT brain and CT cervical spine is normal. She has ligature mark around the neck.**

a. Enumerate hard and soft signs of neck injury for her.
b. Comment upon no-zone targeted diagnostic workup.
c. Explain laryngeal injury grading scale.
d. Give difference between adult and pediatric airway.

Q20. **An 18-year-old man presents to the emergency department after falling over some steps leaving a nightclub. The image shown below.**

a. How would you classify this injury?
b. Draw a labeled diagram of tooth anatomy.
c. Which are the transport media for avulsed tooth?

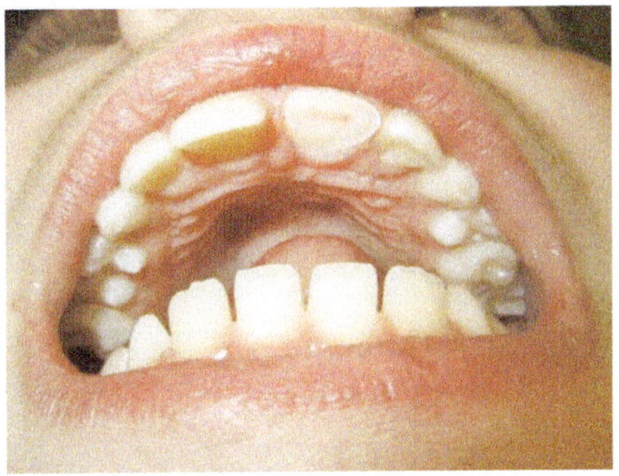

Q21. **A mother brings in her 9-month-old boy with bruising and swelling around his left leg. The child is in obvious discomfort and is crying incessantly. An X-ray of his right lower leg is shown below.**

a. What is the diagnosis?
b. Write radiological findings that should raise suspicion of nonaccidental injury (NAI).
c. Risk factors for NAI.

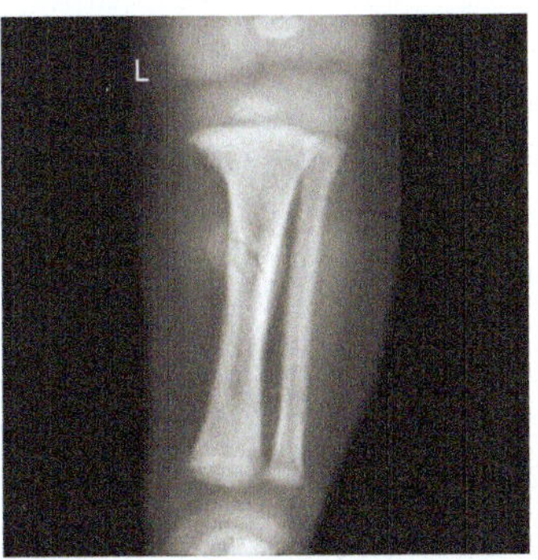

Q22. A 23-year-old medical student presents limping with an injury to his left knee that occurred during a tackle. He tells you that he heard a "pop" when it happened, and he is unable to bear weight due to pain.

a. Which fracture is seen here?
b. Which ligament is most commonly involved in this injury?
c. Which are the diagnostic test to evaluate ligamentous and menisci injury?
d. What is O Donoghue's unhappy triad of knee?

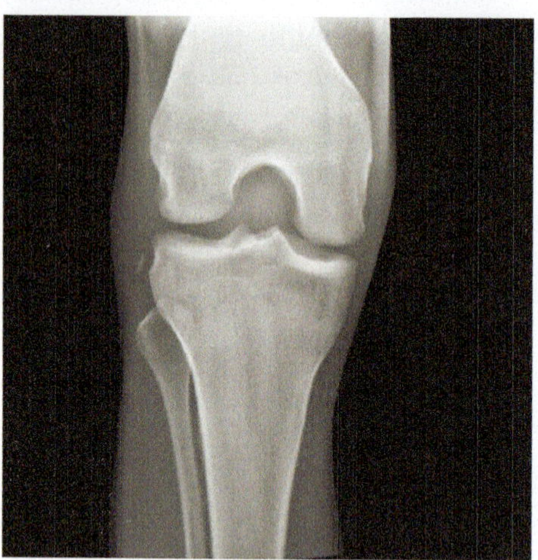

ANSWERS

Ans. 1

a. The indications are all human bite wounds under 72 hours old, even if there is no sign of infection; all cat bites; animal bites to the hand, foot, face, and genitalia; puncture or crush wounds; wounds requiring surgical debridement; wounds involving bones, joints, tendons, ligaments, or suspected fractures; bites on limbs with impaired circulation; wounds that have undergone primary closure; people who are at risk of serious wound infection (i.e., diabetic, cirrhotic, asplenic, immunocompromised, or at extremes of age); patient with a prosthetic valve or joint; and patient with delayed presentation (>8 hours but <24–48 hours).
b. Bite wounds over 24 hours old, infected bite wounds, deep puncture wounds, crush injuries, heavy contamination, and uncertain adequacy of debridement.
c. For both prophylaxis and treatment of an infected human, dog, or cat bite, prescribe amoxycillin with clavulanic acid for 7 days. For people who

are allergic to penicillin, prescribe metronidazole plus clarithromycin or clindamycin for 7 days.

Ans. 2

a. Knee dislocation
b. Although rare, this injury indicates severe disruption of the ligamentous structures and soft tissues of the knee. Look carefully for associated injuries (e.g., femur or lower limb), and document status of distal pulses and sensation—the popliteal artery or nerve are often injured.
c. Obtain X-rays if there is suspected fracture or other significant injury. Ottawa knee rule helps in making the decision about requirement of X-ray (aged between 18 and 55 years). X-rays are only required if any of the following are present:
    - Isolated bony tenderness of the patella
    - Bony tenderness over the fibula head
    - Patient cannot flex the knee to 90°
    - Patient unable to bear weight both immediately after the injury and at the time of examination

Ans. 3

a. Lateral column, right side
b. Incomplete lesions of spinal cord are as follows:
    - *Brown-Séquard syndrome:* Hemitransaction, e.g., penetrating trauma or unilateral compression of the cord, all tracts on one side ipsilateral hemiparesis, ipsilateral loss of proprioception/vibration/fine-touch sensation, contralateral loss of crude touch/pain/temperature sensation, bilateral motor loss, varying degrees of sensory loss, greater loss in upper limbs than lower limbs, and greater loss of motor function than sensory function.
    - *Central cord syndrome:* Hyperextension injury of cervical spine in patient with preexisting cervical stenosis, e.g., forward fall with facial impact in elderly patient (can occur even without cervical spine fracture/dislocation), corticospinal tract and spinothalamic tract, bilateral motor loss, bilateral loss of crude touch/pain/temperature sensation, and cerebellar dysfunction.
    - *Anterior cord syndrome:* Occlusion of anterior spinal artery with infarction of anterior cord by direct anterior cord compression, flexion injuries of the cervical spine, or thrombosis of anterior spinal artery corticospinal, spinothalamic, and spinocerebellar tracts.
    - *Posterior cord syndrome:* Penetrating trauma to the back or hyperextension injury associated with vertebral arch fractures (very rarely occurs in isolation), dorsal column and bilateral loss of proprioception/vibration/light-touch sensation.

Ans. 4

a. Patella fracture
b. This may follow a direct blow or fall onto the patella or sudden violent knee flexion or contraction of the quadriceps muscle.
c. Treat vertical fractures with analgesia; immobilize in a nonweight-bearing above-knee plaster of Paris (POP) back slab; supply crutches, and arrange orthopedic follow-up. Due to the pull of the quadriceps, transverse fractures tend to displace. Treat with analgesia and immobilization in a POP back slab, and refer to the orthopedic team for probable open reduction internal fixation (ORIF) (occasionally, the orthopedic team may treat an un displaced transverse fracture conservatively).
d. *Patella alta, or a high-riding patella,* means position of the patella is considered high. It may be idiopathic or secondary to a patellar tendon rupture. Congenital patella baja refers to a patella distal in relationship to the femoral trochlea and present since an early age. Acquired patella baja may occur secondary to distal positioning of the patella relative to the femoral trochlea or shortening of the patellar tendon, as a result of trauma or surgery.

Ans. 5

a. *Achilles tendon rupture calf squeeze test (Simmonds/Thompson's test):* Kneel the patient on a chair, facing the back, with the feet hanging free over the edge. Alternatively, position the patient to lie prone on a trolley, with the ankles over the end. Gently squeeze mid-calf, and look for normal plantar flexion of the ankle.
b. Patients on ciprofloxacin/fluoroquinolones or oral steroids or those with a history of steroid injection of the Achilles tendon area are at increased risk.
c. The ankle joint is a hinged synovial joint that is formed by the articulation of the talus, tibia, and fibula bones. Together, the three borders form the ankle mortise. The superior portion of the ankle joint forms from the inferior articular surface of the tibia and the superior margin of the talus. 5.49 ± 2.87° in the coronal position and 13.68 ± 6.62° in the sagittal position. This is the normal ankle-bearing negative line of gravity.

Ans. 6

a. Type III Salter–Harris classification
b. Salter–Harris classification
    - Type I (5–7%); fracture plane passes all the way through the growth plate, not involving the bone
    - Type II (~75%); fracture plane passes across most of the growth plate and up through the metaphysis

- Type III (7–10%); fracture plane passes some distance along the growth plate and down through the epiphysis
- Type IV (10%); fracture plane passes directly through the metaphysis, growth plate, and down through the epiphysis
- Type V (<1%); crushing type injury does not displace the growth plate but damages it by direct compression

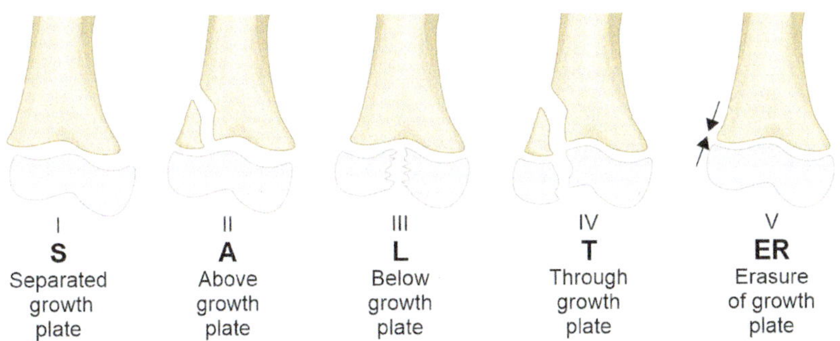

c. Type V fractures are notoriously difficult to diagnose and often complicated by premature fusion.

Ans. 7

a. Tension pneumothorax left side
b. Chest X-ray shows left 2nd–6th rib fracture, tension pneumothorax left side, and left chest subcutaneous emphysema.
c. The most common cause of tension pneumothorax is mechanical positive-pressure ventilation in patients with visceral pleural injury. A simple pneumothorax following penetrating or blunt chest trauma can also complicate to tension pneumothorax (parenchymal lung injury fails to seal), or after attempted subclavian or internal jugular venous catheter insertion. Occasionally, traumatic defects in the chest wall cause a tension pneumothorax when occlusive dressings are secured on four sides or the defect itself constitutes a flap-valve mechanism. Rarely, tension pneumothorax occurs from markedly displaced thoracic spine fractures.
d. The clinical features include chest pain, air hunger, tachypnea, respiratory distress, tachycardia, hypotension, tracheal deviation away from the side of the injury, unilateral absence of breath sounds, unilateral hyperresonant note on percussion, elevated hemithorax without respiratory movement, neck vein distention, and cyanosis (late manifestation).

   Primary management—needle thoracostomy and definitive management—tube thoracostomy.

Ans. 8

a. Basal skull fracture

b. The other clinical signs include periorbital ecchymosis (Raccoon eyes), retroauricular ecchymosis (Battle's sign), cerebrospinal fluid (CSF) leakage from the nose (rhinorrhea) or ear (otorrhea), dysfunction of cranial nerves VII and VIII (facial paralysis and hearing loss), hemotympanum, or bleeding from the ear subconjunctival hemorrhage (with no posterior border seen).

c. The most important contributors to secondary brain injury are cerebral edema, expanding hematoma, hypoxia, and hypotension, seizure, hypoglycemia, hypo- or hypernatremia.

d. Goal-directed therapy-suggested targets

Pulse oximetry ≥90%	CPP ≥60 mm Hg	Serum sodium 135–140 mEq/L
SBP ≥90 mm Hg	ICP <20 mm Hg	INR ≤1.4
MAP ≥80 mm Hg	$PbtO_2$ ≥15 mm Hg	Platelet >75 × 10^3
$PaCO_2$ 35–45 mm Hg	pH 7.35–7.45	Hemoglobin >8 g/dL
Temperature 36°C–38°C	Glucose 8–180 mg/dL	

(CPP: cerebral perfusion pressure; ICP: intracranial pressure; MAP: mean arterial pressure; INR: international normalized ratio; $PaCO_2$: partial pressure of arterial carbon dioxide; $PbtO_2$: brain tissue oxygen tension; SBP: systolic blood pressure)

Ans. 9

a. Anterior shoulder dislocation

b. Patients often present supporting the affected arm with the uninjured arm. Flat shoulder deformity (loss of normal rounded appearance of shoulder). Step-off deformity at the acromion with a palpable gap below the acromion. Humeral head palpable anteroinferior to the glenoid. Evidence of complications.

c. Nerve damage - axillary, radial, brachial plexus vascular damage - axillary artery, associated fracture, e.g., humeral head, greater tuberosity, clavicle, acromion Recurrent shoulder dislocation Rotator cuff injury Hill-Sachs lesion (posterolateral humeral head compression fracture) Bankart lesion (avulsion of the anteroinferior glenoid labrum at its attachment to the anteroinferior glenohumeral ligament complex).

d. External rotation method Modified Kocher's method Modified Milch method.

Ans. 10

a. Diagnosis is pyogenic flexor tenosynovitis. The infection of a finger flexor tendon sheath may follow a penetrating injury.

b. Tenderness over the flexor tendon, symmetrical swelling of the finger, finger held in flexion at rest, and extreme pain on passive extension are features of Kanavel's sign.
c. Consider tetanus prophylaxis; refer urgently for exploration, irrigation, drainage, and intravenous (IV) antibiotics.

Ans. 11

a. Diagnosis is scaphoid fracture and mechanism of action of injury is fall onto an outstretched hand.
b. Examine for tenderness over anatomical snuffbox, tenderness over palmar aspect of scaphoid tubercle, scaphoid pain on compressing the thumb longitudinally (telescoping), scaphoid pain on gentle flexion, and ulnar deviation of the wrist. Complications are nonunion, delayed union, malunion, avascular necrosis, and secondary osteoarthritis.
c. *Anatomical snuffbox borders:*
   - *Ulnar border:* Tendon of the extensor pollicis longus
   - *Radial border:* Tendon of the abductor pollicis longus and extensor pollicis brevis
   - *Proximal border:* Styloid process of the radius
   - *Distal border:* Base of thumb metacarpal floor—carpal bones; scaphoid and trapezium
   - *Roof:* Skin

   Anatomical snuffbox contents:
   - Radial artery
   - Branch of the radial nerve
   - Cephalic vein

Ans. 12

a. Upper limb—9%, head—9%, lower limb—18%, anterior trunk—18%, posterior trunk—18%, groin—1%
b. 18% body surface area (BSA)
c. *Parkland formula:* Fluids required for the first 24 hours = (4 mL) × (patient's weight in kilogram) × (%TBSA burned). Half of the fluid is given over the first 8 hours of burn injury. The second half is given over the remaining 16 hours.
d. Deep partial thickness extends into deep (reticular) dermis; skin is drier, less painful, potentially blistered, red or mottled in appearance, and does not blanch on touch.
e. *Early complications* of burn include respiratory distress (smoke inhalation or a circumferential chest burn), poisoning from inhalation of noxious gases released by burning fluid loss, hypotension, and hypovolemic shock, hypothermia (epidermal damage may lead to problems with thermoregulation), wound infection, and sepsis, toxic shock syndrome (complication of infection caused by *Staphylococcus aureus*), cardiac arrhythmias (electrical shock or electrolyte disturbance),

vascular insufficiency, distal ischemia, or compartment syndrome (from circumferential burn of limb or digit), acute kidney injury (from rhabdomyolysis), limb loss, and death. *Late complications* include wound infection, chronic neuropathic pain, itch, scarring contractures, and psychosocial impact.

Ans. 13

a. Anterior and posterior fat pad sign
b. For adult—radial head fracture; for children—supracondylar fracture of humerus
c. Brachial artery damage
d. *Appearance of elbow ossification centers (CRITOE):* Capitulum: 1-year, radial head: 3 years, internal (medial) epicondyle: 5 years, trochlea: 7 years, olecranon: 9 years, external (lateral) epicondyle: 11 years.

Ans. 14

a. Colles's fracture—dinner fork deformity
b. The complications of this injury are stiffness of wrist and adjacent limb joints, malunion, and cosmetic problems, reflex sympathetic dystrophy (Sudeck's atrophy), carpal tunnel syndrome, and extensor pollicis longus rupture.
c. *Smith fracture* is an unstable distal radius fracture sometimes referred to as a "reverse Colles' fracture" where the distal fragment is impacted, tilted to point anteriorly, and often displaced anteriorly. It usually follows a fall onto a flexed wrist. *Colles' fracture* affects the radius within 2.5 cm of the wrist, such that the distal fragment is angulated to point dorsally. It usually results from a fall onto an outstretched hand.
d. Median nerve

Ans. 15

a. Pubic symphysis diastasis (open book pelvic fracture)
b. REBOA (resuscitative endovascular balloon occlusion of aorta) placement
c. Zone 1—From left subclavian artery above the diaphragm to celiac trunk; zone 2—extends from the diaphragm (celiac trunk) to the lowest renal artery; zone 3—below the level of the renal arteries to aortic bifurcation, including severe pelvic, groin, or proximal lower extremity hemorrhage; the balloon may be inflated within zone 3.
d. Zone 2 extends from the diaphragm to the lowest renal artery and is generally avoided due to the presence of the visceral arteries. Both zone 1 and zone 2 to be deployed for <45 minutes to avoid acute renal ischemia.

Ans. 16

a. Ankle dislocation
b. Examination shows gross deformity of the ankle, severe stretching of the skin (resulting in blisters, ankle fracture, ankle dislocation, skin necrosis, or even converting the injury to a compound fracture), and often associated with deficit in peripheral pulses or sensation.
c. Prompt closed reduction and immobilization in POP usually have to precede X-ray (unless available immediately). Give IV analgesia/ sedation, as needed, with full precautions. Warn that there may be a brief increase in discomfort as the ankle reduces. With the knee flexed and supported, gently grasp the heel with one hand and support the patient's calf with the other. Apply traction smoothly on the heel. Return of normal ankle contours, relief of skin tension, and often dramatic relief of pain suggest successful traction. Once reduced, recheck pulses and sensation, immobilize in a POP slab, and arrange check X-rays. Urgent referral to the orthopedic team is to be done.

Ans. 17

a. Subdural hematoma left fronto-temporoparietal region with mass effect and midline shift due to rupture of bridging veins.
b. The Cushing reflex is a physiological nervous system response to acute elevation of ICP, resulting in Cushing's triad of widened pulse pressure (increasing systolic, decreasing diastolic), bradycardia, and irregular respiration.
c. Formula to calculate: CPP = MAP (mean arterial pressure) – ICP. Normal range of ICP is 7–15 mm Hg; normal range of CPP is 60–80 mm Hg.
d. Management is by ABCD (airway, breathing, circulation, disability) approach. Early intubation to avoid hypoxia and aspiration; prevent increase in ICP and treat it with euvolemia (avoid hypotension) injection 3% hypertonic saline or mannitol, injection antiepileptic; goal-directed therapy early neurosurgical intervention.

Ans. 18

a. Orbital floor fracture—tear drop sign
b. Blowout fracture over left side in Water's view with tear drop sign with fluid seen in left maxillary sinus (hemosinus)
c. Inferior rectus muscle

Ans. 19

a. Hard and soft sign of neck injury and soft sign of neck injury

Hard signs	*Soft signs*
• Airway compromise • Expanding and pulsatile hematoma • Active, brisk bleeding • Hemorrhagic shock • Hematemesis • Neurologic deficit • Massive subcutaneous emphysema • Air bubbling through wound	• Hemoptysis • Oropharyngeal blood • Dyspnea • Dysphagia • Dysphonia • Nonexpanding hematoma • Chest tube air leak • Subcutaneous or mediastinal air • Vascular bruit or thrill crepitus

b. No-zone targeted diagnostic workup

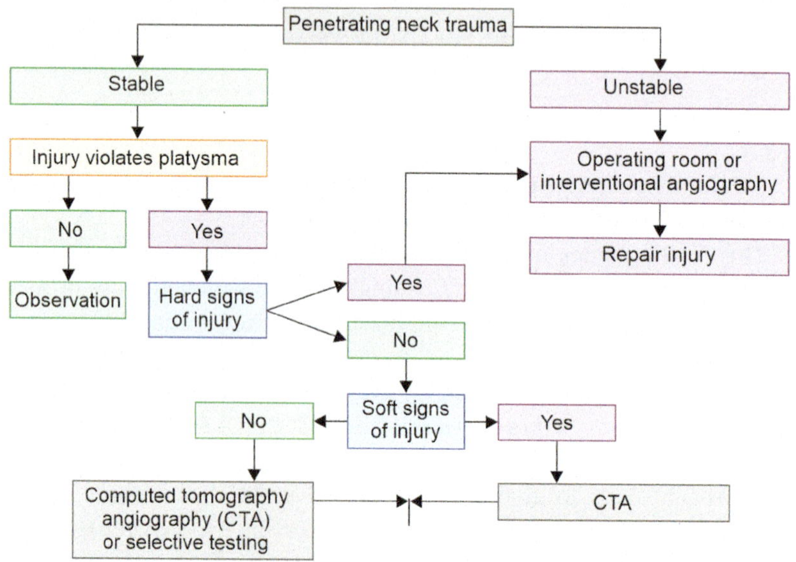

c. *Laryngeal injury grading scale:*

- Grade I—minor endolaryngeal hematoma without detectable fracture
- Grade II—edema hematoma minor mucosal disruption without exposed cartilage nondisplaced fracture
- Grade III—massive edema exposed cartilage vocal fold immobility displaced fracture
- Grade IV—grade III with two or more fracture lines or massive trauma to laryngeal mucosa
- Grade V—complete laryngotracheal separation

d. Difference between adult and pediatric airway

Anatomy/physiology	***Pediatric***	***Adult***
Head and neck	Larger head to body ration	Smaller head to body ratio
Mandibles	Relatively immobile	Mobile
Tongue	Larger with respect to oral cavity	Smaller with respect to oral cavity
Larynx	Higher and anterior	Lower and posterior
Epiglottis	Long, stiff, U-shaped	Shorter, floppy, V-shaped
Narrowest point	Level of cricoid cartilage	Glottic opening
Trachea	Length 4–5 cm, diameter 4 mm funnel-shaped	Length 10–16 cm, diameter 20–25 cm straight tubular-shaped
Respiratory Physiology	Diaphragm dependent lack of "bucket handle"	Diaphragm and "bucket handle" effect of ribs

Ans. 20

a. Complicated crown fracture
b. Diagram of tooth anatomy

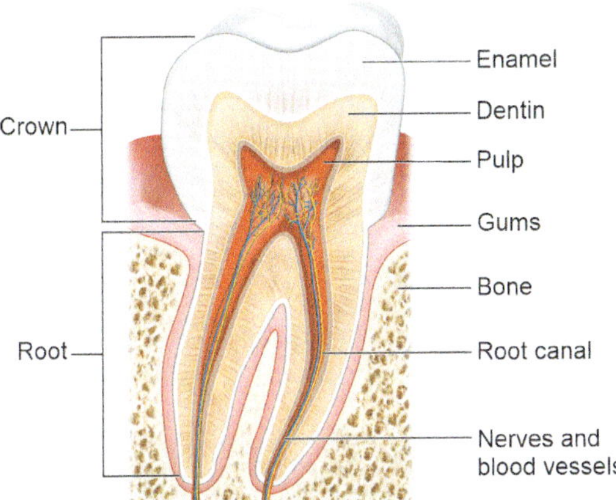

c. The tooth should be held in a physiologically acceptable medium (saline or saliva or milk) before reimplantation within 30 minutes.

Ans. 21

a. *Greenstick fracture of tibia:* This X-ray shows a spiral fracture of the right tibial shaft with subperiosteal new bone formation. The most likely cause of this presentation is NAI.
b. Radiological findings that should raise suspicion of NAI include multiple fractures of different ages, rib and spinal fractures, fractures in children

who are not independently mobile, long bone fractures in children <3 years old; Salter-Harris I and II fractures of knee, wrist, elbow, and ankle (shaking injuries); occipital skull bone fracture; multiple, wide, or comminuted skull fracture.

c. Risk factors for NAI include previous history of child abuse in the family, history of domestic violence, mental illness or disability in the caretaker, drug or alcohol misuse in the caretaker, housing or financial problems, disability in the child, and single parent, especially if immature or unsupported.

Ans. 22

a. *Segond fracture:* This is highly suggestive of complex knee injury, an anterior cruciate ligament (ACL) rupture, and avulsion type fracture of the lateral proximal tibia at the attachment of the anterolateral ligament.
b. ACL
c. *Diagnostic tests:*
    - ACL—anterior drawer test, Lachman test, pivot shift test
    - Posterior cruciate ligament (PCL)—posterior drawer test
    - Menisci injury—McMurray test, Apley grind or compression test
    - Medial collateral ligament/lateral collateral ligament (MCL/LCL)—valgus/varus stress test
d. O'Donoghue's unhappy triad of knee tear of three ligaments of knee joint, which is crucial MCL, ACL, and medial menisci.

Pediatric Trauma: Part II OSCE

Awaneesh Katiyar

QUESTIONS

Q1. Refer to the image and answer the following:

a. What is the name of the tape?

b. Where it is used?

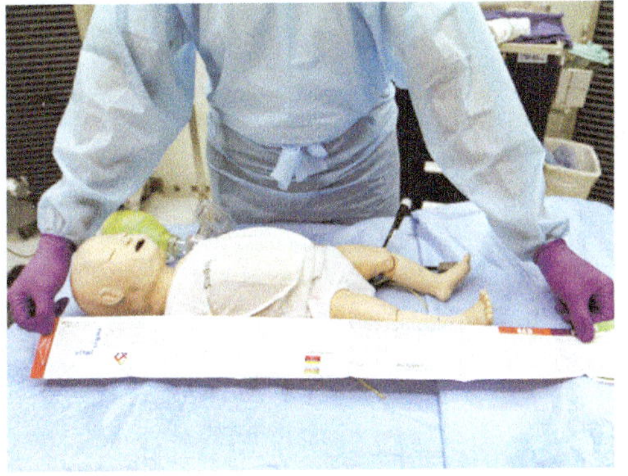

Q2. A 2-year-old child was brought to emergency by their parents after road traffic injury. On arrival, the baby was having pulse rate of 136 beats/min, blood pressure (BP) 68/46 mm Hg, and peripheral oxygen saturation (SpO_2) 86 at room air and was arousable.

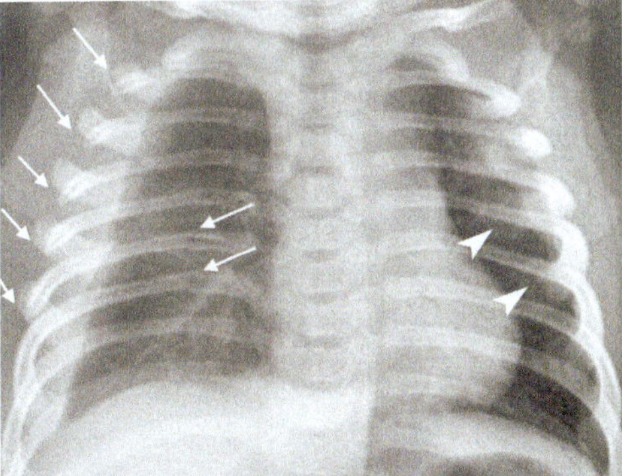

a. What is your diagnosis?

b. What is the management of diagnosis?

Q3. A 5-year-old child fell from 18 feet on hard surface (concrete). At presentation, pulse rate 120 beats/min, BP 90/60 mm Hg, respiratory rate (RR) 24 breaths/min, and SpO_2 98% at room air, Glasgow coma scale (GCS) 12/15. On examination, the patient was having 5 cm lacerated wound over right temporoparietal area.

a. What is your diagnosis?
b. What will be the immediate management protocol in an emergency?
c. What will be the definitive management?

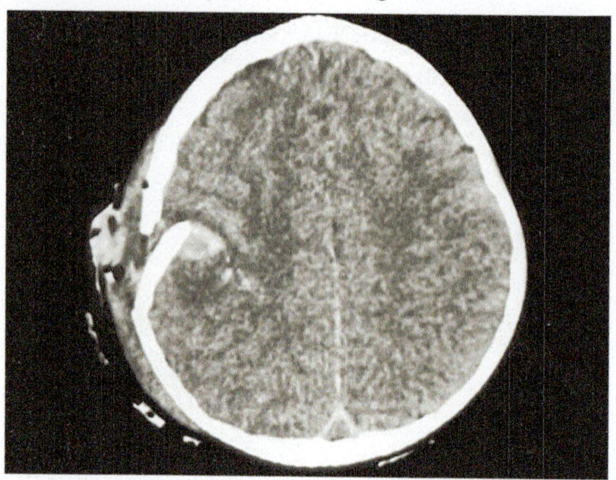

Q4. A 3-year-old child was hit by a wooden stick on head. At presentation, pulse rate 110 beats/min, BP 90/60 mm Hg, RR 20 breaths/min, and SpO_2 98% at room air, and GCS 6/15. No external injury is noted.

a. What is your diagnosis?
b. What will be the immediate management of the patient?
c. What will be the definitive management?

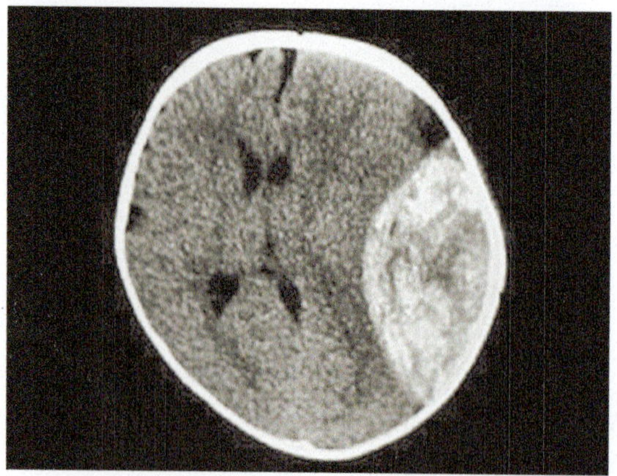

Q5. A 12-year-old child fell from bike and sustained injury to the abdomen. At presentation, pulse rate 134 beats/min, systolic blood pressure (SBP) 60 mm Hg, RR 28 breaths/min, and SpO_2 96% at room air, eye opening noted on localizing pain and patient is confused, A 2 × 3 cm superficial abrasion is noted at right upper abdomen. Abdomen is tender on examination and eFAST (extended focused assessment with sonography in trauma) shows moderate free collection in hepatorenal and perisplenic area.

a. What will be the initial management protocol?
b. What will be the fluid of choice?
c. What will be the next investigation?

Q6. A 15-year-old having blunt trauma abdomen presented in emergency with grade 3 hemorrhagic shock. Computed tomography (CT) shows grade 3 liver injury.

a. How much fluid should be given?
b. What will be the blood product of choice in this patient?
c. What is balanced resuscitation?
d. What is the most crucial parameter to monitor in this patient during resuscitation to see better perfusion?

Q7. A 14-year-old having blunt trauma abdomen, presented in emergency with pulse rate 130 beats/min, SBP 65 mm Hg, peripheral pulse not palpable on arrival, and eFAST positive for abdomen. Warm Ringer's lactate was given with rate of 20 mL/kg, but patient was not responding to the fluid. Balanced resuscitation started but BP was not rising, diagnostic peritoneal lavage (DPL) shows frank blood.

a. What will be the next step?
b. What is the most common solid organ injured in abdomen after blunt trauma?

Q8. A 15-year-old boy sustained blunt trauma after a car crash. He was wearing a lap belt. On presentation, he was having pain in abdomen, primary survey is normal, and no external injury is noted. eFAST shows mild collection in hepatorenal pouch.

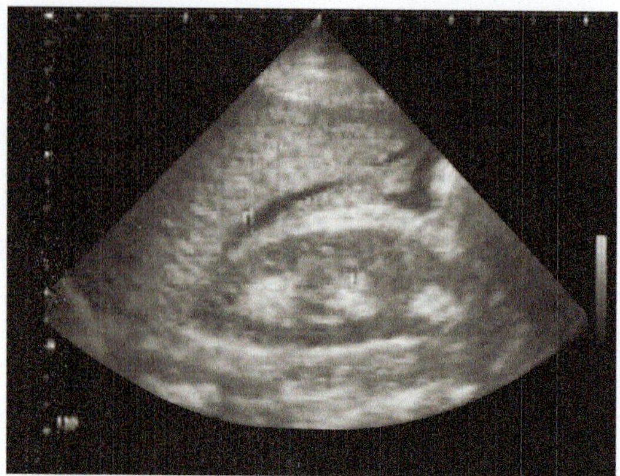

a. What is the most common injury that occurs due to a lap belt?
b. What will be the next step of management?

Q9. A 7-year-old child fell from height (18 feet). At presentation, pulse rate 120 beats/min, BP 92/60 mm Hg, RR 18 breaths/min, and SpO_2 98% at room air. The child was opening eyes on painful stimuli, was restless and agitated, and showing normal flexion on pain.

a. What is the GCS of the child?
b. What is the next investigation of choice?

Q10. A 10-month-old male baby who fell from height of 12 ft was crying and active, with right raccoon eye present.
On arrival pulse rate was 98 beats/min, BP 100/60 mm Hg, SpO_2 96% on 2 L of oxygen. There was no history of seizure and loss of consciousness.

a. According to PECARN (Pediatric Emergency Care Applied Research Network), should CT be indicated or not?
b. What are the CT findings?
c. What will be the management protocol?

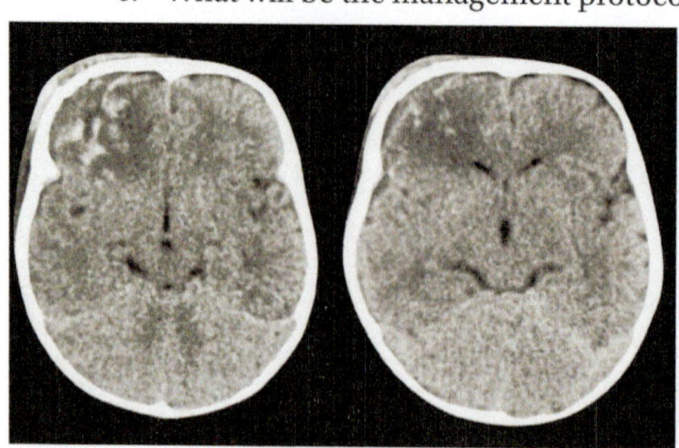

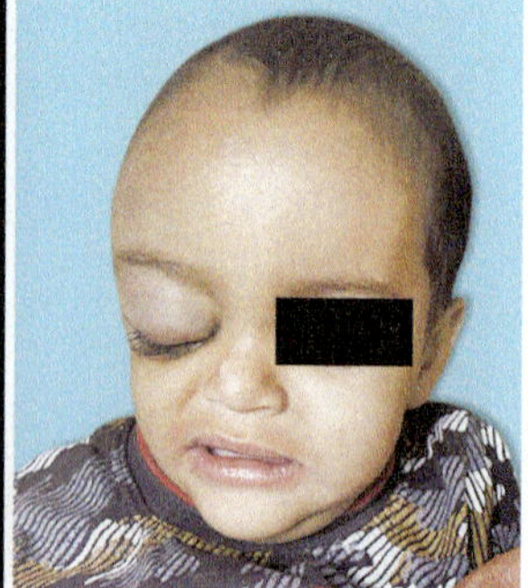

Q11. A 3-year-old child was having blunt trauma abdomen, with clinical features of peripheral shock.

a. What is the fluid of choice?
b. What is the full form of eFAST?
c. How many areas are examined?

Q12. A 7-year-old child sustained whiplash injury showing quadriparesis.

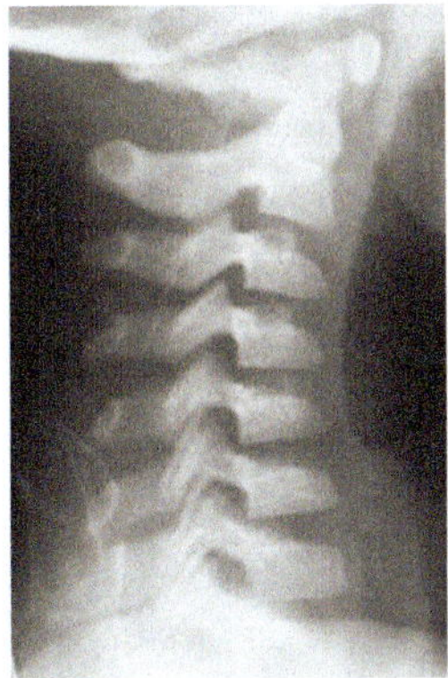

a. What abnormality is seen in the cervical spine X-ray?
b. What is this condition called?
c. What is the level of spine most commonly involved?

Q13. A 12-year-old child who sustained blunt trauma was having pain in abdomen, was in the shock, and no distal pulse is palpable. No external injury is noted. eFAST shows collection in the abdominal cavity. Veins are not visible. Intraosseous (IO) cannula is secured.

a. What are the sites of intravenous (IV) cannula?
b. What are the complications of IO cannula?

Q14. PECARN head CT rule widely utilized to choose whether CT is needed or not, to reduce X-ray exposure of radiation in children.

a. What is the predictability of fatal cancer in children who underwent CT?
b. What is ALARA?

Q15. A 2-year-old baby sustained blunt trauma chest. Chest X-rays show no fracture of the ribs, but pneumothorax is seen on the right side of the chest. Baby is breathless and saturation is 70% at room air and 90% on 4 L/min oxygen.

a. What is the management of choice?
b. Why rib fractures are not common in children?
c. What is the management of choice for tension pneumothorax?

ANSWERS

Ans. 1

a. Broselow® Pediatric Emergency Tape
b. Emergency (for quick pediatric drug dosing and size analysis)

Ans. 2

a. Right hemothorax
b. Right intercostal chest tube placement

Ans. 3

a. Depressed skull fracture with underlying contusion
b. ABCDE (airway, breathing, circulation, disability, exposure) protocol
c. Immediate decompression and elevation of bone

Ans. 4

a. Extradural hematoma (EDH)
b. ABCDE—primary survey
c. Decompression and evacuation of EDH

Ans. 5

a. Follow ABCDE protocol
b. Warm Ringer's Lactate
c. Contrast-enhanced CT of abdomen

Ans. 6

a. 20 mL/kg warm Ringer's lactate
b. Packed red blood cells (PRBC) with rate of 10–20 mL/kg
c. *PRBC:* Fresh frozen plasma (FFP): Platelets—1:1:1
d. Urine output

Ans. 7

a. Exploratory laparotomy
b. Liver

Ans. 8

a. Mesenteric injury
b. Exploratory laparotomy

Ans. 9

a. E2V2M3
b. Noncontrast CT (NCCT) head

Ans. 10

a. Yes
b. Right frontal contusions with edema
c. Conservative treatment—Mannitol and antiepileptics

Ans. 11

a. Warm Ringer's lactate
b. Extended focused assessment with sonography in trauma
c. Pericardial cavity, hepatorenal space, splenorenal space, perivesical space, and bilateral pleural cavity

Ans. 12

a. Normal
b. SCIWORA (spinal cord injury without radiological abnormality)
c. Occiput or C3

Ans. 13

a. Proximal and distal tibia
b. Early complication—leakage of fluid; late complication—osteomyelitis

Ans. 14

a. 1:1000
b. ALARA refers to as low as reasonably achievable

Ans. 15

a. Warm Ringer's lactate
b. Children are more elastic and malleable
c. Decompression of chest

Environmental Emergencies OSCE

Olita Shilpakar

Q1. **A 40-year-old tourist who went for hiking was brought to the emergency room (ER) in an unresponsive state with the alleged history of drowning in a lake in the cold winter. On examination, he had no pulse or breathing.**

a. List the different stages of hypothermia.
b. Mention the important points to be considered while you perform cardiopulmonary resuscitation (CPR) in a hypothermic patient.
c. What is the electrocardiogram (ECG) finding in a hypothermic patient?

Q2. **A 65-year-old man suddenly develops one episode of generalized tonic–clonic seizure (GTCS) while standing in a line for the bus in the scorching heat of summer. On examination, after regaining consciousness, his skin is dry and red and he is confused. He has been taking medications for a heart condition.**

a. What is your diagnosis?
b. What are the risk factors for this condition?
c. How will you manage this condition?

Q3. **A 35-year-old male is brought to the emergency department with the complaint of sharp pain over the joints and more severe pain in the bilateral shoulders. He gives history of underwater diving a day back.**

a. What is your provisional diagnosis?
b. What are the clinical manifestations of this condition?
c. What is the definitive management of this disease?

Q4. **A 10-year-old boy fell into a lake and was rescued within 10 minutes of drowning. The child was brought to the ER and was responsive to pain only. On examination, he had crepitations in all the lung fields and was in shock.**

a. Discuss the pathophysiology of drowning.
b. What is the prehospital care management of drowning?
c. What is your management and disposition plan for this patient?

Q5. A 35-year-old tourist while hiking in the mountains developed mild headache at 2,800 m. At 3,000 m he complained of having difficulty to walk, since he seemed to lose balance and was feeling dizzy. His friends then noticed him talking irrelevantly following which he was unresponsive.

a. What is your diagnosis?
b. List the important high-altitude illnesses.
c. What could be the differential diagnoses in this case?
d. Discuss the management of this case.

Q6. A 30-year-old female gives history of hiking trip to the Himalayan region. She ascended rapidly to an altitude of 3,800 m (12,467 ft) within a couple of days. After reaching this elevation, she began experiencing symptoms such as severe shortness of breath (SOB), persistent cough, and fatigue.

a. What is your diagnosis?
b. What could be the computed tomography (CT) chest findings in high-altitude pulmonary edema (HAPE)?
c. Discuss the management.

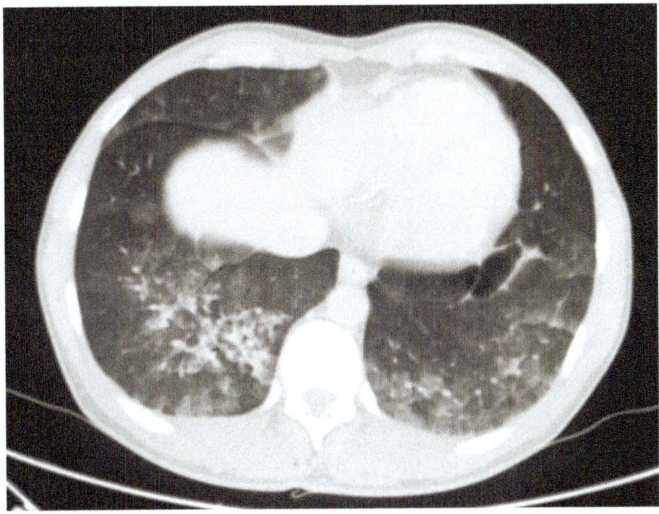

Q7. An electrician gives alleged history of being thrown away while mending wires of a high-tension electricity pole. He has second-degree burns in bilateral upper limbs and complains of pain.

a. Discuss fluid and pain management in this patient.
b. What are the factors determining the magnitude of such injuries?
c. List the complications of electrical injuries.

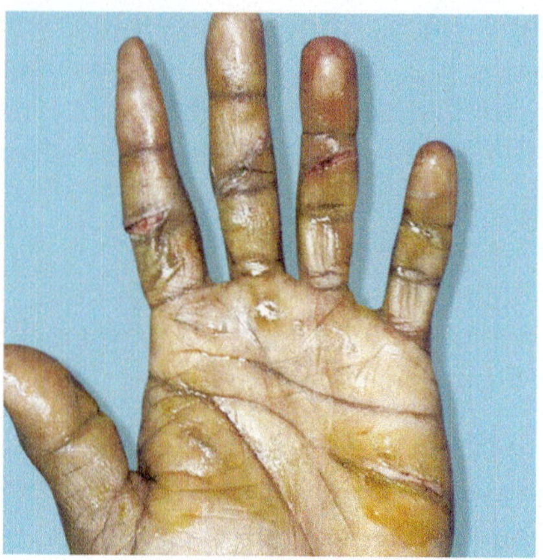

Courtesy: Dr Gaurav B Shetty

Q8. **A 35-year-old farmer was struck by lightning and was unresponsive. He was immediately brought to the ER. On examination, he had a fine branching rash resembling the branches of a tree over his back as shown in the image.**

a. What is your diagnosis?
b. What are the clinical features of this condition?
c. How will you manage this case?

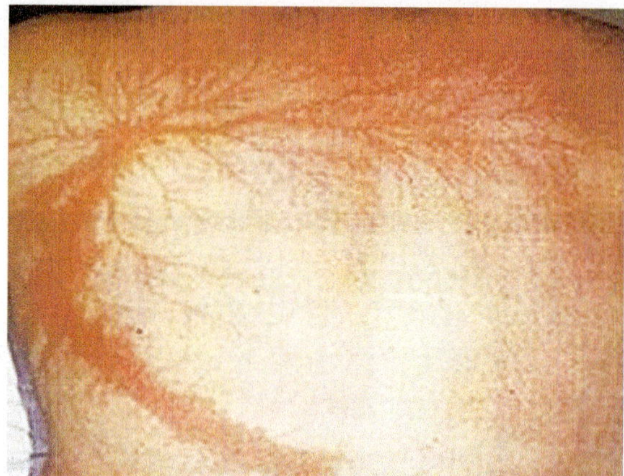

Q9. **A 25-year-old female is bitten by a snake on the right ankle while collecting firewood in the forest. She was rushed to a nearby hospital where she suddenly started having SOB, ptosis, profuse sweating, and developed one episode of GTCS.**

a. What kind of snake could have been the culprit in this case?
b. List the clinical features suggestive of this type of snakebite.
c. What is the specific treatment for this condition?

Q10. A 30-year-old man was bitten by a snake on his hand 3 hours back and presented to the emergency department with fluid filled hemorrhagic blisters. His investigations show a prothrombin time of >60 seconds and INR of >5.

a. Mention the type of snakebite in this case.
b. How will you perform 20WBCT (20-minute whole blood clotting test)?
c. Discuss in brief the prehospital management in this patient.

Q11. A 38-year-old female is brought to the emergency with the history of being stung by a dozen wasps 4 days back over the face and the upper limbs. She was taken to a local health center where she received some medications to relieve her pain, however, she complained of decreased urine output which was concentrated dark in color. Her arterial blood gas (ABG) revealed severe metabolic acidosis.

a. What are the complications of wasp sting?
b. Mention the pathophysiology of wasp sting.
c. Outline the management of this case.

Q12. A 25-year-old female presented to the ER with the complaint of being stung by a jellyfish 1 hour back.

a. What are the important features of jellyfish sting?
b. Discuss the management in brief.

Q13. A 40-year-old male has been working in construction sites as a worker since the past few years. He gives history of SOB and dry cough on and off since the past 6 months, which is progressively increasing to such an extent that it is getting difficult to continue his daily work now. He presented to the ER with increased SOB followed by fever. On examination, he has clubbing of his fingers and his echo revealed pulmonary artery hypertension.

a. What is your provisional diagnosis?
b. What are the symptoms and signs of asbestosis?

Q14. A 30-year-old male presented to the ER with the alleged history of being stung by a scorpion 2 hours back. He is complaining of sudden onset of SOB which is worsening. He is agitated and feeling intense pain at the sting site.

a. Mention the classification and clinical consequences of scorpion sting.
b. What could be the chest X-ray findings in scorpion sting in this case?
c. Discuss in brief the management of scorpion sting.

Q15. A person works in a laboratory where he has to deal with body fluid samples and chemicals. The X-ray room is right next to the laboratory. He keeps getting unwell frequently since the time he joined work.

What could be the potential health hazards in this case?

ANSWERS

Ans. 1

a. *Different stages of hypothermia:*
   - *Stage 1:* Clear consciousness with shivering: 35°–32°C
   - *Stage 2:* Impaired consciousness without shivering: 32°–28°C
   - *Stage 3:* Unconsciousness: 28°–24°C
   - *Stage 4:* Apparent death: 24°–13.7°C
   - *Stage 5:* Death due to irreversible hypothermia: <13.7°C

b. *CPR in a hypothermic patient:*
   - Rewarming should start prehospital.
   - Extended CPR should be performed since hypothermic patients can have excellent outcomes despite long hours of CPR. Brief pauses in CPR patients have been revived, because hypothermia protects the brain from injury.
   - Transport to an extracorporeal membrane oxygenation (ECMO) center may be beneficial.
   - Medications may fail to be metabolized and accumulate so avoid repeated doses of medications.
   - Defibrillation may not be successful until the patient is rewarmed. Thus, serial shocks for VT/VF (ventricular tachycardia/ventricular fibrillation) arrest are unlikely to add benefit. As the patient rewarms, further attempts may be made at defibrillation.

c. *ECG finding in a hypothermic patient:* Bradyarrhythmia J waves also known as Osborne waves prolonged PR, QRS, and QT intervals, shivering artifact, and ventricular ectopic.

Ans. 2

a. Heat stroke
b. Risk factors for heat stroke condition are age >65 or <15 years, cognitive impairment, cardiac or pulmonary comorbidities, obesity, drugs, and excess physical activity in high temperature.
c. *Management heat stroke:* Maintain airway, breathing, circulation (ABC) with strict hemodynamic monitoring. Rapid mechanical cooling with resuscitative measures, if necessary, should be considered. The body temperature must be lowered quickly for which the patient needs to

be moved to a cool area and the clothing should be removed. Active cooling methods should be considered which include immersion in cold water, hyperthermia vest, cold compresses to the body, and use of fan or dehumidifying air conditioning unit to bring the core temperature down. Aggressive ice water immersion is the gold standard for life-threatening heat stroke.

Ans. 3

a. Decompression illness
b. *Clinical manifestations of decompression illness:*
    - *Skin:* Itching, rashes, mottling
    - *Lymphatics:* Lymphedema, localized pain
    - *Musculoskeletal:* Periarticular pain, muscular pain
    - *Respiratory:* Dyspnea, tachypnea, frothy sputum, cough
    - *Central nervous system (CNS):* Headache, dizziness, visual loss, ataxia, nausea, vomiting, confusion, visual field defect, focal neurological deficits
    - *Spinal cord:* Back pain, numbness, paresthesia, urinary retention, loss of anal tone, loss of deep tendon reflexes
c. *Definitive management of this decompression illness:* Hyperbaric oxygen therapy is the definitive management of decompression illness. Recompression therapy in a hyperbaric chamber reduces the volume of bubbles. It also improves the delivery of oxygen to ischemic tissues and blood vessel permeability, thus reducing tissue edema.

Ans. 4

a. *Pathophysiology of drowning:* Drowning begins with a period of panic, loss of the normal breathing pattern, breath-holding, air hunger, and struggling to stay above the water. Reflex inspiratory efforts occur which lead to aspiration of water, laryngospasm, and coughing when water contacts the lower respiratory tract. Hypoxemia followed by loss of consciousness and apnea develops and within minutes. Cardiac arrest occurs from hypoxemia and is preceded by bradycardia and pulseless electrical activity.
b. *Prehospital care management of drowning:* Rescue and immediate resuscitation by bystanders and emergency medical personnel improves the outcome of drowning victims. The need for CPR is determined as soon as possible without compromising the safety of the rescuer or delaying the removal of the victim from the water. In a patient with cardiac arrest due to drowning, bystander CPR improves outcomes compared with no CPR; conventional CPR with rescue breaths is preferable.
    - Check for pulses
    - Begin chest compressions

- Automated external defibrillator (AED) when available and appropriate
- Manage the airway
- Keep the victim warm
- Cervical spine immobilization is not routinely needed

c. *Management and disposition plan for drowning patient:* Advanced airway management with orotracheal intubation and mechanical ventilation with positive end-expiratory pressure (PEEP) should be done. Administration of crystalloids followed by vasopressors should also be started to manage shock. The patient should then be disposed in the intensive care unit for close hemodynamic monitoring.

Ans. 5

a. HACE (high-altitude cerebral edema)

b. *Important high-altitude illnesses:* AMS (acute mountain sickness), HACE, HAPE (high-altitude pulmonary edema)

c. Acute psychosis, brain tumor, carbon monoxide poisoning, CNS infection, cerebrovascular bleed or infarct, cerebrovascular spasm, diabetic ketoacidosis, hypoglycemia, hyponatremia, ingestion of drugs, and seizure disorder

d. The mainstay of treatment is the immediate descent of at least 1,000 m or until symptoms improve. Minimize physical exertion, which may otherwise worsen the patient's condition. If descent is not possible, a portable hyperbaric chamber with supplemental oxygen can be used, but this should never replace or delay evaluation/descent when possible. Dexamethasone 8 mg stat followed by 4 mg every 6 hours should be considered in adults via PO, intramuscular (IM), or IV routes. Acetazolamide 250 mg PO twice daily may also have beneficial effects as an adjunct treatment modality.

Ans. 6

a. HAPE

b. *CT chest findings in HAPE:*

- *Ground-glass opacities (GGOs):* The CT scan may show bilateral GGOs, which represent areas of increased lung density without obscuring the underlying vascular markings. These opacities are indicative of fluid accumulation in the lungs.
- Interstitial thickening with thickening of the interlobular septa and intralobular lines may be observed, reflecting the presence of interstitial edema.
- Consolidation of lung parenchyma
- Enlarged pulmonary arteries due to vasoconstriction and increased pulmonary vascular resistance

c. *Management of HAPE:*
   - Immediate descent to lower altitudes is the definitive management. This reduces the hypoxic stress on the lungs and allows for the resolution of pulmonary edema.
   - Supplemental oxygen via portable oxygen concentrator or high-flow oxygen to alleviate hypoxia.
   - Nifedipine is a calcium channel blocker to reduce pulmonary artery pressure.
   - Corticosteroids may be considered to reduce inflammation.
   - Adequate bed rest to minimize physical exertion and reduce the workload on the heart and lungs
   - Adequate hydration

Ans. 7

a. *Fluid and pain management in electric burn patient:* Adult patients with deep-partial and full-thickness burns involving >20% of the total body surface area (TBSA) should receive initial fluid resuscitation of 2 mL of lactated Ringer's/%TBSA. Target fluid resuscitation is calculated as 4 mL/kg/%TBSA for electrical burns.

   Half of the fluid is given over the course of 8 hours and the remaining half is provided over a span of 16 hours. The rate of fluid administration should be titrated to effect using a target urine output of 0.5 mL/kg/h in adults or 1 mL/kg/h in children who are hemodynamically normal.

   For pain management, a short-acting opioid such as fentanyl (1 μg/kg IV) can be started as a continuous infusion and can be titrated as per the requirement.

b. Voltage source resistance offered by the victim, course traversed by the electric current, and time duration of the contact.

c. Sepsis secondary to infection, compartment syndrome, rhabdomyolysis, associated injuries like long bone fractures, spinal fractures, lacerations, pneumothorax, and cardiac complications like fatal arrhythmias.

Ans. 8

a. Lightning injury

b. *Clinical features of lightning injury:*
   - Burns like arc burns, flash burns, superficial or deep burns
   - *Lichtenberg figures:* Branching rash resembling a tree branch is unique for lightning injuries.
   - Retinal detachment
   - Rupture of tympanic membrane
   - Ischemic stroke
   - Hemorrhagic bleed
   - Spinal cord injury

- Myoglobinuria
- Rhabdomyolysis

c. *Management of lightning injury:*
- Maintain ABC
- Look for the types of injuries sustained and provide treatment accordingly
- In case of any burns, fluid resuscitation and antimicrobial therapy should be provided.
- Cardiac monitoring and consultation in case of arrhythmias
- Adequate pain management with proper analgesia

Ans. 9

a. *Type of snake in this case on the basis of clinical features:* Neurotoxic snake, e.g., cobra or krait

b. *Clinical features:*
- *Ptosis:* Inability to retract upper eyelids on looking up
- *Ophthalmoplegia:* Double vision (perception of two images of a single object), blurred vision and inability to move eyes in the instructed direction
- *Pupillary dilatation:* Often nonresponsive to light; inability (or limitation) to open mouth
- *Tongue extrusion:* Inability to protrude the tongue beyond incisors teeth; inability to swallow
- *Broken neck sign:* Patients cannot hold their neck straight when sitting up (active or passive) from supine position.
- *Skeletal muscle weakness:* Limb weakness, flaccid paralysis, and loss of deep tendon reflexes
- Loss of gag reflex leading to inability to clear secretion and drooling of saliva
- *Paradoxical breathing:* Outward protrusion of abdomen during deep inspiration
- Respiratory failure

c. Administration of an antivenom (monovalent or polyvalent as per the availability) in line with the national guidelines of the country

Ans. 10

a. Hematotoxic snakebite most likely due to vipers

b. *Steps to perform 20WBCT:*
- With normal blood, a clot is seen at 20 minutes after sample collection
- Incoagulable blood at 20 minutes, from a patient with Russell's viper envenoming
- Place 3 mL of freshly sampled venous blood in a small, new, dry glass tube

- Leave the tube standing undisturbed for 20 minutes at ambient temperature
- Gently tip the tube once; if the blood is still liquid (unclotted) and runs out, the patient has uncoagulable blood

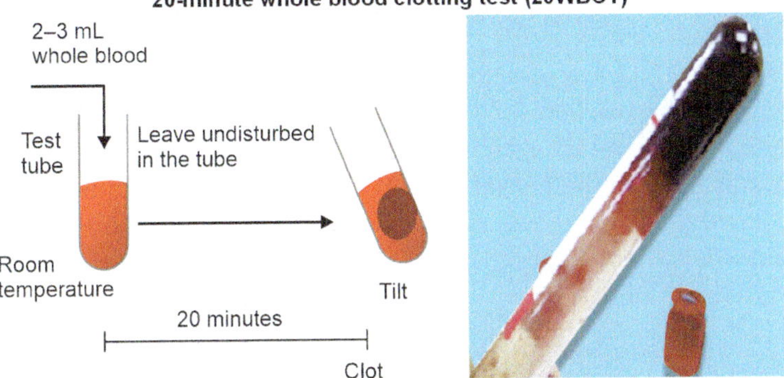

c. *Prehospital management of hematotoxic snakebite patient:*
   - *Reassurance:* The victim may be very frightened and anxious. Reassure victim that most of the suspected snakebites are caused by nonvenomous snakes and that snakebite is a treatable condition.
   - *Immobilization:* Immobilize the bitten limb with a splint or sling. Any cloth or bandage may be used for this purpose. Any form of movement causing muscle contraction like walking and undressing will increase absorption and spread of venom by squeezing veins and lymphatics.
   - *Rapid transport:* The victim should be transported to the hospital where he can receive the medical care. The most common cause of death due to snakebite envenoming is due to respiratory paralysis.

Ans. 11

a. *Complications of wasp sting:*
   - Local and systemic allergic reactions
   - Cardiovascular complications like myocardial infarction, myocarditis, and atrial fibrillation
   - Neurological complications include ocular myasthenia gravis, optic neuritis, limb numbness, trigeminal neuralgia, and encephalopathy
   - Acute renal failure
   - Rhabdomyolysis
   - Acute pancreatitis
   - Disseminated intravascular coagulation
   - Multiorgan dysfunction

b. Wasp venom is a vasoactive inflammatory substance containing amines and thrombogenic peptides such as histamine, leukotrienes, and thromboxane. The venom also contains allergic proteins such as phospholipase A2, antigen 5, acid phosphatases, and hyaluronidases, which elicit immunoglobulin E response and mast cell activation. This mast cell activation causes the release of vasoactive amines such as histamines, acetylcholine, serotonin, several kinins, leukotrienes, thromboxane, proteins, and *de novo* synthesis of other mediators, and cause vasospasm and vasoconstriction of the vasculature, causing ischemic complications. Phospholipases in wasp venom may cause an anaphylactic reaction.

c. Adequate pain management is an important aspect of management of this case. In the background of decreased urine output with dark-colored urine and severe metabolic acidosis shown by the ABG reports, immediate hemodialysis should be initiated and the patient should be closely monitored.

Ans. 12

a. *Important clinical features of jellyfish sting:*
   - Mild skin rash with pricking or burning sensation
   - Pruritis
   - Paresthesia
   - Throbbing pain
   - Blistered dark edematous skin
   - Anaphylaxis
   - SOB, respiratory failure
   - Nausea, vomiting, abdominal cramps
   - Fatal arrhythmias
   - Seizures, loss of consciousness

b. *Management jellyfish sting:*
   - Following a jellyfish sting, the skin should be decontaminated immediately with a generous application of vinegar, rubbing alcohol, baking soda, fresh lemon juice, or olive oil, together with shaving the skin to help remove the remaining nematocysts and effectively control the initial reaction.
   - For the sting of the venomous box jellyfish, local application of heat (up to 45°C) by immersion in hot water is considered effective.
   - Topical application of an anesthetic ointment (lidocaine, benzocaine), an antihistamine (diphenhydramine), or a glucocorticoid (hydrocortisone) may be helpful.
   - Persistent severe pain after decontamination may be treated with narcotic analgesics.
   - Muscle spasms may respond to diazepam given intravenously.
   - An ovine-derived antivenom is available for stings from the box jellyfish found in some countries.

- In case the patient develops compartment syndrome, urgent fasciotomy should be performed to relieve vascular impairment.

Ans. 13

a. Asbestosis
b. SOB, persistent dry cough, chest tightness and pain, fatigue, loss of weight and appetite, crackling sounds when breathing, clubbing of fingers and toes, pulmonary artery hypertension, and mesothelioma.

Ans. 14

a. *Classification and clinical consequences of scorpion sting:*
    - *Class I:* Local manifestations—Burning sensation, necrosis, paresthesia, pain, petechiae
    - *Class II:* Minor systemic manifestations—Not life-threatening (abdominal distension, hypertension, thirst, hyperthermia, urinary retention, hypothermia, vomiting)
    - *Class III:* Major systemic manifestations—Wheezing, hematuria, pancreatitis
    - *Class IV:* Lethal envenomation—Cardiogenic, respiratory, and neurologic failure
b. Diffuse, fluffy, bilateral infiltrates, which are predominantly in the right hemithorax features suggestive of acute pulmonary edema
c. *Management of scorpion sting:*
    - First aid
    - Supportive management
    - Pain management
    - Management of wound
    - Antivenom
    - Prazosin

Ans. 15

Potential health hazards in person handling with body fluid samples and chemicals:

- *Biological hazards:* Exposure to bacteria, virus, fungi, and other living organisms
- *Chemical hazards:* Harmful chemical in the form of solid, liquid, or gas exerting toxic effects by inhalation, absorption, and ingestion
- *Physical hazards:* Ionizing and nonionizing radiation exposure, noise radiation
- *Air contaminants:* Dust, fumes, mist, aerosols, gas and vapor contaminants

SECTION 2 MCQs in Emergency Medicine

Sample MCQs Emergency Medicine

Examples of type "A" questions require the candidate to select the SINGLE best answer from the options presented. In some cases, the other options are clearly wrong, but in others the distinction will be less clear-cut. The accompanying referenced notes should clarify the reasoning behind the correct answer.

Q1. Regarding the fluid resuscitation of the trauma patient which statement is False?

a. Resuscitation with large volumes of crystalloid increases the incidence of abdominal compartment syndrome
b. Hypertonic saline has been shown to increase survival compared with crystalloid
c. Arterial base deficit is a better indicator of adequacy of fluid resuscitation than urine output
d. Serum lactate is a better indicator of adequacy of fluid resuscitation than urine output
e. Rate of clearance of base deficit is correlated with survival

Ans. b. A correlation exists between the magnitude of crystalloid resuscitation and the development of the abdominal compartment syndrome. Although the use of hypertonic saline may reduce the chances of this complication, evidence that it improves trauma survival rates compared with standard fluid resuscitation is lacking. Both arterial base deficit and serum lactate are better indicators of the adequacy of volume resuscitation than clinical markers such as blood pressure and urine output. Both initial base deficit and rate of improvement of base deficit are correlated with survival—failure to normalize a base deficit within 2 days of injury is associated with a poor prognosis.

Reference

Deitch EA, Dayal SD. Intensive care unit management of the trauma patient. Crit Care Med. 2006;34(9):2294-301.

Q2. Which of the following is the most useful measure in the early management of a patient with rhabdomyolysis following a crush injury?

a. Intravenous crystalloid
b. Acetazolamide
c. Mannitol
d. Sodium bicarbonate
e. Pentoxifylline

Ans. a. Retrospective analysis has shown that vigorous intravenous fluid administration is associated with a reduced incidence of acute renal failure in patients with rhabdomyolysis. While mannitol has several theoretically useful properties in the management of rhabdomyolysis including a free radical-scavenging action, improved renal blood rheology, and a "flushing out" effect on the renal tubules, it has not been shown to improve outcome compared with fluids alone in a large retrospective study. Bicarbonate or acetazolamide is often given to alkalinize the urine, allowing more (acidic) myoglobin to be dissolved and excreted. However, bicarbonate may have deleterious effects including worsening systemic hypocalcemia, and has not been shown to confer any benefit over fluid resuscitation alone. Pentoxifylline is one of several free radical scavengers which have theoretical but largely unproven benefits in the management of this condition.

References

1. Brown CV, Rhee P, Chan L, Evans K, Demetriades D, Velmahos GC. Preventing renal failure in patients with rhabdomyolysis: do bicarbonate and mannitol make a difference? J Trauma. 2004;56(6):1191-6.
2. Huerta-Alardín AL, Varon J, Marik PE. Bench-to-bedside review: Rhabdomyolysis—an overview for clinicians. Crit Care. 2005;9(2):158-69.

Examples of type "K" questions consist of a statement followed by four statements, EACH requiring a "True" or "False" answer.

Q1. The following may be signs of hypomagnesaemia:

a. Trousseau's and Chvostek's signs
b. Hyperreflexia
c. Flushing
d. Ataxia

Ans. a. True, b. True c. False, and d. True

Normal serum magnesium levels are 0.6–1 mmol/L. Absorption of dietary magnesium occurs in the terminal ileum, and excretion is via the kidney; most is reabsorbed in the proximal tubule and thick ascending limb of the loop of Henle. Hypomagnesemia occurs through malabsorption, diarrhea, malnutrition, renal disease and a variety of drugs (diuretics, cisplatin, pentamidine). Diabetics lose magnesium through osmotic diuresis, alcoholics through a combination of osmotic diuresis and malnutrition. The prevalence of hypomagnesemia is 2% in the general population but 50–60% in intensive care unit (ICU) patients. Symptoms and signs are legion and nonspecific; flushing is a sign of hypermagnesemia.

Reference

Dubé L, Granry JC. The therapeutic use of magnesium in anesthesiology, intensive care and emergency medicine: a review. Can J Anaesth. 2003;50(7):732-46.

Q2. The following features favor a diagnosis of encephalopathy over encephalitis in a patient presenting with an altered sensorium:

a. Meningism
b. Normal cerebrospinal fluid analysis
c. Gradual steady deterioration in mental status
d. Seizures

Ans. a. False, b. True, c. True, d. False

Encephalopathy is a noninflammatory diffuse brain dysfunction, caused by intoxication or metabolic dysfunction. Encephalitis is an infection of brain tissue, which is a medical emergency. It is characterized by an acute deterioration in mental status, the presence of focal neurological signs and seizures, and peripheral manifestations of the infectious agent (most commonly viral, e.g., parotitis, myocarditis, and lymphadenopathy). Cerebrospinal fluid is rarely normal in encephalitis. A lymphocytic pleocytosis may indicate tuberculosis, while polymerase chain reaction (PCR) testing is extremely sensitive for the detection of viral agents. Herpes simplex is the most common cause of encephalitis.

Reference

Polhill S, Soni N. Encephalitis in the ICU setting. Curr Anaesth Crit Care. 2007;18(2):107-16.

Basic Concepts of Emergency Medicine MCQs

Devendra Richhariya

Q1. All are the good qualities of the emergency physicians, *except*:

a. Multitasking
b. Team leader
c. Good communicator
d. Association with patient

Ans. d. Emergency physicians must have professional qualities and should be calm, approachable, passionate, knowledgeable, enthusiastic leaders, reliable mentors, efficient learners, and facilitators emergency physicians should avoid advertising, Association with drug manufacturers, association with patients, adultery, addiction, alcohol consumption on duty.

Q2. Which of the following are the components of professionalism at work?

a. Reliability
b. Integrity
c. Competency
d. Work focused
e. All

Ans. e. Professionalism is expected without even an iota of a doubt, their act of professionalism says a lot and spreads very easily through word of mouth. Displaying confidence as the head of the family or head of the hospital in that scenario is again very important.

Q3. Emergency physicians should perform all except which of the following?

a. Attend and manage all types of emergencies
b. State authorities should be informed in case of epidemic and fatal communicable diseases
c. Attend court for medicolegal cases
d. Association with the drug manufacturer

Ans. d. Emergency physicians should avoid advertising, association with drug manufacturers, association with patients, adultery, addiction, and alcohol consumption on duty.

Q4. Which of the following are the components of the infrastructure of a new emergency department (ED)?

a. Resuscitation area
b. Triaging areas
c. Treatment areas
d. All

Ans. d. There are a number of factors that must be considered when structuring an ED department. This will include both staff requirements and patient needs and demographics.

Q5. Which of the following are the deciding factors for staffing in an emergency?

a. Patient volume
b. Patient length of stay (LOS)
c. The capabilities of physicians
d. The hospital's expectations
e. All

Ans. e. Correct staffing is the key to delivering timely and high-quality care in the ED. Correct staffing in EDs results in safer care with improved quality, better performance, increased efficiency, and a happy and resilient workforce.

Q6. Which of the following are the types of observation units?

a. Open unit
b. Closed unit
c. Hybrid unit
d. All

Ans. d. While designing the observation unit in the ED, clinical effectiveness and financial viability are the top priorities. Various types of observation unit designs are described by Ross and colleagues. The first type of observation unit is protocols driven which is termed type 1 observation unit. Another type of observation unit is those managed by the clinical direction given by individual clinicians (not based on protocols) termed a type 2 observation unit. In type 3 observation unit patients can be observed in any hospital bed, but care is protocol based. Type 4 If the patient is observed in a nonprotocolized manner in any hospital bed. Another classification of observation units is closed or open observation units. In a closed observation unit, the patient is managed under a single group or specialty like an emergency medicine specialist in the open observation unit the patient is managed by individual clinician directives.

Q7. Following are the types of isolation rooms, *except*?

a. Class S
b. Class N
c. Class P
d. Class A
e. Class K

Ans. e. Isolation rooms are broadly classified into 4 classes. Class-S standard pressure rooms—for patients with contact and droplet isolation. A normal air condition room is appropriate. Class-N negative pressure rooms are used for airborne droplet nuclei isolation. Also known as "airborne infection isolation" or "infectious isolation unit." The negative pressure gradient is maintained from the room to the anteroom and the ambient air. The air change rate of 12 air changes per hour. Class P positive pressure room-rooms are positive pressure relative to ambient air used for immunocompromised and transplant patients. Class A-alternating pressure (negative/positive)—room with alternate negative and positive pressure. Usually not recommended as difficulty in maintaining the appropriate airflow.

Q8. What are the benefits of the implementation of clinical decision rules in the observation area of ED?

a. Reduce practice variability
b. Maximize use of resources
c. Help identify and diagnose high-risk conditions
d. All

Ans. d. Clinical decision rules (CDRs), also known as decisions, are evidence-based tools or protocols to assist emergency physicians/clinicians in decision-making for common complaints in ED. These clinical decision rules are often helpful in the ED setting, to identify patients that might be at higher risk for serious conditions such as pulmonary embolism (PE) or subarachnoid hemorrhage (SAH), or they are used to prevent overuse of unnecessary testing.

Q9. Which of the following are the five-tier triage scales, *except*?

a. Australasian triage scale
b. Manchester triage scale
c. Simple triaging and rapid treatment (START)
d. Canadian triage scale
e. Emergency severity index

Ans. c. START (Simple triage and rapid treatment) system allow first responders to triage multiple victims within 30 seconds, based on 3 primary observations like Respiration, Perfusion and mental status and categorized them into Minor, Delayed, Immediate, Expectant categories.

Q10. Parameters for Modified Early Warning Score (MEWS) scores are all, *except*:

a. Respiratory rate
b. Weight
c. Heart rate
d. Systolic blood pressure (BP)

Ans. d. *Modified Early Warning Score (MEWS):* The MEWS score is based on blood pressure, heart rate, respiration, oxygen saturation, and alertness.

Q11. Triaging methods used for mass causality are:

a. START
b. Sort, assess, lifesaving intervention, treatment/transport (SALT)
c. Both
d. None

Ans. c. In mass casualty situations the number of patients and their severity are much more than the existing capability for management. In this critical situation, simple triaging format START and SALT triaging should be used.

Q12. How do you calculate the fall rate in ER?

a. Number of falls × 1,000
b. Number of falls/number of beds in ED × 1,000
c. Number of falls/month × 100
d. Number of patient falls/number of patient bed days × 1,000

Ans. d. Count the number of falls in the month. Figure out how many bed days were occupied. Add the total occupied beds each day for the month (patient bed days). Divide the number of falls by the number of patients' bed days for the month. Multiply by the results by 1,000 to get the fall rate per 1,000 bed days.

Q13. What are the "structure" and "process" components to be measured to reduce acquired nosocomial infection due to poor hand hygiene practices of doctors and staff?

a. Number of staff, number of patients
b. Number of bedside hand rubs/hand wash facility, steps of hand wash/hand rub
c. Hand wash opportunities and staff-patient ratio
d. Staff ratio, training on handwash

Ans. b. Structure + process = outcomes. To improve outcomes (in this case to reduce the number of infections) we need to measure the structure component (availability of hand wash/rub) at all times and + the process component (all staff are following hand wash technique/steps). Mere training/retraining (focus on people without system or process improvement) alone will not help improve outcomes.

Q14. Which of the following is ED "throughput"?

a. Door to needle time
b. Nurse to doctor assessment
c. Patients LOS in emergency room (ER)
d. Doctors handover during shift change

Ans. c. Patient's LOS in ER. Includes increments of time between the arrival to and departure from the ED. Reducing an ED's LOS promotes quality care and patient safety and is often used as a key performance indicator for hospital EDs.

Q15. A 67-year-old diabetic patient on insulin was treated for hypoglycemia in the ER due to a missed meal. He was advised not to skip his meal while on insulin and discharged from the ED. Which of the following is the best method to assess this patient's understanding of the teaching?

a. Patient satisfaction survey
b. Written demonstration by the patients
c. Ability to reverbalize the instructions by the patient
d. Postdischarge home call to check if he is following instruction

Ans. c. Studies have shown that the average verbal communication between a doctor and patients is only about 73 seconds and up to 65% of the written instructions are never read out or explained to the patients. To ensure patient safety, instructions, and advice to the patients are provided in a written manner and it is recommended to verbalize the same to the patient and check reverbalization in the patient's own language to check to understand.

Q16. Which of the following statements is false?

a. Health QUEST National guidelines of the Society for Emergency Medicine India (SEMI), Indian Society of Critical Care Medicine (ISCCM), and Indian Space Research Organisation (ISRO) provide a focused guideline for patient safety in the ED and intensive care unit (ICU).
b. Accreditation for EDs is available from the National Accreditation Board for Hospitals and Healthcare Providers (NABH) and the Quality Accreditation Institute in India.
c. The World Health Organization (WHO) has introduced a trauma safety checklist similar to the surgical safety checklist which can be adapted in all EDs.
d. Accreditation is mandatory for all EDs.

Ans. d. Accreditation is still a voluntary process in India.

Q17. What is the most crucial step in standard precaution?

a. Gloves
b. Mask
c. Hand hygiene
d. Gown

Ans. c. *Hand hygiene:* Hand hygiene is the single most crucial method in standard precautions of IPC. It provides the first line of defense in the prevention of transmission of microorganisms in healthcare facilities. They are not an alternative to hand hygiene. Hands should be decontaminated thoroughly with soap and water or alcohol-based hand rub (ABHR).

Q18. Mention True or False for each statement with regard to the usage of gloves.

a. Gloves are an alternative to hand hygiene
b. Gloves are multiuse and can be decontaminated
c. Gloves should be changed for different procedures on the same patient
d. Gloves may not be changed for the same procedure on different patient

Ans. a. False, b. False, c. True, and d. False

Gloves should be changed between patient encounters and when they get torn or visibly contaminated, namely between each patient and between different procedures on the same patient to prevent cross-contamination of body sites or contamination of medical equipment. Gloves are single-use and should never be decontaminated, washed, reused, or shared with another user.

Q19. What is the right sequence of doffing personal protective equipment (PPE) as per the Centers for Disease Control (CDC)?

a. Gown, mask, goggles, gloves
b. Gloves, gown, goggles, mask
c. Mask, goggles, gown, gloves
d. Gloves, goggles, gown, and mask

Ans. b. Gloves, gown, goggles, mask

The sequence for removing PPE is gloves, face shields or goggles, gown, mask or respirator, and hand hygiene.

Q20. Mention True or False for each statement against the criteria for selecting the right PPE.

a. Clinical presentation of the patient
b. Suspected or identified infectious agent
c. Diagnosis of the medical condition
d. Transmission route of infectious agent

Ans. a. False, b. True, c. False, and d. True

Appropriate PPE is selected according to the risk assessment done, which is not based on the clinical presentation or diagnosis of the patient but rather on the suspected or identified infectious agent, transmission route of the infectious agent, patient care setting, and tasks or procedures undertaken.

Q21. Which of the following aerosol-generating procedures (AGPs) does not warrant N99/FFP3 respirator?

a. Nebulization
b. Postintubation with closed circuit ventilation
c. Tracheostomy
d. Cardiopulmonary resuscitation (CPR) with bag-mask ventilation (BMV)

Ans. b. For all AGPs use level 3 PPE in any circumstances (nebulization, tracheal intubation, noninvasive ventilation, tracheotomy, cardiopulmonary resuscitation, manual ventilation before intubation, and bronchoscopy).

Q22. Mark the statement True or False regarding high-consequence infectious diseases (HCIDs).

a. HCID transmitted by contact, droplet, or an airborne route or a combination of any of these
b. Typically has a low case-fatality rate
c. May not have effective prophylaxis or treatment
d. Is easy to recognize and detect
e. Is able to spread in the community and within healthcare settings
f. Requires an enhanced individual, population, and system response to manage effectively, efficiently, and safely.

Ans. **a. True, b. False, c. True, d. False, e. True, and f. True**

High-consequence infectious diseases (HCIDs) typically have a high case-fatality rate. It is often difficult to recognize and detect rapidly.

Q23. AGPs are:

a. Intubation, extubation, and other procedures
b. Tracheostomy
c. Manual ventilation
d. Bronchoscopy
e. All of the above

Ans. e. Aerosol-generating procedures are intubation, extubation, and other procedures, tracheostomy, manual ventilation, open suctioning, bronchoscopy, noninvasive ventilation, high-frequency oscillating ventilation, and high-flow nasal oxygen.

Q24. The following are device-related infections, *except*:

a. Catheter-associated urinary catheter infections (CAUTI)
b. Central line-associated bloodstream infections (CLABSI)
c. Ventilator-associated pneumonia (VAP)
d. Community-acquired pneumonia (CAP)

Ans. d. Device-associated infections are one of the largely preventable sources of healthcare-associated infections. Care bundles have been formulated based on evidence-based research work and best-considered practice.

Q25. VAP prevention strategies are all, *except*:

a. Head elevation of the bed to 30–45°
b. Oral care with chlorhexidine
c. Avoid sedation for patient
d. Subglottic suctioning

Ans. c. Ventilator-associated pneumonia is defined as the diagnosis of a new pneumonia after >48 hours of mechanical ventilation, not present at the time of intubation. Endotracheal intubation in the ED and prolonged ED stay have also been related to high VAP rates in comparison with the ICU. Daily sedation and vacation are important strategies for the prevention of VAP.

Q26. A 72-year-old female patient is being planned for discharge from the hospital. During her stay, she acquired a nosocomial infection, Clostridium difficile in preparing a teaching plan for the patient and caretaker, which priority point would the nurse include?

a. Report any constipation to your physician immediately
b. Clostridioides difficile causes diarrhea accompanied by flatus and abdominal discomfort.
c. The client should consume a diet high in fiber and low in fat
d. No special cleaning or disinfection will be required in the home

Ans. b. Clostridium difficile infection (CDI) is due to a toxin-producing bacteria that causes a more severe form of antibiotic-associated diarrhea. The disease ranges from mild diarrhea to severe colon inflammation that can even be fatal. Clostridium difficile is a gram-positive bacterium.

Q27. A patient has an infection that spreads through droplets. Which of the following is vital for the nurse to use while taking patient vitals?

a. Gloves
b. Goggles
c. A gown
d. A mask

Ans. a. Droplet transmission travels only short distances (usually <2 m) before settling. They may also fall on surfaces and then be transferred onto someone's hand who then rubs their eyes, nose, or mouth.

Q28. An educator is teaching her newly joined nursing staff about ways of preventing the spread of infection. The breaking of the cycle of this infectious process was also included, which may be attained through:

a. Hand washing before and between providing client care.
b. Thoroughly cleaning the environment.
c. Wearing infection control-approved protective equipment when providing client care.
d. Using medical and surgical aseptic techniques at all times.

Ans. a. The way to stop germs from spreading is by interrupting this chain at any link.

Q29. A nurse discusses the procedure for protective isolation with the wife of a patient who has been hospitalized for neutropenia and is receiving chemotherapy. Which statement made by the wife indicates the teaching was effective?

a. "Protective isolation helps prevent the spread of infection from my wife to healthcare personnel and visitors."
b. "Protective isolation helps prevent the spread of infection to my wife from the outside environment."
c. "Protective isolation helps prevent the spread of infection from my wife by using special techniques to destroy infectious fluids and secretions."
d. "Protective isolation helps prevent the spread of infection to my wife by using special sterilization techniques for her linens and personal items before use."

Ans. b. The patients who are immunocompromised are usually kept in isolation rooms with positive pressure, such that opportunistic infection does not have a chance to infect the weakened immune system.

Q30. Mrs Lakra is being transported for special procedures for a PICC line placement. The patient is kept under droplet precautions. What are the nursing actions to ensure proper transport of the patient?

a. Inform the receiving department and provide the patient with an N95 mask.
b. Place a surgical mask on the patient and inform the receiving department.

c. Cancel transport and notify the physician for further orders.
d. Report to the receiving department and place goggles, gown, and mask on the patient.

Ans. b. Droplet transmission occurs usually when bacteria or viruses travel on relatively large respiratory droplets when people sneeze, cough, or exhale. They travel only short distances (usually <2 m) before settling. Respiratory hygiene/cough etiquette should be used when a patient has signs/symptoms of a respiratory infection. This infection control technique includes, (1) covering the nose and mouth when coughing or sneezing and (2) offering a surgical mask to anyone who is symptomatic. A surgical N95 respirator is recommended if airborne precautions are required for coughing, etc.

Recent Concepts in Emergency Medicine MCQs

Devendra Richhariya

Q1. Digital Health Technology can revolutionize the way care providers. (Mark each statement True/False).

a. Retrieve and view a medical record
b. Initiate diagnostic and procedure orders
c. Stay away from the patient's complaints
d. Get real-time alerts and notifications
e. Adjust treatment plans on various devices at the point of care or on the move

Ans. a. True, b. True, c. False, d. True, and e. True

Digital Health Technology enhances patient engagement and helps them connect with care providers. Hence answer (c) is false.

Q2. A single-screen command center view for the emergency room (ER) automatically retrieves key medical information of the patients to enable. (Mark each statement True/False)

a. Quick decision making
b. Dispatching appropriate category of ambulance
c. Track the ambulance through global positioning system (GPS)
d. Drop the patient home

Ans. a. True, b. True, c, True, and d. False

ER command center may be responsible for all ambulance movements including dropping the patient home, however, retrieving key medical information is not vital for dropping the patient home.

Q3. A well-designed and structured clinical documentation format. (Mark each statement True/False).

a. Mandates every department to create their own document format
b. Saves time required for documentation
c. Promotes standardized clinical documentation
d. Help in analyzing recorded data for further improvements

Ans. a. False, b. True, c. True, and d. True

Digital clinical documentation does not mandate departments to create their own document format. In fact, it promotes standardization of clinical documentation across the organization.

Q4. Digital documentation. (Mark each statement True/False)

a. Saves environment
b. Saves cost
c. Increases the need of porters to carry the documents
d. Promotes access anytime, from anywhere

Ans. a. True, b. True, c. False, and d. True

Digital documentation enables real-time access anytime, from anywhere. It does not require porters to carry the documents from one care provider to another. Therefore, it decreases the need for porters to carry the documents.

Q5. Benefits of digitally enabled standardized care are: (Mark each statement True/False)

a. Improved patient safety
b. Reduces redundancy of work
c. Increases compliance
d. Reduces cost
e. Increases the workload

Ans. a. True, b. True, c. True, d. True, and e. False

Digitally enabled standardized care typically reduces the workload over a period as it reduces the redundancy of work and captures the data automatically via various integrations with software and medical equipment.

Q6. Barcode technology is *not* useful in reducing:

a. Patient identification errors
b. Incident of patient falls
c. Medication administration errors
d. Blood transfusion errors

Ans. b. Barcode technology is extremely useful in reducing patient identification errors by scanning barcoded wristbands, medicine administration errors by checking the five rights of medication administration, and blood transfusion errors by scanning patient wristbands and blood bags. However, it has no role in reducing the incidents of patient falls.

Q7. Benefits of using a mobile device in quality-of-care delivery are all, *except:*

a. Capturing images and videos
b. Easily connected with social media
c. Used as barcode scanner
d. Reduced training needs
e. Access anytime, from anywhere

Ans. b. Using mobile helps capture the images and videos for further review between clinicians. The use of mobile cameras as barcode scanners goes a long way in preventing medication and transfusion errors. The widespread use of mobile devices reduces the training effort and it allows access of medical records anytime, from anywhere. Connectivity with social medical platforms has no direct benefit in the care delivery process.

Q8. The latest digital health initiatives being implemented across the globe are all, *except:*

a. Digitally smart ambulances
b. Artificial intelligence (AI)-based electronic medical records
c. Achieving national and international quality accreditations
d. Dynamic clinical decision support system

Ans. c. Digital Health Initiatives may help in getting national and international quality accreditation, but Quality accreditation such as Joint Commission International (JCI), and National Accreditation Board for Hospitals and Healthcare Providers (NABH), etc., by itself is not a digital health initiative. It has been in existence for many decades.

Q9. Digital health technology tools are designed only for care providers.

a. True
b. False
c. Partially true
d. None

Ans. b. Many digital health technology tools, such as web portals, patient apps, and telemedicine platforms are made available not only to care providers but to the patients as well, enabling increased patient engagement in the care delivery process.

Q10. Which could be the best option from the following for the best results from implementing digital health technology?

a. Care delivery process should be automated first
b. Care delivery process should be made stable and robust first
c. Either way benefits of digital health technology can be achieved
d. None

Ans. a. For any process automation to work effectively and efficiently, it is necessary to have a robust and stable process. Only a stable process can give rise to meaningful data which can then be processed and converted into information to make smart decisions.

Q11. Which of the following are the advanced technologies that are helpful in the smooth functioning of the emergency department?

a. Patient flow software
b. Barcode Scanner
c. Realtime location
d. Online check-in
e. All of the above

Ans. e. Technology has revolutionized the way medical professionals work, communicate, and process information. Nowhere is this more apparent than in the emergency department. Digital communication tools allow nurses and clinicians to uncover and track data in real time and adjust the course of treatment.

Q12. Which of the following is not an observational study?

a. Cross-sectional design
b. Longitudinal design
c. Randomization
d. Cohort design

Ans. c. Randomization comes under experimental studies. In an observational study, the natural history of treatments (standard of care) is studied.

Q13. To avoid bias in the study which of the following is applied in the study?

a. Blinding
b. Cohort
c. Randomization
d. None

Ans. a. To avoid any bias in the study, blinding is resorted which means concealing or masking of the subject's assignment to a study group (control or treatment) from those participating in the study. The blinding could be single-blinded, double-blinded, or triple-blinded.

Q14. Simulation-based education in medicine is supported by which of the following approaches?

a. Adult learning theory
b. Constructivism
c. Experiential learning model of Kolb
d. Dewey's experiential learning theory
e. All of the above

Ans. e. Simulation-based education in medicine is supported by various pedagogical and andragogical approaches, as well as learning theories ranging from the Adult Learning Theory, Constructivism, Experiential Learning Model of Kolb, Dewey's Experiential Learning Theory, Deliberate Practice, and Mastery Learning. A combination of these approaches and learning theories helps develop a learner's knowledge and skills needed to successfully perform and practice medicine.

Q15. Simulation-based education in emergency medicine. (Mark the true statement)

a. It helps improve the attitude, confidence, and comfort of the trainees.
b. It advances knowledge and skills, changes in behavior, and application of the skills in the workplace.
c. Simulation also helps to reduce medical errors, complications, and to improve clinical and patient outcomes.
d. Provide a safe environment for learners to apply clinical knowledge and practice skills for low to high-risk scenarios and skills.
e. All of the above

Ans. e. Simulation-based education in emergency medicine helps improve the attitude, confidence, and comfort of the trainees. It advances knowledge and skills, changes in behavior, and application of the skills in the workplace. Simulation also helps to reduce medical errors, complications, and to improve clinical and patient outcomes. Some uses of simulation-based training are Procedural skills training code blue response and resuscitation skills, human factors, and crisis resource management (CRM) training to improve problem-solving skills. Nontechnical skills training to address professionalism, interprofessional collaboration, team dynamics, communication, and ethics. Overcrowding and patient flow management and multitasking, testing of process and system to identify errors.

Special Situations in Emergency Medicine MCQs

Devendra Richhariya

Q1. In dealing with difficult patients which of the following statements is True/False?

a. I will never have a difficult patient
b. I will never let any patients or family get angry in my practice
c. Patients and families become arrogant only because of expenses
d. Most difficult patients can be managed by just talking to them in a calm and collected manner

Ans. a. False, b. False, c. False, and d. True

We all will have patients with different mind frames. At times it may not be possible to anticipate a developed difficult patient scenario, even on post-hoc evaluation, and most of the time it is a cumulative effect of more than one trigger or experience that leads to a difficult patient. Medical expenses can be a factor in aggravating the relationship, but the real concern and start of anguish in patients and families would be multifactorial. The tried and tested method that helps in resolving many difficult situations is to listen to patients' concerns and talk to them in a calm and collected manner.

Q2. The following type of patients could become difficult to deal with: (Mark the sentence True or False)

a. Manipulative patients
b. Patients who somatize
c. Frequent flyers
d. Critically ill patients

Ans. a. True, b. True, c. True, and d. False

Manipulative patients: These patients often play on the guilt of others, threatening rage, legal action, or suicide. They tend to exhibit impulsive behavior directed at obtaining what they want, and it is often difficult to distinguish between borderline personality disorder and manipulative behavior.

Somatizing patients: These patients present with a chronic course of multiple vague or exaggerated symptoms and often suffer from comorbid anxiety, depression, and personality disorders. They often have "doctor-shopped" and have a history of multiple diagnostic tests.

Frequent fliers: These patients may stand out due to the sheer bulk of their medical charts. They may be lonely, dependent, or too afraid or embarrassed to ask the questions they really want answered. They may also be patients with a large number of perfectly rational questions, the "worried well" or simply patients who have been given misinformation that needs clarification. Hence these patients can be difficult to manage.

Q3. The following clinician attributes contribute toward patient-clinician discord: (Mark each below statement True/False)

a. Dogmatic or arrogant
b. Fatigued doctor
c. Angry or defensive
d. Calm and patient-clinician

Ans. a. True, b. True, c. True, and d. False

Dogmatic or arrogant physicians. Personal beliefs and values, as well as our beliefs and values about medical care, can lead us to overemphasize our own beliefs and emotions in ways that disempower patients or prevent them from providing us with adequate information about their care. Fatigued or harried physicians. Most of us have been overworked, sleep-deprived, or generally busier than we needed to be at one time or another. It is important that we be sensitive to the impact of physician fatigue on medical errors and patient safety and set reasonable limits for ourselves. Angry or defensive physicians. Physicians who are burned out, stressed, and generally frustrated over near-term crises or long-term concerns are more likely to react negatively to patients. Being calm and patient while dealing with our patients helps in developing a good rapport between clinician and patient. This relationship goes a long way toward having a healthy relationship with patients.

Q4. Factors which would help diffuse a difficult situation: (Mark each below statement True/False)

a. Talk to patient and family patiently
b. Asking the attendees to go out of department
c. Making the patients and family wait to be seen unnecessarily
d. Showing care and concern toward the patient

Ans. a. True, b. False, c. False, and d. True

Showing care and concern for our patients is one of the basic attributes of the clinician. When in tough times with patients and family it always sticks to basics. It will help fulfill our primary responsibility and also work toward gaining patient's and family's trust and confidence. When there is a misunderstanding or difficult situation, talk to the patient and family. Do not ignore either of them.

Involve them in the discussion and make them feel listened to. Asking the family and attendees to leave the department or not attending to them in a timely manner will only make the situation worse.

Q5. After dealing with a difficult patient what should you do?

a. Carry on with your work
b. Keep thinking about the incident for the rest of the day
c. Avoid seeing any patients with similar complaints
d. Take a break and cool off

Ans. d. Dealing with difficult patients is a very stressful and draining experience. There will be a lot of emotions involved in these situations and can linger in one's mind. It is advisable to take some time to sit down and "cool off." This will give time and opportunity to draw a line under the incident and recompose to start to carry on working.

Q6. Regarding dealing with difficult patients which of the following is incorrect?

a. Successfully handling difficult patients will lead to greater respect for your practice
b. Successfully handling difficult patients will lead to increased staff morale
c. Successfully handling difficult patients will lead to better patient confidence
d. Dealing with difficult patients always ends up in losing the patient's confidence

Ans. d. Handling difficult patients is seen as an opportunity rather than trouble, you may find that you can strengthen your patient service skills while retaining their business. Your ability to successfully handle difficult patients will lead to greater respect for your practice, more patients, higher revenue, and increased staff morale.

Q7. The following physician characters contribute to difficult situations, *except:*

a. Dogmatic or arrogant physicians
b. Patient and calm physicians
c. Fatigued or harried physicians
d. Angry or defensive physicians

Ans. b. Being calm and patient while dealing with our patients helps in developing a good rapport between clinician and patient. This relationship goes a long way toward having a healthy relationship with patients. Dogmatic or arrogant physicians. Personal beliefs and values, as well as our beliefs and values about medical care, can lead us to overemphasize our own beliefs and emotions in ways that disempower patients or prevent them from providing us with adequate information about their care. Fatigued or harried physicians. Most of us have been overworked, sleep-deprived, or generally busier than we needed to be at one time or another. It is important that we be sensitive to the impact of physician fatigue on medical errors and patient safety and set reasonable limits for ourselves. Angry or defensive physicians. Physicians who are burned out, stressed, and generally frustrated over near-term crises or long-term concerns are more likely to react negatively to patients.

Q8. Which of the following is True of manipulative patients?

a. It is often difficult to distinguish between borderline personality disorder and manipulative behavior
b. It is always better to meet the expectations of manipulative patients
c. It is usually better to share your own emotional experience with these manipulative patients
d. You should never say "no" to manipulative patients

Ans. a. Manipulative patient. These patients often play on the guilt of others, threatening rage, legal action, or suicide. They tend to exhibit impulsive behavior directed at obtaining what they want, and it is often difficult to distinguish between borderline personality disorder and manipulative behavior. The keys to managing encounters with manipulative patients are to be aware of your own emotions, attempt to understand the patient's expectations (which may actually be reasonable, even if his or her actions are not), and realize that sometimes you have to say "no."

Q9. Mark the below sentences as True/False.

a. The person helping the road traffic accident victim is bound to give his personal details while dropping the victim off at the hospital
b. If a medicolegal case (MLC) is not prepared at the time of admission, it cannot be prepared later on even if needed
c. Postmortem of an MLC cannot be done without relatives' permission
d. Consent is not needed to examine a victim of rape or sexual assault

Ans. **a. False, b. False, c. False, and d. False**

A bystander who is helping the trauma victim is not bound to give personal information to the hospital. Medicolegal case reports can be prepared whenever the facts are brought to the notice of the treating doctor.

Q10. The following are the types of grievous injury. (Mark as True or False)

a. Multiple contused lacerated wound (CLW) over left arm
b. Dislocation of tooth
c. Blunt trauma to abdomen
d. Multiple CLW over the face

Ans. **a. False, b. True, c. False, and d. True**

Dislocation of the tooth and facial injuries are grievous injuries.

Q11. Following are the scores for assessing the emergency department (ED) overcrowding except for

a. Emergency Department Crowding Score
b. Emergency Department Work Index (EDWIN)
c. Real-Time Emergency Analysis of Demand Indicators (READI) Scores
d. National Emergency Department Overcrowding Study (NEDOCS)
e. Emergency Department Workforce Score

Ans. e. Emergency Department Crowding Score, EDWIN, READI scores, and NEDOCS are the scores for assessing overcrowding in ED.

Q12. What are the strategies used for dealing with the ED overcrowding situation?

a. Input strategies
b. Throughput strategies
c. Output strategies
d. Reverse triaging
e. All

Ans. e. Overcrowding of ED can be overcome by Input strategies, throughput strategies, output strategies, and reverse triaging.

Q13. Which of the following are bioethical issues relevant to end-of-life care?

a. Autonomy and self-determination
b. Futility
c. Justice
d. Declaration of death and organ donation.
e. All

Ans. e. There are various bioethical issues for end-of-life care.

Q14. ABCDE of death declaration is:

a. Advance preparation
b. Build a therapeutic environment/relationship
c. Communicate well
d. Deal with patient and family reactions
e. Encourage and validate emotions
f. All

Ans. f. Death declaration is one of the important aspects of ED.

Q15. Essential steps mandatory for brain death determination are all, *except:*

a. Documentation of irreversible coma due to a known proximate cause
b. Documentation of absence of brainstem reflexes
c. Documentation of apnea—The Apnea Test
d. Documentation of fixed dilated pupil

Ans. d. Documentation of irreversible coma due to a known proximate cause, documentation of the absence of brainstem reflexes, and documentation of apnea—The Apnea Test are the steps mandatory for the determination of brain death, not the fixed dilated pupil.

Q16. Which of the following is most responsible for improving solid organ transplant viability during the past 20 years?

a. Better infection control
b. Improved techniques for immunosuppression
c. Improved technique in transplantation
d. Improved technology in obtaining the organ
e. More aggressive organ harvesting

Ans. b. The single most important factor in organ survival has been the improvement in immunosuppressive technology. This improvement has allowed transplanted organs to maintain their viability and function. Unfortunately, as immunosuppression has improved, the biggest challenges in organ survival currently include infection and malignancy.

Q17. Regarding the effect of death on survivors, which of the following statements is True or False?

a. Surviving spouses of many years of marriage are at a lower risk of dying after a short while
b. Most common symptoms of relatives of deceased patients include visual or auditory hallucinations of a deceased person, denial, prolonged hysteria, and anger

c. Suicidal intentions are not of much importance in the close family members
d. The members of the family may be under threat from criminal gang members if involved in the death of the deceased person

Ans. **a. False, b. True, c. False, d. True**

Surviving spouses of many years of marriage are at a higher risk of dying after a short while. They have an undying attachment to each other. Suicidal intentions must be taken seriously as the loss of a near and dear one can produce a sense of survivor's guilt. These are more common in situations where the patient dies of committing suicide.

Q18. Which of the following statements are false regarding the viewing of the deceased person in ED?

a. Life support such as endotracheal tubes, central lines, and cardiac monitor must be disconnected and kept away from the patient
b. Make sure the secretions or blood spills are wiped off
c. Addressing the deceased body as "it" or "that" is important
d. Ensure that emotionally weak relatives are not allowed to view the deceased person as they may suddenly collapse and hurt themselves due to sudden emotional outbursts

Ans. c. Addressing the deceased body as "it" or "that" must be avoided. Respect the dead and acknowledge the loss of the family.

Q19. Regarding organ donation, which of the following statements is True or False?

a. Skin, bone, cornea, fascia, cartilage, heart valves, and cornea can be harvested for up to 48 hours if the deceased body was preserved for 4 hours after death
b. All patients up to the age of 80 years are suitable for organ donation
c. Members from the organ procurement team should counsel the patient's family about organ donation and necessary arrangements should be made
d. Organs such as lungs, heart, liver, and pancreas should be recovered only if adequate tissue perfusion is preserved

Ans. **a. False, b. False, c. True, d. True**

Skin, bone, cornea, fascia, cartilage, heart valves, and cornea can be harvested up to 24 hours, if the deceased body is preserved for 4 hours after death. All patients up to the age of 80 years are suitable for organ donation, excluding patients with oncological ailments, organ damage, and/or infectious ailments.

Q20. Which statement is false regarding Rabow & McPhee's patterned mnemonic for communicating with family members of deceased patients?

a. Prior mental preparation about how to deliver the news to the family may help in maintaining a calm and composed conversation
b. Disregard the initial reactions of family members and hurry up the process of handing over the body without allowing family members to think
c. Allocate a separate room where disruptions in conversation can be prevented
d. Acquainting oneself of all clinical findings and carrying additional documents as a method of proof while communicating with patients

Ans. b. Response to any bad news must be expected. Initial cognitive coping mechanisms such as denial, anger, disbelief, and intellectualization are likely to occur. Empathy toward family members is essential, and allowing time and space to acknowledge the bad news is essential.

Q21. Which of the following statements is not true regarding the organ donation of a deceased child?

a. The size of the organ does not play a role in organ donation
b. Parents are more appreciative than overwhelmed when discussing organ donation if they are approached at the right time and by skillful team members
c. It is advisable if the organ procurement team member directly counsels the parents of the deceased child after giving them adequate time for grieving
d. Handling of the death of a child should be handled critically and by skillful staff

Ans. a. In pediatric patients, the size of the organ poses a major concern for organ procurement teams.

Q22. Which of the following is true regarding the evaluation of a patient with injuries that have potential forensic implications?

a. During evidence collection, hematomas, unlike lacerations, do not need to be photographed
b. During strangulation, a period of 6 minutes is required for compression of blood supply to the brain to cause irreversible neuronal death and damage
c. Irrigate and explore all wounds prior to documentation and photographs

d. The death certificate must be completed by the physician who last attended to the deceased within 24 hours of the death
e. Unlike the entrance wound, the exit wound of a bullet is surrounded by a circumferential rim of abrasion

Ans. d. The death certificate must be completed by the physician who last attended to the deceased within 24 hours of the death. The type of wound, location, and recovery of particles from inside a wound can give important forensic information; therefore, wounds should never be irrigated and explored prior to documentation and photographs. Photographs should be taken of all wounds, including hematomas, to help determine the weapon. Unlike the exit wound, the entrance wound from a bullet is surrounded by a circumferential rim of abrasion. This is produced by friction from the bullet on the skin margins. During strangulation, a period of 4 minutes is required for compression of the blood supply of the brain to result in neuronal death. Bruising or ligature marks on the neck and pinpoint hemorrhage, especially in the conjunctival lining of the eyes, are also markers of strangulation.

Q23. Which of the following should include medical treatment of sexual victims in ED?

a. Preventive measures for sexually transmitted diseases and treatment of wounds
b. Emergency contraception
c. Prophylaxis for tetanus, hepatitis B, and human immunodeficiency virus (HIV)
d. Counseling and psychological support
e. All

Ans. e. All above are required to start as medical therapy.

Q24. All are the types of emergency contraceptive pills, *except:*

a. Ulipristal
b. Progestin-only
c. Combined pill
d. Testosterone only

Ans. d. *Ulipristal*—more effective than progestin-only or combined pill in preventing unprotected pregnancy, approved in 2010 and can be taken up to 120 hours after unprotected intercourse.

Progestin only—progestin levonorgestrel 1.5 mg single dose or 750 μg 12 hours apart in two doses, can be taken up to 72 hours. The combined pill contains both estrogen and progestin in higher doses. It delays the ovulation most effectively within 3 days of unprotected intercourse.

Q25. All are the steps of the apnea test, *except:*

a. Preoxygenation
b. Arterial blood gas analysis
c. Allow partial pressure of carbon dioxide ($PaCO_2$) to rise
d. Check the methemoglobin level

Ans. d. Preoxygenation, arterial blood gas analysis, allow $PaCO_2$ to rise then repeat arterial blood gases.

Q26. Mark the below sentences as True/False.

a. In the case of an unconscious victim emergency surgery cannot be performed until relative or guardian consent is obtained
b. One identification mark is enough in a medical-legal report
c. Personal belongings of suspected homicidal or suicide victims should be immediately handed over to the relatives

Ans. **a. False, b. False, c. False**

Belongings should be handed over to police personnel in cases of medicolegal cases. Emergency surgery can be performed if the victim is unconscious.

Q27. Potential harms of ED overcrowding are all, *except:*

a. Medication errors and adverse events
b. High mortality
c. Compromised quality of care
d. Rapid assessment and rapid treatment of the patient

Ans. d. Medication errors compromised quality of care and high mortality are the harmful effects of overcrowding. Rapid assessment and rapid treatment cannot be performed.

Q28. Boarding time in ED is defined as:

a. Waiting time in the ambulance
b. Time of arrival in ED to the time of initial assessment
c. Time of initial assessment to the time of admission
d. Time from admission decision until the patient leaves the ED
e. Time of total stay in ED

Ans. d. Boarding time is the time from admission decision until the patient leaves the ED.

Q29. At what percentage of the hospital census, do the admissions from ED begin to accumulate from prolonged boarding?

a. 75–80%
b. 80–85%
c. 85–90%
d. 90–95%
e. Above 95%

Ans. c. When the census is <85%, hospitals can typically function efficiently (Green). Hospitals become stressed as census increases beyond 85% and admissions from the ED begin to accumulate from prolonged boarding (yellow) filling the ED to capacity. Most hospitals cannot overcome inefficiencies when the hospital census is above 90%.

Q30. The various goal-directed solutions toward overcoming ED crowding include all, *except:*

a. Input
b. Throughput
c. Shortput
d. Output

Ans. c.

Q31. Among the various strategies, which is least beneficial in overcoming the issue of ED overcrowding?

a. Ambulance diversion
b. Smoothing of elective cases
c. Weekend discharges
d. Full capacity protocol

Ans. a. There is scant evidence that ambulance diversion actually works. Rather there is evidence for delayed care in the face of ambulance diversion. In this regard, Nicholl, et al., demonstrated an increased mortality rate with prolonged transport times.

Q32. Fallouts of ED overcrowding are

a. Increases patient waiting time
b. Increases ambulance diversion
c. Results from non-urgent ED visits by patients
d. Can be tackled by critical measures in ED alone
e. Can increase the risk of human error leading to patient morbidity and mortality

Ans. **a. True, b. True, c. False, d. False, e. True**

Overcrowding of the ED is caused by institutional overcrowding, with the resultant boarding of admitted patients in the ED. There is no evidence that overcrowding results from excess poor patients or nonurgent visits. ED overcrowding causes multiple problems for ED patients and staff, including increased waiting times, increased ambulance diversion, increased length of stay, increased medical errors, increased patient mortality, and increased harm to hospitals due to financial losses.

Prehospital and Disaster MCQs

Devendra Richhariya

Q1. Every prehospital healthcare worker must know the following concepts to improve the patient outcome:

a. Golden 10 minutes
b. Silver 10 minutes
c. Platinum 10 minutes
d. Diamond 10 minutes

Ans. c. The "platinum 10 minutes" was proposed as the ideal amount of time that should be taken to move a casualty to an ambulance. In the first 10 minutes, the ambulance and medical personnel must work in harmony with the police and fire service to secure the scene. Patient outcomes will be desirable if a trained prehospital care professional maximizes the first 10 minutes. Medical direction of a critical patient, if occurs within first 10 minutes after the paramedic reaches the scene, is also an ideal situation.

Q2. Which of the following ground medical transport model is often followed in India and other developing countries?

a. Scoop and stay
b. Scoop and run
c. Stay and stabilize
d. None of the above

Ans. a. The Anglo-American model is also known as "load and go" or "scoop and run". In this model, ambulances are staffed by paramedics and/or emergency medical technicians. They have specialized medical training, but not to the same level as a physician. The physicians who work in EMS provide oversight for the work of the ambulance crews. This may also include on-line medical control, in which the physician is contacted to provide advice and authorization for various medical interventions.

Q3. In the context of ground medical transport services offered to emergency patient in public-private partnership (PPP) mode select the appropriate from the following:

a. Chargeable
b. ₹ 20/KM
c. Free
d. All of the above
e. None of the above

Ans. c. Government of India under National Health Mission (NHM) provides funds to state government on capital expenditure and supports the state government for the first 4 years in operational expenditure. State governments have to follow National Ambulance Service (NAS) norms and National Ambulance Code (NAC) norms. Services offered under NAS and in PPP mode are free of cost to the emergency victim.

Q4. Correct full form of "SBAR" abbreviation applied in patient handover has the following components, *except:*

a. Severity
b. Background
c. Assessment
d. Reassurance

Ans. d. Healthcare organizations implement a standardized approach to handover communication between staff, change of shift, and between different patient care units in the course of a patient transfer. Suggested elements of this approach include: use of the SBAR (Situation, Background, Assessment, and Recommendation) technique.

Q5. State whether following statements are True or False in case of types of road ambulances in India:

a. *Medical first responder:* Will not have the capability to transport patients in a supine state or provide them with medical care inside the vehicle
b. *Basic life support (BLS) ambulances:* For the transport of patients who are not expected to become emergency patients
c. *Patient transport vehicle:* For the transport and treatment of patients requiring noninvasive airway management/basic monitoring
d. *Advanced life support ambulance:* For the transport and treatment of emergency patients requiring invasive airway management/intensive monitoring

Ans. a. True, b. False, c. False, and d. True

Q6. State whether following statements are True or False in case of air medical transfer of the patient:

a. A "donut model" has been created to display the benefits of using different modes of transport for air transfer over variant distances
b. Physiological changes cause direct impact on air transfer patient care: Trapped air will increase 20% in size
c. Physiological changes cause direct impact on air transfer patient care: Arterial oxygen pressure will increase by 23%
d. Alveolar CO_2 pressure will decrease by 6.5%

Ans. a. True, b. True, c. False, and d. True

Q7. Use of a ground emergency medical services (EMS) unit is preferred to an air EMS unit in the following situation:

a. Bad weather
b. Long transport distance
c. Need for advanced airway procedure
d. Obstetric patient
e. Urban environment

Ans. a. Bad weather is a major limitation to the use of aeromedical EMS. Weather issues can present a serious threat to safety. A long distance between the scene and the receiving facility generally favors the use of aeromedical EMS.

Q8. Weakest part of most disaster responses is:

a. Access to care
b. Communications
c. Documentation
d. Personnel
e. Transportation

Ans. b. Communication has historically been the weakest component of disaster responses, which has led to a focus on communication redundancy as a key to effective response. Transportation and manpower are generally sufficient.

Q9. What is the key defining characteristic of a disaster?

a. Location
b. Mismatch between available and required resources
c. Number of patients
d. Types of injuries involved
e. Use of chemical, biological, or radiological agents

Ans. b. A disaster by definition is an event that overwhelms the available resources to immediately manage the event. The number of patients, location, and types of injuries involved may contribute to this resource mismatch but are not the defining characteristics.

Q10. What is the main goal of triage during a disaster?

a. Determine who needs comfort care rather than resuscitation
b. Identify the sickest patients first
c. Obtain primary insurance authorization for treatment
d. Optimize individual patient outcome
e. To do the most good for most of the people

Ans. e. The main goal of disaster triage is to do the best for the most people. This is in contrast to the main goal of routine emergency department triage, which is to identify the sickest patients first; in a disaster, the sickest patients may not be salvageable with the available resources, requiring a change in how priorities for patient care are assigned.

Q11. What deficit is uniformly present in postdisaster communities?

a. Inability to access healthcare facilities
b. Lack of clean water
c. Limited law enforcement capability
d. Loss of resources
e. Poor access to prescription medications

Ans. d. Although many specific problems can occur in postdisaster communities, such as inability to access healthcare facilities, lack of clean water, limited law enforcement capability, and poor access to prescription medications, the underlying and constant theme is loss of resources.

Q12. Which of the following is frequently a major health threat in disaster-affected populations?

a. Cadaver-transmitted infections
b. Exacerbation of chronic diseases
c. Malaria
d. Tuberculosis
e. Yellow fever

Ans. b. Inability to access regular sources of healthcare frequently leads to exacerbations of chronic diseases, such as hypertension and diabetes.

Q13. What is the "universal" decontamination agent?

a. Bleach
b. Decontamination foam
c. Fuller's earth
d. Neutralizing alkali
e. Water

Ans. e. Tepid water, often used with a mild soap and a brush, is the preferred decontamination agent for almost all chemicals.

Q14. A patient presents with urinary and fecal incontinence, drooling, vomiting, and irritated eyes after exposure to an unknown vapor. Which of the following antidotes should be empirically given?

a. Atropine
b. Diazepam
c. Hydroxocobalamin
d. N-acetylcysteine
e. Sodium thiosulfate

Ans. a. This patient is suffering from exposure to an organic phosphorus (or organophosphate) agent, and is demonstrating key features of the "SLUD" (salivation, lacrimation, urination, and defecation) or

"SLUDGE" syndrome (salivation, lacrimation, urination, defecation, gastrointestinal upset, and emesis). Atropine and pralidoxime are indicated to help relieve these symptoms.

Q15. Which of the following protective methods is appropriate for most infectious agents of concern for bioterrorism?

a. Airborne precautions
b. Contact precautions
c. Droplet precautions
d. Patient isolation
e. Standard precautions

Ans. d. Standard precautions are sufficient for the majority of biological agents. Agents that are contagious through airborne or droplet transmission are requiring droplet precautions and patient isolation, viral hemorrhagic fevers (requiring droplet precautions), and smallpox (requiring airborne precautions, contact precautions, and patient isolation).

Q16. Which of the following organ systems is most sensitive to the effects of ionizing radiation?

a. Cardiovascular
b. Hematopoietic
c. Musculoskeletal
d. Nervous
e. Respiratory

Ans. b. The hematopoietic system, along with other systems containing rapidly proliferating cells with high turnover rates such as the gastrointestinal and reproductive systems, is highly sensitive to the effects of ionizing radiation.

Q17. Which of the following should be monitored as an indicator of the extent of radiation injury?

a. Erythrocytes
b. Lymphocytes
c. Neutrophils
d. Platelets
e. Schistocytes

Ans. b. Lymphocytes are rapidly destroyed and slowly replenished after acute radiation injury, causing a rapid decline, which is a hallmark of the hematopoietic syndrome and an excellent indicator of the extent of radiation injury.

Q18. Which symptoms are most likely to be the first encountered with acute radiation syndrome?

a. Altered mental status
b. Fever and fatigue
c. Hypotension
d. Nausea and vomiting
e. Seizures

Ans. d. Nausea and vomiting, along with other gastrointestinal symptoms, are part of the prodromal phase that occurs first in the progression of acute radiation syndrome.

Q19. What constitutes the vast majority of blast injuries?

a. Aircraft incidents
b. Fireworks-related incidents
c. Industrial incidents
d. Motor vehicle collisions
e. Terrorist bombings

Ans. e. Terrorism-related bombings using conventional explosives comprise the vast majority of blast injuries.

Q20. What is the most common fatal primary blast injury?

a. Compartment syndrome
b. Intestinal perforation
c. Pulmonary barotrauma
d. Shrapnel injuries

Ans. c. Pulmonary barotrauma including parenchymal disruption, hemorrhage, hemopneumothorax, and eventual acute respiratory distress syndrome is the most common fatal primary injury associated with blast injuries.

Resuscitation MCQs

Devendra Richhariya

Q1. The nasopharyngeal airway can be used in:

a. A patient who is semiconscious
b. A patient with trismus
c. A patient with jaw wiring
d. A patient with coagulopathies
e. A patient with suspected base of skull fracture

Ans. a. True, b. True, c. True, d. False, and e. False

Nasopharyngeal airway is contraindicated in a patient with coagulopathies and suspected fracture of base of skull.

Q2. An endotracheal tube can be passed through:

a. I-gel
b. Cobra perilaryngeal airway
c. Combitube
d. Fastrach
e. All of the above
f. None of the above

Ans. a.

Q3. The first supraglottic airway device was developed by:

a. Sir Ivan Magill
b. Robert Macintosh
c. Michael Frass
d. Archie Brain
e. Francis Murphy

Ans. d. Dr Archie Brain has developed first supraglottic airway device.

Q4. Noncuffed supraglottic airway devices are:

a. Combitube
b. Classic laryngeal mask airway (LMA)
c. Proseal LMA
d. I-gel
e. LMA Supreme

Ans. d.

Q5. Advantages of a LMA are:

a. Ease of insertion
b. Less sore throat as compared to endotracheal intubation

c. Better oxygenation than bag valve ventilation
d. Less chances of gastric distension than a cuffed endotracheal tube
e. It is a definitive airway

Ans. **a. True, b. True, c. True, d. False, and e. False**

Q6. What caused the majority of fatal dysrhythmias leading to sudden cardiac death?

a. Brugada syndrome
b. Commotio cordis, related to blunt trauma during athletics
c. Congenital heart disease
d. Dilated and hypertrophic cardiomyopathies
e. Structural coronary artery abnormalities including coronary atherosclerosis

Ans. e. Structural coronary artery abnormalities and their consequences (e.g., myocardial ischemia and infarction) are associated with 80% of fatal arrhythmias.

Q7. The key to survival following cardiac arrest is:

a. Depth of chest compression to 2 inches
b. Early defibrillation
c. Prolonged single rescuer cardiopulmonary resuscitation (CPR)
d. Sodium bicarbonate therapy
e. Ventilation with 100% oxygen

Ans. b. Ventricular tachydysrhythmias are the most common cause of sudden cardiac death in adults. Defibrillation is the most effective treatment for VT and VF.

Q8. The outcome of resuscitation and the likelihood of survival are greatest when the initial cardiac rhythm is which of the following?

a. Agonal rhythm
b. Asystole
c. Idioventricular rhythm
d. Pulseless bradycardia
e. Ventricular fibrillation (VF)

Ans. e. The likelihood of survival is relatively high (up to 60%) if the initial rhythm is VT or VF, especially if the VF is "coarse.

Q9. When approaching a collapsed victim in the out of hospital setting, after assessing the level of responsiveness, the next step should be:

a. Administer ventilations
b. Call for help (C) and initiate an intravenous (IV)

c. Stabilize the cervical spine
d. Start chest compressions

Ans. b. If the individual does not respond, get help first before starting ventilations and chest compressions.

Q10. Which of the following is the current recommended drug for the treatment of supraventricular tachycardia (SVT) in children?

a. Adenosine
b. Amiodarone
c. Calcium
d. Magnesium
e. Sodium bicarbonate

Ans. a. Adenosine (0.1 mg/kg) is the current recommended drug for SVT in children. This dose can be doubled if the first dose is unsuccessful.

Q11. A 75-year-old man is diagnosed with sick sinus syndrome. What is the most important and appropriate initial therapy?

a. Atropine
b. Diltiazem
c. Increase fluids and acetaminophen as needed
d. Metoprolol
e. Permanent pacemaker placement

Ans. e. Sick sinus syndrome is an indication for a permanent pacemaker. Pharmacologic treatment of atrial tachyarrhythmias carries the risk of aggravating preexisting AV block or sinus arrest.

Q12. The most common medical cause of maternal death in pregnant women is:

a. Homicide
b. Infection
c. Motor vehicle accidents
d. Pregnancy-induced hypertension
e. Pulmonary embolism

Ans. e. Pulmonary embolism is the most common medical cause of death in pregnant women. Trauma (homicide) is the most common overall cause of maternal death.

Q13. A 23-year-old woman suffers a cardiac arrest in your emergency department (ED) from a suspected pulmonary embolism. She is 34 weeks pregnant. Resuscitative efforts are not going well. Which of the following is True regarding perimortem cesarean section?

a. Maternal CPR should be stopped as soon as the procedure is considered to avoid trauma to the infant

b. Perimortem cesarean section should not be considered after 4 minutes of maternal cardiac arrest
c. Prognosis for intact survival of the infant is best if delivery occurs within 5 minutes of cardiac arrest
d. The patient should be moved to an operating suite before the procedure is performed

Ans. c. Prognosis for intact survival of the infant is best if delivery occurs within 5 minutes of cardiac arrest. If the 5-minute time frame has been exceeded, a perimortem cesarean section is still recommended. The patient should not be moved to an operating suite, as this wastes time.

Q14. A 47-year-old man suffers a right ventricular and inferior wall infarction. Which of the following is *most likely* to occur as a complication of this heart attack?

a. Aortic valve failure
b. Flash pulmonary edema
c. Left bundle branch block
d. Right bundle branch block
e. Second-degree atrioventricular (AV) block

Ans. e. Common occurrence of AV conduction disturbances with acute inferior wall MI. The AV node receives its blood supply from the right coronary artery in 90% of individuals or from left circumflex artery in the other 10%.

Q15. According to the latest advanced cardiac life support (ACLS) manual, the first-line drug for the treatment of ventricular tachycardia (VT) or VF is:

a. Amiodarone
b. Lidocaine
c. Procainamide
d. Propranolol
e. Sodium bicarbonate

Ans. a. Lidocaine is used in the treatment of ventricular arrhythmias and ectopy. In the most recent ACLS guidelines, it is considered second line to amiodarone for the treatment of VF and pulseless VT.

Q16. Long-term oral therapy with amiodarone is associated with which of the following side effects?

a. Adrenal insufficiency
b. Corneal deposits
c. Impotence
d. Retroperitoneal fibrosis
e. Torsades de pointes

Ans. b. Long-term oral therapy is associated with thyroid disorders, pulmonary fibrosis, skin discoloration, hepatic dysfunction, corneal deposits, and other conditions. Before long-term treatment, patients need baseline ophthalmologic and pulmonary function tests.

Q17. Which of the following is the best choice regarding a diagnostic test to perform in a pregnant woman at 32 weeks of gestation with a suspected pulmonary embolism?

a. Arterial blood gas (ABG)
b. Chest radiograph
c. CT scan or ventilation-perfusion scan
d. D-dimer
e. No diagnostic test is acceptable; simply treat the patient and admit for the duration of the pregnancy.

Ans. c. When pulmonary embolism is suspected, empiric treatment with heparin should be started immediately, especially if the patient is hypoxic or hemodynamically unstable. Once treatment has begun, a CT scan or ventilation-perfusion scan should be obtained to confirm the diagnosis. D-dimer concentrations increase progressively throughout normal pregnancy and an elevated D-dimer level is not a helpful screen for the diagnosis of venous thromboembolic disease during pregnancy. Chest radiograph and ABG are not sensitive and are nonspecific.

Q18. The postcardiac arrest syndrome consists of:

a. Postcardiac arrest brain injury
b. Postcardiac arrest myocardial dysfunction
c. Systemic ischemia/reperfusion response
d. Persistent precipitating pathology
e. All of the above

Ans. e. Duration and cause of cardiac arrest determine the severity of this syndrome. If the cardiac arrest is brief, it may not occur at all. Postcardiac arrest brain injury may present as coma, seizures, myoclonus, varying degrees of neurocognitive dysfunction, and brain death.

Q19. Mark the following statement True or False about targeted temperature management (TTM)

a. TTM is indicated for adults after out-of-hospital cardiac arrest (OHCA) who remain unresponsive after return of spontaneous circulation (ROSC)

b. Temperature is maintained between 22°C and 26°C with temperature control monitoring system
c. Minimum duration of TTM should be at least 6 hours
d. Methods of inducing and/or maintaining TTM include simple ice packs and/or wet towels, cooling blankets or pads, and water or air circulating blankets

Ans. **a. True, b. False, c. False, and d. True**
Temperature is maintained between 32°C and 36°C with temperature control monitoring system. Minimum duration of TTM should be at least 24 hours. Following the TTM trial, many intensive care clinicians elected to use 36°C as the target temperature for postcardiac arrest temperature control.

Q20. The tests for prognostication in postcardiac arrest are as follows, *except:*

a. Clinical examination
b. Neurophysiological studies
c. Biochemical markers
d. Histopathological studies
e. Imaging studies

Ans. d. When predicting poor prognosis about patients who are comatose after resuscitation from cardiac arrest, tests should have 100% specificity or zero false positive rate (FPR). Prognostication of the comatose postcardiac arrest patient should involve multiple types of tests of brain injury, and should be done after 72 hours from cardiac arrest. By this time, any neurological recovery and full clearance of sedatives can occur. *Clinical examination*—GCS score, pupillary response to light, corneal reflex, and presence of seizures. *Neurophysiological studies*—somatosensory evoked potentials (SSEPs) and electroencephalography (EEG). *Biochemical markers*—neuron-specific enolase (NSE) is the most commonly used. *Imaging studies*—brain CT and magnetic resonance imaging (MRI).

CHAPTER 28 Intensive Care Management MCQs

Devendra Richhariya

Q1. Following are the high-flow oxygen delivery system, *except:*

a. Air entrainment (venturi) mask (AEM)
b. Air entrainment nebulizer
c. Blending system
d. Nonrebreathing circuit (closed)

Ans. d. Nonrebreathing circuit (closed) is low flow oxygen delivery system.

Q2. What is the most common complication of hyperbaric oxygen therapy (HBOT)?

a. Barotrauma of the ear
b. Cataract
c. Exacerbation of preexisting infection
d. Sensorineural hearing loss

Ans. a. Barotrauma is usually due to pressure of the gas characterized by ear pain and discomfort. Cataract per se does not happen but a possibility of increased opaqueness of lens has been noted in patients with preexisting cataract. HBOT is used in treatment of other two conditions.

Q3. Medicines with absolute contraindications to HBOT include all, *except*:

a. Bleomycin
b. Cisplatin
c. Doxorubicin
d. Sulfamethoxazole

Ans. d. Bleomycin causes interstitial pneumonitis, cisplatin leads to impaired wound healing, and doxorubicin causes cardiotoxicity.

Q4. Off label indications for HBOT include all, *except:*

a. Cerebral palsy
b. Migraine
c. Multiple sclerosis
d. Idiopathic sudden sensorineural hearing loss

Ans. d. It is an ECHM (European Committee on Hyperbaric Medicine) approved indication of HBOT.

Q5. HBOT is used because—mark the below sentences True/False.

a. It suppresses bacterial growth
b. It helps in angiogenesis
c. It is bacteriostatic for anaerobes
d. It enhances the effects of antibiotics

Ans. a. True, b. True, c. False, and d. True

Hyperbaric oxygen therapy enhances leukocyte killing activity thereby suppressing bacterial growth and enhancing antimicrobial effects. It promotes neovascularization and is bactericidal for anaerobic organisms.

Q6. For patients in hyperbaric chambers—mark the below sentences True/False.

a. Intravenous (IV) infusions should be given in glass bottles
b. Syringe pumps operated by battery can be used
c. Defibrillators are safe to be used in case of sudden cardiac arrest
d. All balloon devices should be filled with fluid in place of air

Ans. a. False, b. True, c. False, and d. True

Intravenous infusions should be given by flexible bags only. Battery operated syringe pumps are safe to use. Defibrillation inside chamber is controversial and chamber should be decompressed before using it. Fluids in place of air in balloon devices will prevent their rupture due to air expansion.

Q7. Which of the following is not the indication for noninvasive ventilation (NIV)?

a. Acute hypoxemic respiratory failure
b. Obstructive sleep apnea-hypopnea syndrome
c. Obesity hypoventilation syndrome
d. Severe hemodynamic instability of the patient

Ans. d. Severe hemodynamic instability of the patient is a contraindication for the NIV.

Q8. Noninvasive positive pressure ventilation (NIPPV) works by:

a. Decreasing inspiratory work of breathing (WOB)
b. Decreasing inspiratory muscles work
c. Decreasing "pressure-time product" (PTP) of inspiratory muscle
d. Increase in preload and afterload

Ans. d. Positive pressure application in NIV reduces the WOB by 60% through several mechanisms; similarly pressure support (PS) application also reduces the WOB by decreasing the inspiratory transpulmonary pressure. Positive end-expiratory pressure (PEEP) and PS helps in improving ventilation perfusion mismatch, oxygenation, and removal of carbon dioxide removal.

Q9. Which of the following are the causes of high peak pressure but normal of low plateau pressure in mechanically ventilated patient?

a. Bronchospasm
b. Mucous plugging
c. Acute respiratory distress syndrome (ARDS)
d. Foreign body aspiration

Ans. c. Acute respiratory distress syndrome associated with high peak pressure but high plateau pressure

Q10. What are the ideal qualities for sedative-analgesic for mechanically ventilated patient?

a. Rapid onset
b. Short acting
c. Adequately controls the symptoms
d. No immediate or late adverse effects
e. All

Ans. e. Unfortunately, no ideal medication is present. Medications are typically divided into two classes first for analgesia and second those for sedation.

Q11. To standardize the level of a patient's consciousness in mechanically ventilated patient, which of the following scales are used?

a. Richmond agitation-sedation scale (RASS)
b. Riker sedation-agitation scale
c. Both
d. None

Ans. c. *The Richmond agitation-sedation scale and the Riker sedation-agitation scale* are most commonly used and helpful to standardize the level of a patient's consciousness. Sedation scoring scales also helpful to standardize communication between healthcare workers and specifies targets for medication titration.

Q12. Which parameter is the best predictor of a successful spontaneous breathing trial (SBT)?

a. Respiratory rate 30 breaths/min
b. Heart rate 50 beats/min

c. Tidal volume 3 mL/kg ideal body weight
d. Absent altered mental status
e. High Rapid Shallow Breathing Index (RSBI)

Ans. d. The evaluation should be a holistic assessment which consists of a patient's general clinical stability and hemodynamic parameters, i.e., heart rate (between 60 and 140 beats/min), ability to manage secretions, respiratory effort (respiratory rate between 8 and 30 breaths/min), oxygen saturation >92%, PaO_2 >70 mm Hg, and spontaneous tidal volume >5 mL/kg ideal body weight. It is also important to ensure the absence of severe anxiety or altered mental status.

A high RSBI indicates the patient's inability to tolerate independent breathing.

Q13. Which of the following condition requires continuous mechanical ventilation?

a. Multifocal stroke
b. Thoracolumbar spinal injury
c. Chronic obstructive lung disease
d. Interfacility transfer
e. Postendoscopic procedure

Ans. d. A clinician has to ensure no other anticipated factors which will require continuous mechanical ventilation, e.g., intracranial pathologies (severe brain injury or brainstem stroke), cervical spine injury, acute airway trauma, acute lung injury, pneumonia, drowning, or interfacility transfer and transport. Extubation under strict monitoring can be considered in chronic obstructive lung disease.

Q14. What is the mainstay of treatment for postextubation cardiopulmonary dysfunction?

a. Intravenous nitroglycerin
b. Nebulize salbutamol
c. Intravenous infusion norepinephrine
d. Venturi mask oxygen
e. Intravenous furosemide

Ans. a. Postextubation cardiopulmonary dysfunction is similar to acute cardiogenic pulmonary edema. The signs and symptoms include tachypnea, increased WOB, hyperdynamic responses, and progressive hypoxemic respiratory failure.

Point-of-care lung ultrasound will demonstrate new B-lines to suggest "wet lungs". NIV and intravenous nitroglycerin remain the mainstays of acute management. Diuretics may also be helpful in removing excess fluid and decrease pulmonary congestion.

Q15. What is the best modality to reduce reintubation rate in patients with postextubation hypoxemic respiratory failure?

a. Noninvasive ventilation
b. High-flow nasal cannula (HFNC)
c. Nonrebreather mask
d. Bag mask ventilation
e. Nasopharyngeal airway

Ans. b. High-flow nasal cannula has potential benefits in reducing reintubation rate in patients with postextubation hypoxemic respiratory failure safely and effectively. It can improve ventilation-perfusion mismatch and gas exchange, as well as preventing shunt, recruiting the lungs and preventing atelectasis.

Q16. What is the best method to assess the risk for postextubation laryngeal edema?

a. Arterial blood gas
b. Flexible endoscopy
c. Airway ultrasound
d. Computer tomography (CT) of the neck
e. Lateral cervical radiograph

Ans. c. The airway patency can be assessed by using ultrasonography. The difference of air column width at the level of the vocal cords between pre- and postendotracheal cuff deflation can be measured. A lower air column width difference and air column width during endotracheal cuff deflation were found in patients who developed postextubation stridor.

Q17. Indicators which are feasible for emergency department (ED) extubation are all, *except:*

a. Documentation of a challenging airway
b. Good cough reflex
c. Low ventilator setting
d. Improved mental status

Ans. a. Patient should not have any known or documented glottic swelling, upper airway obstruction, or difficult laryngoscopic intubation at the initial ED or prehospital care (PHC) airway management.

Q18. Regarding SBT, which statement is not true?

a. Absence of altered mental status predicts successful SBT
b. Continuous positive airway pressure (CPAP) is the mode of setting
c. High RSBI shows the patient's ability to tolerate independent breathing
d. Pressure support SBT is the recommended screening method for extubation

Ans. c. High rapid shallow breathing index (RSBI) indicates patient's inability to tolerate independent breathing.

Q19. Regarding postextubation complications, which statement is false?

a. Cuff leak test (CLT) identifies risks for laryngeal edema
b. Clinical features are similar to acute cardiogenic pulmonary edema
c. Nonrebreather oxygen has benefit in reducing reintubation rate
d. The airway patency can be assessed by ultrasonography

Ans. c. High-flow nasal oxygen (HFNO) is an alternative modality to reduce risk of reintubation as compared to standard oxygen therapy in intensive care unit (ICU) patients.

Q20. Regarding palliative extubation in ED, all statements are true, *except:*

a. It would be an appropriate indication in a patient whom aggressive care is not beneficial
b. Clinical decision making is ethically challenging
c. Opioid infusion is part of a standard palliative care
d. It should be indirectly communicated with the patient's family

Ans. d. Ethical decision making in regards of palliative extubation should be communicated directly to the patient's family and it should involve all members of a care team. Moreover, palliative extubation is an important skill set for emergency physicians.

Q21. Conditions that can be considered for ED extubation include:

a. Cervical spine injury
b. Clinically improved drug intoxication
c. Myasthenia crisis
d. Acute epiglottitis

Ans. b. Cervical spine injury Myasthenia crisis. Acute epiglottitis are the clinical conditions may potentially require prolonged invasive mechanical ventilation. The risk of extubation failure should also be anticipated.

Q22. Regarding peripheral catheters, which statement is true?

a. Peripheral catheters are appropriate for treatment of central compatible medications
b. Volume <900 mOsm/L
c. Peripheral catheters are appropriate for vesicant or irritant
d. Duration of treatment >10 days
e. A high risk of infection

Ans. b. Peripheral catheters are considered appropriate for treatment of peripherally compatible medications and solutions (<900 mOsm/L, not vesicant or irritant) and duration of treatment <6 days with transition to midline or peripherally inserted central catheter (PICC) when duration is extended. Peripheral catheters need access into the veins and arteries of the arms and legs for pediatric or neonatal applications. Peripheral access has a lower risk of infection (0.5/1,000 catheter days).

Q23. Which statement for using a central venous catheter (CVC) is false?

a. Ideal for administering inotropes
b. Can monitor central venous pressure (CVP)
c. Jugular access has less complication than subclavicle vein
d. Can be used for cardiac catheterization
e. Commonly used for transvenous cardiac pacing

Ans. c. In the emergency department, CVCs are inserted for a large number of different indications: administering drugs (vasopressors/inotropes and antibiotics), monitoring CVP, measurement of central venous oxygen saturation ($ScvO_2$), poor peripheral venous access, cardiac catheterization, and transvenous cardiac pacing.

Q24. Mark the below statement True/False regarding indications for PICC:

a. Hemodynamically unstable patients where cardiac monitoring or use of vasopressors is necessary
b. Continuous infusions of vesicant, chemically irritating
c. For cyclic chemotherapy where treatment is <3 months
d. Patients receiving frequent phlebotomy
e. For burn patients where early implementation of PICC increases risk of bacteremia

Ans. **a. False, b. True, c. False, d. True, and e. False**

Hemodynamically unstable patients where cardiac monitoring or use of vasopressors is necessary in cases <14 days and >15 days (CVCs favored over PICCs).

For use with continuous infusions of vesicant, parenteral nutrition, chemically irritating, or nonperipherally compatible solutions for any duration.

For cyclic chemotherapy with active cancer where treatment is >3 months. Consideration given to discontinuation of PICC when each cycle complete (peripheral catheter preferred when >3 months).

Use with patients receiving frequent phlebotomy of every 8 hours or more often with duration of 6 days or more.

For burn patients where early implementation of PICC decreases risk of bacteremia.

For use in patients in palliative treatment, actively dying or in hospice requiring IV solutions.

Q25. All are the complications of femoral artery access, *except:*

a. Bleeding at the puncture site (hematoma)
b. Thrombosis and occlusion
c. Venous thrombosis
d. Pseudoaneurysm
e. Injury of a nerve

Ans. c. Femoral artery access complications are bleeding at the puncture site (hematoma), thrombosis and occlusion of the radial artery (1.5–35%), local or general infection from the catheter, pseudoaneurysm (mean incidence 0.09%), injury of a nerve causing pain or transient functional impairment, obstruction of the arterial catheter with a clot, atheroma thrombus with arterial ischemia, and arterial spasm.

Q26. Mark the statement True or False regarding contraindications of intraosseous (IO) access.

a. Fractures in the same extremity as the targeted bone
b. Previous surgery in the bone
c. Cutaneous infection
d. Local vascular compromise
e. Previous failed IO insertion within 1 month in the targeted bone

Ans. a. True, b. True, c. False, d. True, and e. False

Contraindications to IO access: Fractures in the same extremity as the targeted bone; Previous surgery involving hardware in the bone targeted for IO access; Infection at the insertion site or within the targeted bone; Local vascular compromise; Previous failed IO insertion within 24 hours in the targeted bone; Inability to locate the landmarks.

Q27. Preferred resuscitation fluid in a patient with traumatic brain injury (TBI) is:

a. Albumin
b. Ringer's lactate
c. 5% dextrose
d. 0.9% saline

Ans. d. Fluids which are hypotonic to plasma including Ringer's lactate, PlasmaLyte, and 5% dextrose should be avoided in patients with raised intracranial pressures (including patients with TBI). Albumin when compared to 0.9% saline in patients with (TBI) lead to worse outcomes and should be avoided in this population.

Q28. Which of the following is a false statement regarding balanced salt solutions?

a. Lactate in Ringer's lactate solution can raise plasma lactate making it harder to use trends in lactate to guide fluid management
b. PlasmaLyte contains acetate and gluconate as buffers instead of lactate
c. Sterofundin contains acetate and maleate as buffers
d. Ringer's lactate contains higher sodium and lower chloride and thus resembles the electrolyte composition of plasma more closely than PlasmaLyte

Ans. d. PlasmaLyte contains higher sodium and lower chloride and thus resembles the electrolyte composition of plasma more closely than Ringer's lactate. PlasmaLyte contains acetate and gluconate as buffers instead of lactate and claims to eliminate the problems with the use of lactate. In spite of these, no studies have proven it to be superior to much cheaper Ringer's lactate in terms of clinical outcomes.

Q29. Mark the statement True or False—transfusion of large volume of normal saline to a patient may lead to:

a. Acidosis
b. Alkalosis
c. Increase in strong ion difference (SID)
d. Worse renal outcomes

Ans. **a. True, b. False, c. False, and d. True**

Transfusion of large volume of normal (0.9%) saline will lead to a decrease in SID and hyperchloremic metabolic acidosis. Several observational trials show an association of saline resuscitation and adverse renal outcomes.

Q30. Synthetic colloids are associated with following adverse effects: mark the statement True or False.

a. Renal injury
b. Pruritus
c. Coagulopathy
d. Anaphylactic reactions

Ans. **a. True, b. True, c. True, and d. True**

Several large multicenter randomized controlled trials have suggested that use of hydroxyethyl starch (HES) is associated with increased incidence of acute kidney injury and probably mortality in critically ill patients in general and septic patients in particular. Synthetic colloids are also associated with other important adverse effects, such as coagulopathy, anaphylactoid reactions, and pruritus.

Q31. Regarding maintenance fluid therapy in hospitalized patients: mark the statement True or False.

a. The goal of maintenance fluid therapy is to sustain normal water and electrolyte balance and volume status
b. All hospitalized patients must receive IV fluids even if they are able to take adequate oral intake
c. Maintenance fluids are typically hypotonic but isotonic fluids may be used if there is risk of hyponatremia
d. Requirements increase by 100–150 mL/day for each degree of body temperature elevation above 37°C

Ans. **a. True, b. False, c. True, and d. True**

The goal of maintenance fluid therapy is to sustain normal water and electrolyte balance and volume status. It should only be undertaken if oral or enteral feeding is not possible and must be distinguished from fluid resuscitation. Additional fluid and electrolyte supplements may be needed to replace the extra ongoing losses like diarrhea or rise in body temperature. Serum sodium concentration must be monitored and maintenance fluids must be switched to isotonic crystalloids, if possibility of hyponatremia exists.

Q32. A pulmonary artery catheter must be wedged in which of the following locations?

a. Zone 1
b. Zone 2
c. Zone 3
d. Does not matter

Ans. d. The lung can be divided into three vertical zones with varying pressure changes. For pulmonary capillary wedge pressure (PCWP) to be reliable, the catheter tip must lie in zone 3. Pulmonary artery pressure (P_{pa}) is greater than pulmonary venous pressure (P_{pv}), which is greater than alveolar pressure (P_{alv}) at end-expiration. In zones 1 and 2, P_{pw} reflects P_{alv} if P_{alv} is greater than P_{pv}.

Q33. In spontaneously breathing patient, the method of choice for assessment of fluid responsiveness is:

a. Pulse pressure variation
b. MAP (mean arterial pressure)
c. Passive leg raise
d. Bioreactance

Ans. c. In fully mechanically ventilated patients, dynamic measurements of heart-lung interaction such as stroke volume variation are superior to static measures of preload in assessing whether a patient is volume-responsive. For patients who are not fully mechanically ventilated, pulse contour analysis allows real-time assessment of increases in cardiac output in response to passive leg raising.

Q34. All conditions decrease $SvO_2/ScvO_2$, *except:*

a. Hemorrhagic shock
b. Malignant hyperthermia
c. Vasodilatory shock
d. Cardiogenic shock

Ans. c. Hemorrhage, severe anemia, and heart failure, all these conditions decrease tissue oxygen supply thereby decreasing venous oxygen as well. Hyperthermia, fever, exercise, etc. increase tissue oxygen extraction as venous oxygen saturation is decreased as well. In vasodilatory shock tissue oxygen supply is increased and in certain conditions like cytopathic hypoxia and severe sepsis, tissue utilization of oxygen is also hampered and therefore venous oxygen saturation is increased.

Q35. Regarding hemodynamic monitoring: mark the statement True or False.

a. Ultrasonic cardiac output monitor (USCOM) is a bedside and noninvasive technique
b. The pulse contour cardiac output [pulse-induced contour cardiac output (PiCCO)] system requires lithium indicator dilution
c. Esophageal Doppler uses pulse contour analysis
d. Use of the pulmonary artery catheter in critical care is associated with improved patient outcome.
e. The noninvasive cardiac output monitor (NICOM) system uses bioreactance.

Ans. **a. True, b. False, c. False, d. False, and e. True**

Pulmonary catheter was a standard CO monitor for many years and widely adopted but pulmonary artery catheter (PAC) was introduced without any clinical trials establishing benefit in critically ill patients, and after several years of use concerns over its safety and efficacy were raised. In clinical trials, major clinical outcome benefit was not found rather it was found to increase mortality and morbidity. LidCO and not PiCCO uses lithium indicator dilution, PiCCO uses thermodilution. Esophageal Doppler assesses aortic flow and not pulse contour. Bioreactance is one of the methods of NICOM, USG-guided assessment of hemodynamics or also known as USCOM is also a noninvasive technique which can easily be done at the bedside.

Q36. Regarding fluid responsiveness assessment in critically ill patient: mark the statement True or False.

a. Static and dynamic variables are equally useful
b. Stroke volume variation/pulse pressure variation (SVV/PPV) measurement requires the patient to be mechanically ventilated at 8 mL/kg tidal volume
c. PPV <8% is suggestive of volume responsiveness
d. Dynamic variables working principle is based on heart-lung interaction
e. Atrial fibrillation is not a contraindication for PPV calculation

Ans. a. False, b. True, c. False, d. True, and e. False
Dynamic variables are found to be superior to static variables for fluid responsiveness assessment. In dynamic variables, PPV/SVV are very commonly use. They need placement of an arterial line and pulse contour analysis is used for CO monitoring. Variation of pulse pressure with respiratory cycle in mechanically ventilated patient, at least with 8 mL/kg of tidal volume, correlates well with volume responsiveness. PPV >12% is categorized as cut off for volume responsiveness. They should not be used in isolation. Limitations such as irregular heart rhythms or low tidal volumes must be recognized.

Q37. Which of the following is not a clinical manifestation of hypernatremia?

a. Hypotension
b. Hypothermia
c. Tachycardia
d. Oliguria
e. Confusion

Ans. b. Clinical findings are based on volume deficiency, hypertonicity, and dehydration in the cells in central nervous system. Hypotension, orthostatic hypotension, tachycardia, oliguria, dryness of the skin and mucous membranes, and turgor tonus decrease occur due to hypovolemia. In addition, lethargy, irritability, cloudiness, confusion, widespread weakness, myoclonic jerks, seizures, and coma are neurological signs and symptoms.

Q38. Which of the following is incorrect for the treatment of hypernatremia?

a. In acute hypernatremia, serum sodium should be reduced to 2–3 mEq/L/hour and not >12 mEq/L/day
b. In patients with asymptomatic or mildly symptomatic chronic hypernatremia, serum sodium should be reduced by 0.5 mEq/hour and not >8–10 mEq/24 hours

c. In patients with hypervolemic hypernatremia, hemodialysis treatment is planned for patients with loop diuretics and, if necessary, severe loading findings
d. If hypernatremia has acute or life-threatening symptoms, treatment with isotonic fluids and loop diuretics should be initiated immediately
e. During the hypernatremia treatment, the patients are followed-up with hourly neurological examination and serum and urine electrolyte measurements

Ans. d. The goal is to decrease serum sodium by not >12 mEq in 24 hours. Close serial monitoring of serum sodium every 2–4 hours is essential during the acute phase of correction. Seizures occurring during correction of hypernatremia are a sign of cerebral edema due to rapid shifts in osmolality, and the administration of hypotonic fluids should be halted. The estimated free water deficit should be corrected over 48–72 hours with a decrease in serum sodium not exceeding 0.5 mEq/hour. Patients should be carefully monitored for the rate of correction, urine output, and ongoing losses. During the treatment, the patient is followed up with hourly neurological examination, serum, and urine electrolyte measurements. If hypernatremia has acute or life-threatening symptoms, treatment with hypotonic fluids should be initiated immediately. In patients with hypervolemic hypernatremia, hemodialysis treatment is planned for patients with loop diuretics and, if necessary, severe loading findings.

Q39. Which of the following is a laboratory test used in the differential diagnosis of hyponatremia?

a. Serum and urine osmolality
b. Coagulation tests
c. Ketonuria and ketonemia
d. Complete blood count
e. Arterial blood gases

Ans. a. Urinary sodium, serum, and urine osmolality together with serum sodium level are important tests for diagnosis. Urine osmolality is <100 mOsm in primary polydipsia. Urinary osmolality above 100 mOsm shows high antidiuretic hormone (ADH) level. Serum osmolality is important for the differential diagnosis of real and pseudohyponatremia. Due to hyperlipidemia or hyperproteinemia (such as myeloma) in pseudohyponatremia, the protein or lipid ratio of plasma fluid drops from 97 to 80%. For this reason, serum sodium level is measured high. In this state, the patient's osmolality is normal.

Q40. Which of the following is not an ECG sign of hyperkalemia?

a. Peaked T wave
b. Shortened QT interval
c. Loss of P wave
d. Widening of the QRS complex
e. Sinus tachycardia

Ans. e. Typical ECG findings in hyperkalemia progress from tall, "peaked" T waves and a shortened QT interval to lengthening PR interval and loss of P waves, and then to widening of the QRS complex culminating in a "sine wave" morphology and death if not treated.

Q41. Which of the following is used to treat severe hyperkalemia with ECG findings?

a. 1–2 g IV magnesium sulfate
b. IV isotonic fluid resuscitation
c. IV 10% calcium chloride 10 mL is infused with slow push (at 5–10 minutes)
d. 20 unit insulin in 5% dextrose 200 mL
e. 20% mannitol 1–2 g/kg

Ans. c. Patients with severe hyperkalemia, potassium levels above 7 mEq/L, and patients with cardiac rhythm problems in ECG are monitored by immediately opening the airway and vascular access. IV 10% calcium chloride 10 mL is infused with slow push (at 5–10 minutes).

Q42. The following may be signs of hypokalemia. Mark each statement True or False.

a. Nausea and vomiting
b. Muscle weakness
c. Dehydration
d. Ileus

Ans. **a. True, b. True, c. False, and d. True**

Significant muscle weakness occurs at serum potassium levels below 2.5 mmol/L but can occur at higher levels if the onset is acute. Similar to the weakness associated with hyperkalemia, the pattern is ascending in nature affecting the lower extremities, progressing to involve the trunk and upper extremities and potentially advancing to paralysis. Affected muscles can include the muscles of respiration which can lead to respiratory failure and death. Involvement of gastrointestinal (GI) muscles can cause an ileus with associated symptoms of nausea, vomiting, and abdominal distension. Severe hypokalemia can also lead to muscle cramps, rhabdomyolysis, and resultant myoglobinuria. Periodic paralysis is a rare neuromuscular disorder, which is inherited or acquired, that is caused by an acute transcellular shift of potassium into the cells. It is characterized by potentially fatal episodes of muscle weakness or paralysis that can affect the respiratory muscles. Dehydration is not a symptom of hypokalemia.

Q43. The following are important principles of potassium replacement for hypokalemia patients. Mark each statement True or False.

a. Oral potassium tablets are sufficient for mild to moderate hypokalemia
b. IV aggressive treatments are required in patients with cardiac rhythm problems or severe hypokalemia
c. Maximum 20 mEq IV potassium replacement can be performed per hour
d. Maximum IV 220 mEq replacement can be done daily

Ans. a. True, b. True, c. True, and d. False

Mild-to-moderate hypokalemia (2.5–3.5 mEq/L) is usually minimally symptomatic or asymptomatic. Replacing these patients with oral potassium tablets is sufficient. IV and more aggressive treatments are required in patients with cardiac rhythm problems or severe hypokalemia. Potassium can cause phlebitis during IV application. Maximum 20 mEq IV potassium replacement can be performed per hour. Both ECG and serum potassium levels monitoring should be done during replacement. Maximum IV 120 mEq replacement can be done daily.

Q44. The following are symptoms and signs of hypercalcemia. Mark each statement True or False.

a. Diarrhea
b. Fatigue and muscle weakness
c. Disorientation, seizures, and coma
d. Short QT interval, widening PR interval, and QRS complex

Ans. a. False, b. True, c. True, and d. True

Generally, hypercalcemia has serious negative effects on the neuromuscular system, central nervous system, and cardiovascular system. Fatigue, muscle weakness, exhaustion, depression, hallucination at higher blood levels, disorientation, loss of tonus, seizures, and coma may be seen. In severe hypercalcemia, signs of dehydration can be seen, as the kidneys' ability to concentrate urine is affected. Severe hypercalcemia inhibits myocardial depolarization leading to arrhythmias. Cardiovascular effects include prolonged PR interval, short QT interval, widened QRS complex, and bradycardia.

Q45. The following are treatment principle of hypocalcemia. Mark each statement True or False.

a. In severe hypocalcemia, IV 10–20 mL of 10% calcium gluconate is given in 100 mL of 5% dextrose or isotonic sodium chloride in 10 minutes
b. Patients with either severe hypocalcemia, usually <7.5 mg/dL, or with neurological manifestations or stridor (laryngo-/bronchospasm) should receive orally calcium tablets
c. Moderately acute (corrected calcium level 7.5–8 mg/dL or ionized calcium level 1.9–2.1 mEq/L) or chronic hypocalcemia patients should be treated with orally calcium
d. Magnesium deficiency should also be treated when present, since it can attenuate the effect of the treatment by calcium and vitamin D

Ans. **a. True, b. False, c. True, and d. True**

Patients with either severe hypocalcemia, usually <7.5 mg/dL, or with neurological manifestations or stridor (laryngo-/bronchospasm) should receive IV calcium. Calcium gluconate (90 mg calcium per 10 mL) should be given as IV slow pushes, generally one vial over 10 minutes, repeated once with electrocardiographic monitoring. A chronic IV drip is then started if the patient is still symptomatic and oral treatment cannot act rapidly enough. The infusion rate should be guided by signs, symptoms, and calcium measurements checked every 1–2 hours, preferably ionized calcium levels. Magnesium deficiency should also be treated when present, since it can attenuate the effect of the treatment by calcium and vitamin D.

Q46. The following are symptoms of hypomagnesemia. Mark each statement True or False.

a. Ventricular arrhythmias
b. Weakness
c. Convulsion
d. Flask muscle paralysis

Ans. **a. True, b. True, c. True, and d. False**

Signs and symptoms related to the neuromuscular system and cardiovascular system are at the forefront. Tremor, weakness, apathy, irritability, convulsion, tetany, and coma can be seen. In addition, atrial and ventricular arrhythmias related to the cardiovascular system can be observed. Flask muscle paralysis is not a finding in hypomagnesemia. It is seen in magnesium poisoning.

Q47. Which of these should be reliable for the assessment and treatment of pain?

a. Healthcare worker's impression
b. Patient's position, expression, and movement
c. Patient's response to a generous dose of an opioid analgesic
d. Patient's subjective report of pain
e. Vital signs

Ans. d. The patient's subjective reporting of pain, not the healthcare worker's impression, is the basis for pain assessment and treatment. There is poor correlation between vital signs such as tachycardia and tachypnea or changes in patient expression and movement, and the patient's report of pain. The amount of opioids required to treat pain can vary a great deal among different patients. Response to a fixed amount of pain medication does not correlate with the amount of pain an individual is experiencing.

Q48. What is an appropriate endpoint for pain management?

a. Comfortable appearing patient
b. Normalization of vital signs
c. Pain score of 2 or less using a 1–10 numeric rating
d. Sleeping patient
e. Sufficient pain relief as determined by the patient

Ans. e. A value assigned by a patient on a validated pain scale depends on multiple factors including the patient's past personal experiences; therefore, a discrete number cannot be used as an endpoint for acceptable pain management. The endpoint for pain management is the patient's judgment about their pain relief. The interpretation of pain is variable, and the only relevant goal should be that which satisfies the needs of the patient. Vital signs do not correlate well with the subjective rating of a patient's pain.

Q49. Which of the following is true regarding pain management?

a. Anxiolytics should not be combined with narcotics due to the increased risk of respiratory depression
b. Dosing of opioid analgesics is straightforward and most patients of similar size and age require similar doses
c. Opioid agonist-antagonists have no benefit over pure opioid agonists
d. Patients of all ages tend to report pain in similar ways
e. The proper use of opioids requires consideration of side effects, initial dose, route and timing of onset, and frequency of administration

Ans. e. *Proper use of opioids requires consideration of the following:* Route and frequency of administration, desired time of onset of action, initial dose, concurrent use of nonopioid analgesics and adjunctive agents, and incidence and severity of side effects. Acute pain is usually accompanied by anxiety and feelings of loss of control. Anxiolytics should be considered if reassurance is insufficient. Patient response to opioid analgesics depends on age, body mass, and previous or chronic exposure to opioids and can vary greatly between individuals. The elderly often report pain very differently than younger patients for various reasons. Unlike pure opioids, opioid agonists–antagonists have a ceiling on respiratory depression despite higher doses.

Q50. For which of the following conditions is a tricyclic antidepressant considered first-line therapy?

a. Complex regional pain syndrome, type 1, also known as reflex sympathetic dystrophy
b. HIV-related neuropathy
c. Phantom limb pain
d. Postherpetic neuralgia
e. Spinal cord injury pain

Ans. d. In general, tricyclic antidepressants are an effective therapy in patients with neuropathic pain, which includes postherpetic neuralgia; however, antidepressants are not effective for spinal cord injury pain, phantom limb pain, and HIV-related neuropathy. Intranasal calcitonin (but no other therapy studied) was recommended by a meta-analysis for complex regional pain syndrome, type 1.

Q51. Which of these is not considered an indication for emergency procedural sedation?

a. Cardioversion for a wide complex tachycardia in a 78-year-old female with chest pain and dizziness
b. Intractable pain from a dislocated shoulder in a 34-year-old male
c. Obtaining a CT scan in an agitated 15-year-old football player who sustained a head injury
d. Reduction of an elbow dislocation in a 65-year-old female with an absent radial pulse
e. Sexual assault examination in a 6-year-old girl who was assaulted an hour ago

Ans. e. Emergent indications for procedural sedation and analgesia include cardioversion for life-threatening arrhythmias, neuroimaging for head trauma, reduction in fractures or dislocations with soft tissue or vascular compromise, care of contaminated wounds, or intractable pain. Sexual assault examinations require less urgent sedation.

Q52. Which vital sign is recommended to be continuously monitored for all levels of sedation, from minimal to deep?

a. Blood pressure
b. End-tidal carbon dioxide (capnography)
c. Oxygen saturation
d. Pulse
e. Respiratory rate

Ans. c. It is recommended that oxygenation be monitored continuously for all levels of sedation. Pulse, respiration, and end-tidal carbon dioxide should be monitored continuously for moderate to deep sedation, and blood pressure should be monitored every 5 minutes in these cases. For minimal sedation, heart rate, respiratory rate, and blood pressure are monitored every 15 minutes with blood pressure readings after medication boluses as well.

Q53. Which of the following is not the determinant of microcirculatory endpoint of resuscitation?

a. Lactate
b. Mixed and venous oxygen saturation
c. Central venous-arterial CO_2 gradient
d. Capillary filling time

Ans. d. Capillary filling time is clinical assessment of perfusion

Q54. Which of the following statements about the management of tracheostomy tubes is most accurate?

a. Patients with tracheostomies and respiratory distress should first be suctioned through the inner cannula with sterile saline and preoxygenation
b. Patients with tracheostomies and respiratory distress should first have the inner cannula removed and cleaned and be suctioned through the tracheotomy tube
c. Patients with tracheostomies and respiratory distress should first have the tracheostomy tube removed and be suctioned through the stoma
d. Patients with tracheostomies <7 days old can be manipulated by an ED physician if the proper technique is used
e. When pediatric tracheostomy tubes are crusted or clogged, only the inner cannula should be removed for cleaning

Ans. a. Tracheostomy tube obstruction with mucous plugging is common. It is best treated with preoxygenation (as suctioning may cause transient hypoxia) and then placing of sterile saline into the trachea and suctioning through large flexible catheters through the inner cannula. If this does not succeed, remove the inner cannula and clean with hydrogen peroxide and rinse with water. Sometimes, the entire tracheostomy tube needs to be removed and cleaned. Tracheostomy tubes <7 days in maturation should be manipulated only by otolaryngology surgeons. Pediatric tracheostomies do not have inner cannulas.

Q55. Sepsis management essentially includes:

a. Resuscitation and hemodynamic stabilization
b. Infection control
c. Modulation of host response
d. All

Ans. d. Sepsis management starts right in the emergency room with triaging. *Surviving sepsis campaign (SSC) suggests 1-hour bundle for early sepsis management.*

Q56. Objectives of implementing the "Code Sepsis" in ED are:

a. Streamline the medical service response
b. Earliest completion of Hour-1 bundle
c. Reduce mortality related to sepsis
d. All

Ans. d. "Code Sepsis" in emergency department is adopted in many emergency rooms, to streamline the response and rapid deployment of specialized medical service. Code concept revolves around earliest completion of Hour-1 bundle and meeting the targets of resuscitation. This exercise improves compliance to SSC care bundle and has been proven to reduce mortality related to sepsis.

Q57. Which of the following is not an indication for surgical cricothyroidotomy?

a. Uncontrollable emesis
b. Young patient age <12 years
c. Upper airway stenosis
d. Facial muscle spasm

Ans. b. Surgical cricothyrotomy is a relative contraindication in children <5–12 years because of the funnel shape of the pediatric airway and a theoretically increased risk of subglottic stenosis.

Q58. Which of the following is not true regarding cricothyroidotomy?

a. Cricothyroid membrane is situated between thyroid and cricoid cartilage

b. Cricothyroidotomy is contraindicated in age <12 years
c. Position of patient should be in supine with neck in hyperextension
d. Cricothyroidotomy can provide supplemental oxygenation

Ans. c.

Q59. All of the following is false, except:

a. IV cannula is inserted in cricothyroid membrane at 55° angle in caudal direction
b. IV cannula is inserted in cricothyroid membrane at 55° angle in cephalad direction
c. IV cannula is inserted in cricothyroid membrane at 45° angle in caudal direction
d. IV cannula is inserted in cricothyroid membrane at 45° angle in cephalad direction

Ans. c.

Q60. The following is early complication of cricothyroidotomy. Mark True or False.

a. Bleeding
b. Hematoma
c. Laryngeal stenosis
d. Subcutaneous emphysema

Ans. a. True, b. False, c. False, and d. True

Q61. The following is contraindication of cricothyroidotomy. Mark True or False.

a. Infection at site of incision
b. Obstruction distal to cricoid membrane
c. Upper airway stenosis
d. Clenched teeth

Ans. a. True, b. True, c. False, and d. False

Cardiovascular Emergencies MCQs

Devendra Richhariya

Q1. What is the recommended door-to-electrocardiogram (ECG) time in patients presenting with chest pain?

a. 1 minute
b. 10 minutes
c. 15 minutes
d. 20 minutes
e. 30 minutes

Ans. b. The current recommendations are for ECGs to be performed as soon as possible and preferably within the first 10 minutes. This short door-to-ECG time is an effort by the American College of Cardiology (ACC) and the American Heart Association (AHA) to shorten the door-to-intervention time in patients with an acute myocardial infarction (AMI).

Q2. How many hours after a cardiac ischemia event would one expect to reliably find a positive troponin?

a. 2
b. 4
c. 6
d. 8
e. 10

Ans. c. Troponins leak out of damaged myocardium cells after prolonged ischemia. Thus, it takes 6 hours for cellular death and breakdown for these biomarkers to leak into the bloodstream. Myoglobin elevations may be seen earlier (in the 2–4 hours range). Patients who present soon after symptoms may have no elevation in biomarkers.

Q3. A patient presents with a history of hypertension and epigastric and chest pain for 3 hours with negative biomarkers. His ECG is normal. He responds to antacids and feels better. What is your next appropriate response?

a. A prescription for the proton pump inhibitor
b. Admit for cardiac workup
c. An emergent cardiac catheterization
d. Nitroglycerine
e. Repeat biomarkers

Ans. e. It is important *not* to be swayed by response to therapy in patients with chest pain. Antacids provide pain relief in 18–45% of patients with acute coronary syndrome. Lack of pain relief with nitroglycerine should also not be convincing. In one study, 65% of patients with acute coronary syndrome did not respond to nitroglycerine. This type of patient, with an atypical story of chest pain and some risk factors, should at least get a second set of biomarkers.

Q4. Which of the following conditions may lead a patient to the emergency department (ED) with "irregular palpitations?"

a. Atrial fibrillation
b. Ventricular tachycardia (VT)
c. Complete (third degree) atrioventricular (AV) block
d. Fever

Ans. a. Atrial fibrillation is a frequent arrhythmia that may occur at any age. The main feature is a supraventricular arrhythmia so defined as "irregularly irregular" because there is no p-wave and regular sinus impulse but rapid and wandering impulses from the atrium that may pass the atrioventricular node (AVN) in an irregular way. Atrial fibrillation may run asymptomatic but when it is acute and has a high ventricular rate the patient is feeling palpitations and sometimes other symptoms, such as chest pain and dyspnea. The other three conditions may cause "regular palpitations."

Q5. All of the following are considered "red flags" in a patient who presents with palpitations and needs special attention, *except:*

a. Onset after exertion
b. Syncope
c. Polyuria (true)
d. Chest pain
e. Headedness

Ans. c. When palpitation is recurrent, persistent, and provoked by exertion, or accompanied by lightheadedness, syncope, chest pain, and dyspnea, a careful workup is mandatory and if the diagnosis is not evident at the beginning of a period of observation and monitoring is necessary. Polyuria is a frequent symptom accompanying supraventricular tachycardia (SVT).

Q6. SVT may cause the following symptoms associated with palpitations. Mark the below statement as True or False.

a. Sweating
b. Chest pain
c. Polyuria
d. Diarrhea

Ans. **a. False, b. True, c. True, and d. False**

Supraventricular tachycardia is a generally benign arrhythmia caused by a reentry mechanism around the AVN or an accessory pathway, such as the Wolff–Parkinson–White syndrome. It occurs frequently in young patients and is generally well tolerated. The most frequent features are palpitations, anxiety, and polyuria, very seldom chest pain. When recurrent (several episodes in a year), it could be necessary to refer the patient to the cardiologist for ablation.

Reference:

European Society of Cardiology. (2019). 2019 ESC Guidelines for the management of patients with supraventricular tachycardia (for the management of patients with). [online] Available from https://www.escardio.org/Guidelines/Clinical-Practice-Guidelines/Supraventricular-Tachycardia [Last accessed May, 2024].

Q7. Which of the following noncardiac conditions may be the cause of palpitation as presenting symptoms to the ED? Mark the below statement as True or False.

a. Caffeine abuse
b. Hyperglycemia
c. Anemia
d. Hyponatremia

Ans. a. True, b. False, c. True, and d. False

Caffeine and any other exciting drug may cause palpitations. Anemia, in particular when the onset is rapid, or it is really severe is a cause of palpitation. Hypoglycemia causes palpitations. Sodium disorders affect conscience and vigilance but normally are not a cause of palpitations.

Q8. Which of the following arrhythmias need immediate electric cardioversion? Mark the below statement as True or False.

a. Atrial fibrillation started 72 hours before, well tolerated
b. VT
c. SVT, heart rate (HR) 180 beats per minute (BPM), blood pressure (BP) 75/40, with associated chest pain
d. Atrial flutter with an ST elevation in V1 to V4, BP 120/70 HR 100 BPM

Ans. a. False, b. False, c. True, and d. False

There is a need for immediate electric cardioversion when the tachyarrhythmia causes hemodynamic instability and symptoms of low perfusion of vital organs (chest pain, hypotension, cold sweating, low level of consciousness). Any arrhythmia, VT included, when the patient is stable, can be carefully evaluated before deciding the treatment.

Q9. In the Framingham Heart Study, which of the following was the *most* common etiology of syncope?

a. Cardiac
b. Orthostatic
c. Seizure
d. Vasovagal
e. Unknown or indeterminate

Ans. e. The longitudinal Framingham study described 822 reports of syncope in 7,814 patients followed for 17 years. The causes of syncope were vasovagal (21%), cardiac (10%), orthostatic (9%), seizure (5%), neurologic (4.1%), and unknown (37%). Other studies also report an unknown cause in about 40% of cases, despite extensive workups. Limited ED evaluations may not determine a specific cause of syncope in 50–60% of cases. The ED focus is to identify patients at increased risk of immediate decompensation or future serious morbidity or sudden death.

Q10. Which of the following causes of syncope decreases in incidence with age?

a. Cardiac syncope due to dysrhythmia
b. Cardiac syncope due to structural abnormalities
c. Neurologic syncope
d. Orthostatic hypotension
e. Vasovagal syncope

Ans. e. The incidence of vasovagal syncope actually decreases with age due to decreased responsiveness of the autonomic nervous system. Orthostatic hypotension is common in the elderly due to a less-sensitive thirst mechanism, and a decreased endocrine response to volume depletion and increased medication use.

Q11. According to the San Francisco Syncope Rules, which of the following are predictors of an adverse event in a patient with syncope?

a. Age >65 years
b. Elevated thyroid stimulating hormone (TSH) level
c. Guaiac positive stool
d. History of congestive heart failure (CHF)
e. Positive pregnancy test

Ans. d. The acronym CHESS [history of Congestive heart failure, Hematocrit <30%, abnormal ECG, a patient complaint of Shortness of breath, and a triage systolic BP <90 mm Hg] summarizes the San Francisco Syncope Rules' five predictors of adverse events, including arrhythmia and mortality: history of CHF, hematocrit <30, abnormal

ECG, shortness of breath, and systolic BP <90. Unfortunately, the etiology of syncope remains unclear in over half of the patients who presented to the ED.

Q12. Which of the following is most useful in distinguishing a grand-mal seizure from syncope?

a. Orofacial trauma
b. Prodromal symptoms
c. Tonic-clonic movements
d. Transitory wide anion gap
e. Urinary incontinence

Ans. d. Distinguishing grand-mal seizures from true syncope is essential yet very challenging. Trauma with or without defensive injuries to the hands or knees suggests a sudden event without warning, which could occur with dysrhythmia, noncardiac syncope, or seizure, so trauma is not a distinguishing feature. Urinary incontinence could occur with seizure or syncope. A transitory wide anion gap occurs after a grand mal seizure but not after an uncomplicated syncopal event.

Q13. All can result in a widened QRS complex, *except:*

a. Bundle branch block
b. Premature ventricular complex
c. Hypokalemia
d. Ventricular preexcitation

Ans. c. Sequential ventricular activation as a result of early activation of one ventricle [premature ventricular contraction (PVC) or ventricular preexcitation] or late activation of a ventricle (bundle branch block) results in the widening of the QRS complex. Hyperkalemia causes prolongation of action potential duration with resultant QRS widening. However, hypokalemia does not cause QRS widening but results in the inversion of T waves.

Q14. Sinus bradycardia is seen in all the following, *except:*

a. Normally during sleep
b. Athletes
c. Some febrile illnesses
d. Anxiety states

Ans. d. Slowing of sinus rate or sinus bradycardia may be seen physiologically during sleep or in those with high vagal tone like athletes. It is also seen in certain types of fever, e.g., typhoid fever. Anxiety states typically result in an increase in catecholamines that cause an increase in HR or sinus tachycardia.

Q15. ST-segment elevation is a hallmark of:

a. Acute myocardial infarction
b. Digitalis toxicity
c. Myocarditis
d. Hyperkalemia

Ans. a. ST-segment elevation is classically seen in acute myocardial infarction occurring because of sudden occlusion of an epicardial coronary artery and is an indication for reperfusion therapy by angioplasty or thrombolytic therapy. The other listed conditions are usually not associated with ST-segment elevation.

Q16. QT interval prolongation can occur in all the following, *except:*

a. Congenital Long QT syndrome
b. Hypercalcemia
c. Hypomagnesemia
d. Ciprofloxacin

Ans. b. Prolongation of QT interval occurs due to prolongation of repolarization as seen in congenital long QT syndrome, hypocalcemia, hypomagnesemia, and the use of certain drugs, such as fluoroquinolones and macrolides. Hypercalcemia results in the shortening of the QT interval.

Q17. Low voltage QRS complexes can be seen in all the following, *except:*

a. Obesity
b. Left ventricular hypertrophy (LVH) due to amyloidosis
c. Pericardial effusion
d. Hyperthyroidism

Ans. d. Conditions wherein there is an impediment of the flow of electricity from the heart to the surface of the body like thick chest wall, obesity, pericardial effusion, and myxedema result in attenuation of QRS voltage. Left ventricular hypertrophy in most situations causes large voltages except in amyloidosis where low voltages are seen. Hyperthyroidism does not result in low QRS voltage.

Q18. The following may be an example of wide QRS tachycardia. Mark the following statement as True or False.

a. Bundle branch reentry tachycardia
b. Idiopathic left VT
c. Orthodromic reciprocating tachycardia with normal AVN—His-Purkinje conduction
d. Sinus tachycardia in the setting of flecainide toxicity

Ans. **a. True, b. True, c. False, and d. True**

Bundle branch reentry tachycardia is a type of monomorphic VT with the QRS morphology identical to that during sinus rhythm wherein the reentrant circuit involves the left and right bundle branches.

Idiopathic left VT also known as fascicular VT is a monomorphic VT with relatively narrow QRS complexes with right bundle branch block (RBBB) morphology involving either the left posterior fascicle (more common) or left anterior fascicle (uncommon). Orthodromic reciprocating tachycardia is an SVT wherein the retrograde limb of the reentrant circuit is an AV accessory pathway and the AVN—His-Purkinje system (HPS) is the anterograde limb. Since AVN-HPS is the anterograde limb, the QRS complexes are typically narrow. Flecainide toxicity results in the widening of the QRS complexes, especially during exercise where it appears like a wide QRS tachycardia.

Q19. The following may be a feature of digitalis toxicity. Mark the following statement True or False.

a. Second degree Mobitz type II AV block
b. Atrial fibrillation
c. Junctional rhythm
d. Bidirectional VT

Ans. **a. False, b. True, c. True, and d. True**

Digitalis toxicity can result in almost any rhythm disorder except second degree Mobitz type II AV block.

Q20. The following may be a feature of severe hyperkalemia. Mark the following statement True or False.

a. Absent P wave
b. QRS widening
c. QT prolongation
d. Absence of ST segment

Ans. **a. True, b. True, c. False, and d. True**

Hyperkalemia is characterized by ECG changes of absent P waves, bradycardia, QRS widening, sinusoidal QRS-T waves, and absence of ST-segment with the end of QRS merging with the onset of T wave. QT prolongation is not a feature of hyperkalemia.

Q21. The following may be noninfarction causes of ST-segment elevation on ECG. Mark the following statement as True or False.

a. Acute pericarditis
b. Left bundle branch block (LBBB)
c. Hypokalemia
d. Early repolarization syndrome

Ans. **a. True, b. True, c. False, and d. True**

Q22. The following may be a feature of acute pulmonary embolism. Mark the following statement as True or False.

a. Sinus bradycardia
b. RBBB
c. $S_1Q_3T_3$ pattern
d. Right precordial T-wave inversion

Ans. **a. False, b. True, c. True, and d. True**

Acute pulmonary embolism results in right ventricular pressure overload and is characterized by sinus tachycardia, RBBB, right precordial T wave inversion, and $S_1Q_3T_3$ pattern.

Q23. All of the following ECG characteristics will aid in differentiating acute pericarditis from acute myocardial infarction, *except:*

a. Absence of the development of Q waves
b. Concave shape to ST elevations
c. PR depression
d. ST elevation in V2
e. T-wave inversions after the return of the ST segments to the baseline

Ans. d. The ECG in acute pericarditis without massive effusion usually displays changes secondary to acute subepicardial inflammation, in acute myocardial infarction, ST elevations are convex, and reciprocal depression is usually more prominent; these changes may return to normal within a day or two. Q waves may develop, with loss of R-wave amplitude, and T-wave inversions are usually seen within hours before the ST segments have become isoelectric.

Q24. You are evaluating a patient with chest pain in the ED. The ECG shows no Q waves or ST-segment changes. Which of the following biomarkers is the preferred biochemical marker for myocardial infarction (MI)?

a. Creatine kinase
b. CK-MB band
c. Erythrocyte sedimentation rate
d. Lactate dehydrogenase
e. Troponin I

Ans. e. Cardiac-specific troponin T (cTnT) and cardiac-specific troponin I (cTnI) have different amino acid sequences from those of the skeletal muscle forms of these proteins, the measurement of cTnT or cTnI is considered a diagnostic tool for MI.

Q25. The greatest delay between symptom onset and definitive therapy for patients with ST-segment elevation MI usually occurs in what time interval?

a. Between the onset of pain and the patient's decision to call for help
b. Between patient call and emergency medical team arrival
c. Between emergency medical team arrival and arrival at the hospital
d. Between arrival at the hospital and decision to initiation reperfusion therapy
e. Between the decision to initiate reperfusion therapy and the actual initiation of this therapy

Ans. a. Most out-of-hospital deaths from ST-elevation myocardial infarction (STEMI) are due to the sudden development of ventricular fibrillation. Therefore, prehospital care is the major element of patients with suspected STEMI. The greatest delay usually occurs not during transportation to the hospital but, rather, between the onset of pain and the patient's decision to call for help.

Q26. All the following may cause elevation of serum troponin, *except:*

a. Congestive heart failure
b. Myocarditis
c. MI
d. Pneumonia
e. Pulmonary embolism

Ans. d. Troponin elevations are not known to be caused by pneumonia in the absence of myocardial necrosis.

Q27. Which of the following medications should be avoided in stable patients with a history of heart failure?

a. Acetaminophen
b. Angiotensin-converting enzyme (ACE) inhibitors
c. Angiotensin receptor blockers
d. Beta-blockers
e. Nonsteroidal anti-inflammatory agents

Ans. e. Nonsteroidal anti-inflammatory agents inhibit the effects of ACE inhibitors and diuretics and can worsen cardiac and renal function. The emergency physician (EP) should review the medication lists of heart failure patients and also avoid prescribing nonsteroidal anti-inflammatory drugs (NSAIDs) when such patients present for injuries or chronic pain. The main risk of acetaminophen, at excessive levels, is hepatotoxicity. Stable heart failure patients are discharged on ACE inhibitors and beta-blockers because these medications have been conclusively shown to decrease mortality. Angiotensin receptor blockers have fewer side effects than ACE inhibitors but can still cause cough or angioedema.

Q28. Which of the following is the most frequent radiographic finding of left-sided heart failure?

a. Cardiomegaly
b. Dilated upper lobe vessels
c. Enlarged pulmonary artery
d. Interstitial edema
e. Pleural effusion

Ans. b. Normally, vascularity in the lower lung fields is more prominent than in the upper lung fields. The radiographic findings of left-side heart failure are, in decreasing order, dilated upper lobe vessels, cardiomegaly, interstitial edema, enlarged pulmonary artery, pleural effusion, alveolar edema, prominent superior vena cava, and Kerley lines.

Q29. Which of the following chest radiographic findings is the most sensitive for acute heart failure?

a. Alveolar edema
b. Cephalization
c. Cardiomegaly
d. Delayed findings of congestion
e. Interstitial edema

Ans. b. Echocardiography is the gold standard for heart failure, but may not be available in most EDs, Chest radiographs are readily obtainable, but findings lack sensitivity for acute heart failure. Cephalization, interstitial edema, and alveolar edema are common X-ray findings but appear after 6 hours of clinical presentation, but treatment should be started immediately.

Q30. Which of the following is the *least* frequently seen radiographic finding of left-sided heart failure?

a. Alveolar edema
b. Enlarged pulmonary artery
c. Kerley lines
d. Pleural effusion
e. Prominent superior vena cava

Ans. c. The specificities of orthopnea and dyspnea for heart failure are, respectively, 88 and 50%. Rales have a predictive accuracy of 70%. Peripheral edema and weight gain are more likely to occur in normotensive acute decompensated heart failure, which develops over days or weeks. Hypertensive heart failure, which occurs over 48 hours or less, is the most common acute presentation. Hypotensive acute heart failure is the least common presentation of acute decompensated heart failure.

Q31. Bradycardia could be due to either intrinsic or extrinsic causes or a combination of the two. Which of the following statements is False?

a. Age-related degenerative disease is the most important intrinsic cause.
b. Carotid sinus hypersensitivity is one of the possible extrinsic causes.
c. Dyselectrolytemia is the second most important intrinsic cause after age-related degenerative disease.
d. Raised intracranial pressure as an extrinsic cause should be considered while evaluating a case of bradycardia.

Ans. c.

Q32. Sinoatrial (SA) exit block refers to the delay in or the inability of formed impulse to conduct to the right atrium. Which of the following statements is Correct?

a. A first-degree SA exit block is due to an increase in the conduction of the generated impulse to the right atrium.
b. Type I second-degree SA exit block (Wenckebach) is due to a progressive delay in impulse transmission to the atrium.
c. Type II second degree SA exit block is manifested as an abrupt decrease in the P-P interval due to a blocked P wave.
d. In a complete SA exit block only some of the generated impulses is conducted to the atrium.

Ans. b.

Q33. Regarding VTs, which of the following statements is False?

a. VTs are the common cause of sudden cardiac death.
b. Ischemic and dilated cardiomyopathies are the common cause for VT
c. The prognosis of patients with VT depends on the presence of underlying structural heart disease or not.
d. In patients presenting with hemodynamic instability related to myocardial ischemia pharmacological reversion of VT can be attempted as a first step in the management of these patients.

Ans. d.

Q34. Which statement is Correct?

a. Polymorphic VT or Torsades de pointes is always self-limiting.
b. Polymorphic VT or Torsades de pointes always requiring electric cardioversion.

c. Polymorphic VT or Torsades de pointes are often associated with long QT syndrome and Brugada syndrome.
d. Polymorphic VT or Torsades de pointes is rarely occurring in acute cardiac ischemia.

Ans. c.

Q35. Regarding antiarrhythmic drugs, which statement is False?

a. Lidocaine is a class I antiarrhythmic drug.
b. Class I antiarrhythmic drugs are membrane stabilizing agents.
c. Amiodarone is a Class IV antiarrhythmic drug.
d. Adenosine can be used in the treatment of paroxysmal SVT.

Ans. c.

Q36. Intrinsic causes of bradycardia include:

a. Ischemia affecting sinus node or conduction tissue
b. Sarcoidosis of the heart
c. Hyperkalemia
d. Myocarditis

Ans. **a. True, b. True, c. False, and d. True**

Q37. Mark the following statements as True or False. In the treatment of SVT:

a. Carotid sinus massage stimulates baroreceptors triggering a reflexive increase in the activity of the vagal nerve and sympathetic withdrawal.
b. Catheter ablation has a very high success rate (>95%) and a low recurrence rate (<5%) in patients with accessory pathways.
c. Facial flushing, chest pain, and hypotension are common side effects of adenosine
d. Complications of catheter ablation include perforation, bleeding, AV fistula, venous thrombosis, pulmonary embolism, myocardial perforation, valve damage, systemic embolism, and rarely death.

Ans. **a. True, b. True, c. True, and d. True**

Q38. What is True or False regarding the different types of SVT?

a. AV nodal reentry tachycardia has a rate between 150 and 230° beats/min.
b. AV reentry tachycardia is due to a concealed AV bypass tract which creates the re-entrant circuit. The AV bypass tract usually allows retrograde conduction only.

c. Sinus node and intra-atrial reentry tachycardia are rarely seen in postcardiac surgery patients caused by reentry in the sinus node and atria, respectively.
d. In the Wolff-Parkinson-White syndrome preexcitation is caused by activation of ventricular muscle by impulses originating in atria and conducted by bypass tracts.

Ans. **a. True, b. True, c. False, and d. True**

Q39. **What is True or False regarding the acute management of VT?**

a. Patients presenting with hemodynamic instability, myocardial ischemia, and pulmonary edema should be promptly electrically cardioverted.
b. In patients who are hemodynamically stable, electric cardioversion is the first choice of treatment.
c. Reversible causes of VT, such as electrolyte imbalances, acute ischemia, hypoxia, and drug toxicities should be corrected.
d. Lidocaine is the first-line agent and is very useful in the setting of myocardial ischemia.

Ans. **a. True, b. False, c. True, and d. True**

Q40. **Mark the below statement as True or False.**

a. Clinical presentation of arrhythmias may vary from mild, i.e., only irritating symptoms such as an awareness of the heart beating very fast to potentially life-threatening conditions, such as a stroke and cardiac arrest.
b. Emergency physicians must keep in mind that an arrhythmia is only part of a patient's presentation, and before analyzing the arrhythmia the patient should be assessed and airway, breathing, and circulation (ABC) must be maintained.
c. The trickiest aspect in the management of bradyarrhythmia is not implanting a pacemaker (which is possibly the simplest aspect); rather it is reaching an accurate diagnosis and then deciding whether or not to treat the condition in a given patient.
d. SVT is usually seen in a structurally normal heart and in the presence of precipitating factors such as excessive intake of coffee, alcohol, or thyroid dysfunction.

Ans. **a. True, b. True, c. True, and d. True**

Q41. **The temporary cardiac pacing is useful for all the following, *except:***

a. Provide adequate HR in symptomatic bradycardia
b. Deliver a shock during polymorphic VT

c. Overdrive treatment of recurrent supraventricular or monomorphic VT
d. Prevention of episodes of polymorphic VT

Ans. b.

Q42. The output of the delivered electrical pulse in a temporary pacemaker is measured in:

a. Milliamperes
b. Millivolts
c. Milliseconds
d. Ohms

Ans. a.

Q43. Temporary transvenous pacing lead can be placed in an individual patient in:

a. Right ventricular apex
b. Right atrial appendage
c. Coronary sinus
d. Any of the above

Ans. d.

Q44. Temporary transvenous pacing lead insertion can be performed:

a. Guided by fluoroscopy
b. Guided by echocardiography
c. Unguided empirically
d. Any of the above

Ans. d.

Q45. The stimulation of the cardiac tissue occurs primarily via the:

a. Anode of the pacing lead
b. Cathode of the pacing lead
c. Both cathode and anode
d. Neither cathode nor anode

Ans. b.

Q46. Mark the below statement as True/False regarding temporary pacing:

a. Is always needed before permanent pacemaker implantation
b. Is done using epicardial pacing wires in patients undergoing cardiac surgery
c. Can not be done without fluoroscopy or echocardiography
d. Is lifesaving in complete heart block with recurrent bradycardia-related syncope

Ans. **a. False, b. True, c. False, and d. True**

Q47. Mark the below statement as True/False. Temporary transcutaneous pacing is:

a. Not very reliable
b. Painless

c. Done through external defibrillator
d. Well tolerated by the patient

Ans. a. True, b. False, c. True, and d. False

Q48. Mark the below statement as True/False. Temporary pacing can be useful in the management of:

a. Recurrent monomorphic VT
b. Torsade the pointes
c. Complete AV block
d. Atrial fibrillation without bradycardia

Ans. a. True, b. True, c. True, and d. False

Q49. Mark the below statement as True/False. Care and follow-up of a patient on a temporary pacemaker are involved.

a. Assessment of battery status of pulse-generator
b. Assessment of the oxygenation status of the patient
c. Assessment of pacing threshold
d. Assessment of access site for any complications

Ans. a. True, b. False, c. True, and d. True

Q50. Mark the below statement as True/False. Temporary cardiac pacing:

a. Should be used prophylactically in all patients of acute inferior MI with complete AV block
b. Is indicated in patients with acute MI and new bifascicular block
c. Is usually required in patients undergoing alcohol septal ablation
d. May be needed for prolonged periods in patients with permanent pacemaker pocket infection

Ans. a. False, b. True, c. True, and d. True

Q51. Regarding the presentation of essential hypertension, most patients present first with:

a. Severe headache
b. Acute ischemic heart attack
c. Gross hematuria
d. Mild or minimal headache or dizziness
e. Enlargement of the forehead, jaw, and nose

Ans. d. Most patients with essential hypertension may have mild symptoms or none at all. Their elevated BP may be identified at a routine check-up or as an incidental finding. Enlargement of the forehead, jaw, and nose is the presentation of acromegaly, which is one of the secondary causes of systemic hypertension.

Q52. To diagnose mild or moderate hypertension:

a. The emergency room is usually the most suitable facility.
b. Once the measurement exceeds the established standard, it is usually not necessary to repeat the measurement at another time or setting.
c. Home or 24-hour ambulatory blood-pressure monitoring may be used, especially in uncertain cases.
d. There is one universal reference standard in diagnosing adult hypertension.
e. Every patient with elevated BP found at the emergency room, regardless of the presentation or severity, must be treated immediately.

Ans. c. Stress, pain, and many other factors may lead to elevated BP. The emergency room is not an ideal place to label patients with hypertension. Many patients' BP returns to normal once their pain or stress is relieved. Emergency physicians should treat patients with hypertensive urgency or an emergency. The remaining patients should be referred to their family physicians or a community facility. Home or 24-hour ambulatory BP monitoring may be used, especially in uncertain cases (white-coat hypertension or masked hypertension).

Q53. Choose the correct option. To treat mild hypertension.

a. An ACE inhibitor is the best choice for all patients.
b. A combination of ACE inhibitor and ARB is often used.
c. An ACE inhibitor and ARB are preferred in patients with hyperkalemia and renal artery stenosis.
d. Calcium channel blockers are often used in patients with second- or third-degree heart block.
e. Lifestyle modification is usually the very first step in treating hypertension.

Ans. e. Drugs must be chosen according to the patient's background and other medical history. Physicians must be aware of the contraindications or side effects of each type of antihypertensive drug.

Q54. Lifestyle modifications for treating hypertension usually involve the following, *except:*

a. Low-salt diet
b. Regular (aerobic) exercise
c. Avoidance of smoking
d. Avoidance of excessive alcohol
e. Home measurement of BP three times a day for patients with mild or moderate hypertension

Ans. e. Lifestyle modifications include a low-salt diet, regular aerobic exercise, and avoidance of smoking and excessive alcohol. Monitoring one's BP is good. However, the overly frequent regular measurements may lead to stress and may otherwise elevate the BP.

Q55. When treating hypertensive urgency or emergency, the following are usually adopted, *except:*

a. The BP must always be lowered to the normal range.
b. The mean arterial pressure (MAP) in intracerebral hemorrhage patients should be lowered by 20–25%.
c. The MAP in hypertensive retinopathy patients should be lowered by 20–25%.
d. For pregnancy-induced hypertension, the SBP should be kept between 130 and 150 mm Hg, and the diastolic blood pressure (DBP) should be kept between 80 and 100 mm Hg.
e. Different presentations have different target BPs.

Ans. a. Different presentations of hypertensive urgency or emergency have different target BPs. However, the target figures may differ among different authorities.

Q56. Mark the statement as True or False regarding hypertensive emergencies.

a. Systolic BP over 180 mm Hg or diastolic BP over 120 mm Hg alone constitutes a hypertensive emergency.
b. Lowering BP down to normal within 1 hour is imperative in all hypertensive emergencies.
c. Oral antihypertensives can be used to treat hypertensive emergencies.
d. Glyceryl trinitrate (GTN) is the drug of choice for a hypertensive emergency associated with acute pulmonary edema.

Ans. **a. False, b. False, c. False, and d. True**

The definition of hypertensive emergency is the presence of acute end-organ damage in the presence of severely high BP. In most situations, BP should be lowered gradually (by > 25% MAP in the first hour) to avoid any compromising of organ perfusion—exceptions include aortic dissection and preeclampsia when rapid BP reduction is indicated. The intravenous route is preferred to deliver antihypertensive treatment in a hypertensive emergency as titration is easier and absorption variability is not an issue. Nitrate causes the vasodilatation of capacitance vessels, thus reducing the preload, and is a coronary vasodilator.

Q57. Mark the statement as True or False. Signs and symptoms that may be associated with hypertensive emergencies include:

a. Seizure
b. New murmur of aortic regurgitation
c. Anuria
d. Abdominal striae

Ans. a. True, b. True, c. True, d. True

The signs and symptoms of hypertensive emergencies depend on which end organ is acutely compromised. Hypertensive encephalopathy is associated with the classical triad of hypertension, papilledema, and altered mental state. There may also be acute onset headache, vomiting, seizures, and focal neurological deficits. Acute thoracic aortic dissection may give rise to a new-onset aortic regurgitation murmur. The presence of oliguria/anuria may denote acute renal failure. Abdominal striae are often present in patients with Cushing syndrome, which can cause secondary hypertension.

Q58. Mark the statement as True or False regarding—In acute aortic dissection:

a. High BP should be reduced by no >25% within the first hour.
b. Lowering the BP is the definitive treatment for type A aortic dissection.
c. Anterior MI is a more common complication of type A aortic dissection than inferior MI is.
d. ACE inhibitors are the preferred choice of antihypertensive drug.

Ans. a. False, b. False, c. False, and d. False

Aortic dissection is classified as type A (involving the ascending aorta) or type B (not involving the ascending aorta). Rapid reduction of systolic BP to below 120 mm Hg is recommended for both types. The definitive treatment for type A dissection is surgery, while strict BP control is often enough for uncomplicated type B dissection. Type A dissection is sometimes complicated by coronary artery involvement, causing MI. Inferior MI is more common than anterior since the right coronary artery is involved more often. The drug of choice to lower BP in the presence of aortic dissection is beta blockers, which reduce both the afterload and the HR.

Q59. Mark the statement as True or False—In hypertension related to catecholamine excess:

a. Symptoms of catecholamine excess can resemble those of thyrotoxicosis.

b. Beta blockers are the first-line drug for reducing BP in phaeochromocytoma patients.
c. Urine toxicology may be a helpful investigatory tool.
d. BP may be reduced by giving benzodiazepines in some situations.

Ans. **a. True, b. False, c. True, and d. False**

The symptoms of catecholamine excess are tachycardia, sweating, and tremors. The source of catecholamine may be endogenous, such as in phaeochromocytoma and exogenous, such as ingesting certain medications and illicit drugs (urine toxicology). Conditions that may mimic excessive catecholamine include anxiety, thyrotoxicosis, and hypoglycemia. Catecholamines stimulate both alpha and beta sympathetic receptors. Alpha-receptor stimulation causes the vasoconstriction of blood vessels and raises the BP. On the contrary, beta-receptor stimulation causes vasodilatation and increases the HR. In phaeochromocytoma patients, beta-blockers should not be used first because the vasodilation beta effect will be lost, and the unopposed vasoconstriction alpha effect will result in an even higher BP. When lowering the BP of patients with pheochromocytoma-associated hypertension, an alpha-blocker should be started first. After a few days, a beta blocker can be added. When managing symptoms due to abusable drugs such as methamphetamines and cocaine, BP often lowers with sedation by using benzodiazepine.

Q60. Mark the statement as True or False—In treating chronic hypertension:

a. Methyldopa and alpha-blockers are good choices for elderly patients.
b. ACE inhibitors or angiotensin receptor blockers are the first choices for diabetic patients.
c. Combining diltiazem with a beta blocker is advisable.
d. Combination therapy between a beta blocker and a dihydropyridine calcium channel blocker is not favorable.

Ans. **a. False, b. True, c. False, and d. False**

Methyldopa can cause delirium and alpha-blocker postural hypotension in elderly patients and should be the last resort for treating hypertension in this age group. ACE inhibitors and ARBs are the first choice for diabetic patients because they protect against diabetic nephropathy and treat hypertension. Beta-blockers should not be combined with nondihydropyridine calcium channel blockers such as diltiazem and verapamil because doing so can cause potentially serious cardiac conductive defects. However, a combination of a beta blocker and a dihydropyridine calcium channel blocker such as amlodipine is synergistic and well tolerated.

Q61. Reperfusion injury may be suggested by all, *except:*

a. Metabolic acidosis
b. Hypokalemia
c. Increase in creatinine kinase level
d. Myoglobinuria

Ans. b. Reperfusion injury is characterized by hyperkalemia and not hypokalemia.

The rest of the features of reperfusion injury are myoglobinuria, metabolic acidosis, and increased creatinine kinase levels.

Q62. Which of the following about acute limb ischemia is True or False?

a. Metabolic complications are the common causes of death after revascularization
b. Normal signal on Doppler ultrasonography is a biphasic velocity waveform
c. Aspirin should be administered to all patients unless contraindicated
d. Compartment syndrome will further propagate the ischemia

Ans. a. True, b. False, c. True, and d. False

One-third of cases due to occlusive arterial disease occur postrevascularization due to metabolic complications. Normal Doppler ultrasonography shows a triphasic velocity waveform. Aspirin should be administered to all patients with limb ischemia unless contraindicated. Aspirin administration reduces the vascular mortality by 25%. Compartment syndrome. Mechanism of propagation of ischemic injury includes clot extension, compartment syndrome due to ischemia-related distal edema, fragmentation of clot in microcirculation, and edema of microvascular cells.

Q63. Which of the following are the features of acute limb ischemia, *except:*

a. Pulselessness
b. Paresis
c. Paresthesia
d. Rest pain

Ans. d. Acute limb ischemia is characterized by Pain, paresthesia, pallor, pulseless-ness, and paralysis. Rest pain and intermittent claudication are features of chronic arterial insufficiency

Q64. Regarding the management of ischemia, all are true, *except:*

a. Patients with acute limb-threatening ischemia from embolism should undergo Fogarty catheter-directed embolectomy.

b. Patient with acute limb-threatening ischemia from embolism can be managed with IV heparin therapy with activated partial thromboplastin time (aPTT) monitoring
c. Contrast arteriography is the definitive diagnostic test
d. Fibrinolytic therapy is reserved for the patient with nonlimb threatening ischemia

Ans. b. Patients with acute limb-threatening ischemia from embolism should undergo Fogarty catheter-directed embolectomy. Contrast arteriography is the definitive diagnostic test of abnormal arterial anatomy. Fibrinolytic therapy is reserved for the nonlimb-threatening ischemia as the clot takes 6–72 hours to lyse.

Q65. Regarding embolic causes of acute limb ischemia mark the statement True or False.

a. Atrial fibrillation is one of the common causes
b. Demarcation of ischemia is diffuse
c. History of claudication is rare
d. Arteriography suggests a sharp cut-off with few collaterals

Ans. **a. True, b. False, c. True, and d. True**

In embolic causes of acute limb ischemia atrial fibrillation is one the common causes, demarcation of ischemia is sharp, history of claudication is rare, and arteriography suggests sharp cut-off with few collaterals.

Q66. Which of the following can distinguish constrictive pericarditis from restrictive cardiomyopathy?

a. Early diastolic sound 60–120 milliseconds after second heart sound
b. Dip and plateau filling pattern
c. Jugular venous distention
d. Kussmaul sign
e. Square root sign

Ans. a. Pericardial knock, an early diastolic sound, which can be heard at the apex 60–120 milliseconds after the second heart sound but before an S3 is associated with constrictive pericarditis but is clinically very challenging to differentiate from an S3. Both conditions share the signs of jugular venous distention (JVD) and Kussmaul, which is an increase in venous pressure with inspiration. The dip and plateau filling pattern, also known as the square root sign, is seen in both conditions. A marked decrease followed by a rapid rise and plateau in early-diastolic ventricular pressure is seen in hemodynamic studies, such as Doppler echocardiography and cardiac catheterization. Computed tomography (CT) and magnetic resonance imaging (MRIs) of the heart can differentiate constrictive pericarditis from restrictive cardiomyopathy.

Q67. Which of the following is the most common cause of restrictive cardiomyopathy?

a. Amyloidosis
b. Endomyocardial fibrosis
c. Hemochromatosis
d. Idiopathic
e. Sarcoidosis

Ans. d. Most cases of restrictive cardiomyopathy are idiopathic, often with an autosomal-dominant familial pattern. The remainder of the causes are systemic disorders such as those listed earlier, progressive systemic sclerosis (scleroderma), and hypereosinophilic syndrome.

Q68. What is the most common location of pain in patients with aortic dissection?

a. Abdominal pain
b. Back pain
c. Chest pain
d. Left arm pain
e. Neck pain

Ans. c. Patients with aortic dissections, 60% presented with chest pain, 64% stated the pain was "sharp," and 50% stated it was tearing or ripping. Syncope occurred 10% of the time. In all 90% of the patients stated that the pain associated with their dissection was the worst they had ever felt.

Q69. What is the best medication for a patient with a BP of 180/100 and confirmed aortic dissection on CT?

a. Esmolol
b. Hydralazine
c. Lisinopril
d. Nitroglycerine
e. Nitroprusside

Ans. a. Beta-blockers are favored as the first-line agent in patients with aortic dissection. When antihypertensive therapy is warranted, the main issue is to limit the shear wall forces on the aorta. The beta-blocker prevents rebound tachycardia.

Q70. What risk factor is highly predictive of developing an abdominal aortic aneurysm (AAA)?

a. Diabetes
b. Family history
c. Hypercholesterolemia
d. Hypertension
e. Smoking history

Ans. b. While it is important to recognize all factors that increase cardiovascular disease, a family history of a first-degree relative with an AAA has been shown to be highly predictive.

Q71. Which of the following are pathophysiologically the most important risk factors for occlusive arterial disease?

a. Diabetes and hyperlipidemia
b. Diabetes and hypertension
c. Diabetes and smoking
d. Elevated C-reactive protein and hyperhomocysteinemia
e. Hypertension and hyperlipidemia

Ans. c. Diabetes and smoking are the two most important risk factors for occlusive arterial disease.

Q72. What is the most common cause of acute limb ischemia?

a. Atheroemboli
b. Cardiac emboli
c. Mural thrombi in arterial aneurysms
d. Thoracic aortic dissection
e. Thrombotic occlusion

Ans. e. Thrombotic occlusion, of native vessels or bypass grafts, is the most common cause of acute limb ischemia, followed by embolic occlusion.

Q73. Which of the following is considered a late finding of complete arterial obstruction?

a. Hypoesthesia or hyperesthesia
b. Muscle weakness
c. Pain
d. Pallor
e. Paralysis

Ans. e. Paralysis and anesthesia are late findings of ischemic injury while pain can be only and earliest symptom of ischemia in a patient with underlying peripheral vascular disease.

Q74. Which of the following features distinguishes neurogenic claudication from intermittent vascular claudication?

a. Leg and buttock pain
b. Relieved by lumbar flexion
c. Relieved by rest
d. Triggered by exercise
e. Worsened by upright posture

Ans. b. Neurogenic claudication, due to spinal stenosis or lumbar radiculopathy, can mimic intermittent vascular claudication. Patients with neurogenic claudication can have bilateral buttock pain and posterior leg pain triggered by exercise and relieved by rest, but the onset of relief is not as immediate as it is in intermittent claudication. Patients with neurogenic claudication have relief of pain with lumbar flexion and worsening pain with upright posture or lumbar extension.

Q75. Which of the following is the most common cause of rapidly progressing cardiac tamponade?

a. Trauma
b. Connective tissue disorder
c. Uremia
d. Malignancy

Ans. a. The most common cause in which rapid progression occurs is traumatic while other medical causes of cardiac tamponade is gradual and more challenging to diagnose. The most common medical causes of cardiac tamponade include malignancy, renal dysfunction, infection, connective tissue disorder, radiation, chemotherapy, or idiopathic sources.

Q76. Which of the following signs is pathognomonic for cardiac tamponade?

a. Tachycardia, chest pain, and diaphoresis
b. Tachycardia, tachypnea, and hypotension
c. Muffled heart sound, distended jugular vein, and hypotension
d. Diastolic murmur, tachycardia, and hypotension
e. Systolic murmur, faint carotid pulse, and hypotension

Ans. c. *Beck triad*—muffled heart sound, distended jugular vein, and hypotension pathognomonic for cardiac tamponade.

Q77. The most common finding in the ECG of patients with cardiac tamponade is:

a. Electrical alternans
b. Tachycardia and low voltage
c. Sinus tachycardia
d. Normal ECG
e. Trifasciular block

Ans. b. In ECG, common findings are tachycardia and low voltage. Electric alternans may present if large pericardial effusion.

Q78. Regarding the initial management of cardiac tamponade which of the following is correct?

a. The initiation of positive pressure ventilation early on is recommended.
b. The initiation of positive pressure ventilation early on can be lethal.

c. No resuscitation is needed, definitive therapy by pericardiocentesis is the treatment.
d. Vasopressors shall be started early on to raise the BP.
e. Fluid resuscitation can be harmful

Ans. b. The initiation of positive pressure ventilation may result in catastrophic circulatory collapse due to an increase in intrathoracic pressure and worsening venous return. So, mechanical ventilation may prove deadly in patients with cardiac tamponade.

Q79. Which of the following will help identify the patient with immediate need of pericardiocentesis?

a. European Society of Cardiology scoring system
b. Clinical experience
c. Echocardiography signs of tamponade
d. Etiology of tamponade
e. Hemodynamic instability

Ans. a. For treating patients with cardiac tamponade, a three-step scoring system has been developed by the European Society of Cardiology Working Group on myocardial and pericardial disease. This scoring system is based on clinical signs and symptoms and echocardiographic findings. The scoring system can be used to identify the patient with an immediate need for pericardiocentesis. Emergent pericardial drainage is required if the score is 6 or above. Drainage can be postponed up to 48 hours if the score is <6.

Respiratory Emergencies MCQs

Devendra Richhariya

Q1. Common bacterial etiology for community-acquired pneumonia (CAP) are all, *except:*

a. *Staphylococcus aureus* b. Coronavirus
c. *Klebsiella pneumoniae* d. *Haemophilus influenzae*

Ans. b. Corona virus—it is not bacteria, it is virus

Q2. Most common etiological agent for hospital-acquired pneumonia (HAP) or ventilator-acquired pneumonia (VAP) among following is:

a. *Pseudomonas aeruginosa* b. *Mycoplasma*
c. *Legionella* d. *Chlamydophila*

Ans. a. *Pseudomonas aeruginosa;* rest all are causes of atypical pneumonia. For HAP and VAP, the common organisms are predominately gram-negative bacteria such as *P. aeruginosa, Klebsiella,* MRSA (methicillin-resistant *S. aureus*), *Legionella,* and *H. influenzae. Acinetobacter* is a pathogen associated with VAP specifically.

Q3. Following are the etiological classification of pneumonia, *except:*

a. Bacterial b. Viral
c. Fungal d. Nosocomial

Ans. d. Nosocomial is HAP based on empiricist classification such as CAP, HAP, and HCAP (health care-associated pneumonia).

Q4. Community-acquired pneumonia is:

a. Which develops after 48 hours of hospital admission
b. Which develops after 48 hours of mechanical ventilation
c. Acute infection of pulmonary parenchyma contracted outside hospital
d. Acute infection of pulmonary parenchyma contracted inside hospital

Ans. c. Community-acquired pneumonia is an acute infection of pulmonary parenchyma contracted outside hospital. HAP develops after 48 hours of hospital admission, whereas VAP develops after 48 hours of mechanical ventilation.

Q5. Health care-associated pneumonia is acute lung parenchymal infection because of all, *except:*

a. History of repeated or multiple hospitalization includes patient undergoing dialysis or chemotherapy
b. Chronic wound care or home intravenous antibiotics care
c. The immunocompromised patient population, and patients from nursing home facilities
d. Patients from remote and hilly area

Ans. d. Patients from hilly areas do not fit in diagnosis of HCAP. HCAP includes group of patients in whom repeated or multiple hospitalizations is required like patients undergoing dialysis or chemotherapy, chronic wound care or home intravenous antibiotics care, the immunocompromised patient population, and patients from nursing home facilities. So due to parenchymal infections, these patients were hospitalized for 2 or more days in the previous 90 days.

Q6. Pneumonia is lung infection of:

a. Blood vessels
b. Lymphatics
c. Parenchyma including alveolus
d. Pleural space

Ans. c. Pneumonia is an alveolar infection that occurs due to defective and compromised innate immune system and lower airway and alveoli that are unable to clear a pathogen from the respiratory tract. Lung parenchyma is further damaged by local inflammatory factors and cytokines and leads to systemic inflammation. Blood vessels diseases include pulmonary arterial hypertension (PAH) and vasculitis. Lymphatics diseases include chylothorax. Pleural diseases are pneumothorax, pleural effusion, empyema, etc.

Q7. Causes of atypical pneumonia are following, *except:*

a. *S. aureus*
b. *Legionella*
c. *Chlamydia psittaci*
d. *Mycoplasma pneumoniae*

Ans. a. *Staphylococcus aureus* causes typical pneumonia.

Q8. Following blood marker will favor more likely typical bacterial pneumonia rather than atypical:

a. C-reactive protein (CRP)
b. Erythrocyte sedimentation rate (ESR)
c. Serum procalcitonin
d. D-dimer

Ans. c. Serum procalcitonin; procalcitonin guidance for antibiotic had a great impact and it was found that there was reduction in antibiotic exposure without an increase in mortality or treatment failure. Most of the time, procalcitonin is able to differentiate between viral and bacterial infection and is very useful. But the sensitivity of procalcitonin for detection of bacterial infection. The rest of all blood parameters like CRP, ESR, and D-dimer can be raised as like any inflammatory marker.

Q9. Hypoxia is found in lung pathology with all, *except:*

a. Parenchymal involvement b. Vascular involvement
c. Interstitial involvement d. Pleural involvement

Ans. d. Pleural involvement does not cause V/Q (ventilation-perfusion) mismatch hence cannot cause hypoxia. Rest all pathology of parenchyma [acute respiratory distress syndrome (ARDS)], vascular (pulmonary embolism), and interstitium [interstitial lung disease (ILD)] affects diffusion of oxygen through alveo-capillary membrane hence affects V/Q leading to hypoxia.

Q10. Ventilation-perfusion defects leading to hypoxia are more profound with all, *except*:

a. Lobar/segmental pneumonia
b. Atypical pneumonia
c. Bilateral pneumonia with ARDS
d. Pulmonary embolism

Ans. a. Lobar/segmental pneumonia; hypoxia is more profound with interstitial pathology because of V/Q defects. Atypical pneumonia affects more of interstitium with defect in ventilation than small lobar or segmental pneumonia. Pulmonary embolism affects more of perfusion which also leads to V/Q defect leading to hypoxia. Mild pneumonia with small lobe or segmental involvement rarely presents with hypoxia or dyspnea.

11. All except one are severity scoring systems of pneumonia:

a. CURB-65 b. CRB-65
c. PSI d. MRSA

Ans. d. MRSA stands for methicillin-resistant *S. aureus;* it is not a severity scoring system. CURB-65 (*c*onfusion, *u*rea >7 mmol/L, *r*espiratory rate >30 breaths/min, *b*lood pressure (systolic <90 mm Hg or diastolic <60 mm Hg), age >65 years) and PSI stands for pneumonia severity index.

12. Pneumonia severity index includes all, *except:*

a. Age
b. Sex
c. Mechanical ventilator
d. Comorbidities (like neoplastic disease history, liver disease, congestive heart failure (CHF), cerebrovascular disease, renal disease)

Ans. c. Mechanical ventilator is not included in PSI.

13. CRB-65 includes all, *except*:

a. Confusion
b. Blood urea nitrogen (BUN)
c. Respiratory rate
d. Systolic blood pressure and diastolic blood pressure

Ans. b. Blood urea nitrogen is included in CURB-65, not in CRB-65.

14. The first and foremost treatment of pneumonia is:

a. Antibiotic
b. Antipyretics
c. Clear the airway
d. Oxygen therapy, if needed

Ans. a. The first and foremost treatment of pneumonia is antibiotic, but other supportive care also needs to be addressed such as antipyretics, clear the airway, oxygen therapy, if needed, adequate hydration, and nutrition.

15. Type 2 respiratory failure is:

a. Hypoxia
b. Hypercapnia
c. Hypoxia with hypercapnia
d. None

Ans. c. Hypoxia with hypercapnia; *type 1 (hypoxemic)*: Arterial partial pressure of oxygen (PaO_2) < 60: Failure of oxygenation

16. Which of the following is not correctly matched?

a. Type 1 respiratory failure—hypercapnia
b. Type 2 respiratory failure—hypoxia with hypercapnia
c. Type 3 respiratory failure—perioperative
d. Type 4 respiratory failure—shock

Ans. a. *Type 1 respiratory failure is only hypoxia; type 1 (hypoxemic):* PaO_2 < 60. *Type 2 (hypoxia with hypercapnic)*: Arterial partial pressure of carbon dioxide ($PaCO_2$) > 45: Failure to exchange or remove carbon dioxide and decreased alveolar minute ventilation, which is often accompanied by hypoxemia.

Type 3 (perioperative): This is because of increased atelectasis due to low functional residual capacity (FRC) in the setting of abnormal abdominal wall mechanics that may result in type 1 or type 2 respiratory failure and can be ameliorated by anesthetic or operative technique, posture, incentive spirometry, postoperative analgesia, and attempts to lower intra-abdominal pressure.

Type 4 (shock): It is basically due to cardiovascular instability, among patients who are intubated and ventilated in the process of resuscitation for shock. Goal of ventilation is to stabilize gas exchange and to unload the respiratory muscles, lowering their oxygen consumption.

17. Type 1 respiratory failure can be managed by oxygen supplement only with the help of all, *except:*

a. Nasal cannula
b. Facemask
c. Positive-pressure ventilation like bilevel positive airway pressure (BiPAP)
d. Venturi mask

Ans. c. Positive pressure ventilation like BiPAP

The treatment of respiratory failure is oxygen supplement. There are different modalities for oxygen supplement for managing hypoxia in pneumonia. Positive-pressure ventilation like BiPAP is needed only if patient has type 2 respiratory failure with CO_2 retention.

18. For type 2 respiratory failure following is used, *except:*

a. BiPAP
b. Mechanical ventilator
c. Mechanical ventilator
d. Venturi mask

Ans. d. Venturi mask is used for oxygen supplement and has no role in CO_2 retention.

19. Positive-pressure ventilation like BiPAP, cannot be used in:

a. Noncooperative patients
b. Patients with Copious secretion
c. Patients with Neck fracture
d. All of the above

Ans. d. All positive-pressure ventilation such as BiPAP and AVAP cannot be used in noncooperative patients, patients with copious secretion, and patients with neck fracture.

20. The physiological effect of high-flow nasal cannula (HFNC) is all, *except:*

a. Increased fraction of inspired oxygen (FiO_2)
b. Intubation and mechanical ventilation
c. Decreases work of breathing: Counteracts intrinsic positive end-expiratory pressure (PEEP)
d. Development of a continuous positive airway pressure (CPAP) effect

Ans. b. Intubation and mechanical ventilation; the physiological effect of HFNC are:

- Increased FiO_2
- Gas inlet flow prevents secondary room air entrainment
- Provides anatomic oxygen reservoirs using nasopharynx and oropharynx
- Washing out of airway dead space
- Development of a CPAP effect
- Decreases atelectasis
- Improvement in pulmonary V/Q
- *Decreases work of breathing:* Counteracts intrinsic PEEP
- Greater patient comfort
- Warmed and humidified nasal oxygen can be better tolerated, especially with flows >6 L/min.

21. Write True or False for each statement in the question.

a. Growth hormone is increased locally at the fingertips in patients with clubbing
b. Megakaryocytes are found trapped in pulmonary capillaries in patients with clubbing
c. Platelet-derived growth factors are increased locally in patients with clubbing
d. Vascular endothelial growth factor is increased locally in patients with clubbing

Ans. a. False, b. False, c. True, and d. True

22. Which one of these factors has not been established as a causative agent for clubbing?

a. Vascular endothelial growth factor
b. Platelet-derived growth factor
c. Basic fibroblast growth factor
d. Prostaglandin E2

Ans. c.

23. Which of these is considered a red flag sign in clubbing?

a. Lovibond's angle >180°
b. Increased fluctuation at the nailbed
c. Digital index >10.2
d. Hypertrophic osteoarthropathy

Ans. d.

24. Which of these is not a cause of isolated peripheral cyanosis?

a. Raynaud's disease
b. CHF
c. Hypovolemic shock
d. Arteriovenous (AV) malformations

Ans. d.

25. Methylene blue is given to treat cyanosis in which of these?

a. Deoxyhemoglobin
b. Methemoglobin
c. Sulfhemoglobin
d. All of these

Ans. b.

26. Which of the following represent increased dead space ventilation?

a. ARDS
b. Cyanide toxicity
c. Pulmonary embolus
d. Pulmonary hemorrhage
e. Pneumonia

Ans. c. With a pulmonary embolism, there is increased dead space ventilation with a relatively higher proportion of V/Q ratio. An area of the lung receives oxygen, but due to thrombotic obstruction of pulmonary vessel, there is an area of underperfusion.

27. In distinguishing a chronic obstructive pulmonary disease (COPD) exacerbation from CHF, which of the following clinical or laboratory features is helpful?

a. B-type natriuretic peptide level
b. Body habitus
c. Distended neck veins
d. History of COPD
e. Peripheral edema

Ans. a. Given the overlapping epidemiology of patients with COPD and CHF, distinguishing between patients with both comorbidities can be challenging for the emergency physician. B-type natriuretic peptide is a useful noninvasive adjunct to differentiate between COPD and CHF due to its release by the left ventricle in response to cardiac stress. When the levels are decreased, it makes CHF very unlikely.

28. Which of the following is NOT a cause of chronic cough of >8 weeks?

a. Asthma
b. Bronchiectasis
c. Gastroesophageal reflux disease (GERD)
d. Pulmonary embolism
e. Upper airway cough syndrome

Ans. d. A chronic cough by definition is a cough that lasts >8 weeks. Choice (d) is correct as pulmonary embolism usually manifests with rapid-onset chest pain and acute respiratory distress. The cough seen with pulmonary embolism may manifest as hemoptysis and usually signifies pulmonary infarct.

29. A patient presents with massive hemoptysis. Which of the following is most likely the source of the bleeding?

a. Alveolar vessel
b. Bronchial vessel
c. Intercostal artery
d. Intercostal vein
e. Internal mammary artery

Ans. b. The answer "bronchial vessel" is correct, as they are under systemic pressure and thus are more likely to bleed briskly.

30. What is the primary reason that patients with brisk hemoptysis require emergent airway management?

a. Asphyxiation
b. Aspiration
c. Exsanguination
d. Infection
e. Nausea and subsequent vomiting

Ans. a. Massive hemoptysis can lead to asphyxiation from obliteration of airspaces due to blood. Aspiration, choice (b), is plausible and may occur to varying degrees depending on the patient's level of consciousness and position, but it is not the primary reason airway management is needed.

31. A patient taking warfarin arrives to the emergency department (ED) with severe hemoptysis. Which of the following would be best initial management?

a. Administer fresh frozen plasma (FFP)
b. Check complete blood cell count
c. Cryoprecipitate
d. Transfusion of uncross matched red blood cells
e. Withhold warfarin for 1 day

Ans. a. Warfarin depletes vitamin K-dependent coagulation factors II, VII, IX, X, and proteins C and S. FFP contains all of these plus several other coagulation factors

32. Which of the following is LEAST efficacious in the treatment of an acute exacerbation of COPD?

a. Albuterol
b. Ipratropium
c. Magnesium
d. Steroids
e. Supplemental oxygen

Ans. c. There is currently no data to support administration of magnesium for acute exacerbation of COPD. Albuterol is the mainstay of acute pharmacologic management of acute exacerbation of COPD.

33. A patient with a long-standing history of COPD on home oxygen supplementation was admitted to the ED for an exacerbation. The patient improved significantly with treatment. The patient is currently comfortable and is no longer requiring frequent breathing treatments and is back to his baseline requirement of 2 L/min of supplemental oxygen. Upon discharge, which of the following is warranted?

a. Increased home oxygen flow to 3 L/min per nasal cannula
b. Magnesium supplementation
c. Physical rehabilitation
d. Steroid taper
e. Switching from metered dose inhaler to nebulizer for albuterol administration

Ans. d. The GOLD (Global Initiative for Chronic Obstructive Lung Disease) does not recommend chronic oral corticosteroids use for COPD, but for acute exacerbation a 10-day course of prednisone 40 mg/day may decrease recurrence of exacerbations, and or hospitalization.

34. A thoracostomy tube was inserted into a 30-year-old male with a large pneumothorax. There was a gush of air noted with the insertion. Which of the following complications should you watch for in this patient?

a. Hemothorax from injury to intercostals vessels
b. Infection of thoracostomy site
c. Mucous plugging of thoracostomy tube
d. Persistent air leak and re-expansion pulmonary edema
e. Tension pneumothorax

Ans. d. Re-expansion pulmonary edema is more often seen in younger patients aged 20–39 years, and with larger pneumothoraces present for >72 hours that are rapidly expanded with suction. Pulmonary edema generally occurs on the side of the re-expanded lung. Treatment is supportive with aggressive volume resuscitation and sharply differs from treatment for cardiogenic pulmonary edema.

35. All of the following conditions have an elevated A–a gradient. Which one of the following not be corrected by supplemental oxygen administration?

a. Age-related decrease A–a gradient due to decreased PaO_2
b. AV shunt
c. CHF
d. Lobar pneumonia
e. Pleural effusion

Ans. b. An AV shunt will not have an appreciable difference in PaO_2 by providing supplemental oxygen.

Gastrointestinal Emergencies MCQs

Devendra Richhariya

Q1. Most common cause of acute nausea and vomiting is:

a. Central nervous system tumor
b. Diabetic ketoacidosis
c. Nonsteroidal anti-inflammatory drugs (NSAIDs)
d. Pregnancy
e. Viral gastroenteritis

Ans. e. Acute nausea and vomiting can be a symptom of many disorders. Viral gastroenteritis is the most common cause.

Q2. Acute constipation can be caused by which one of the following conditions?

a. Amyloidosis
b. Hyperparathyroidism
c. Hypomagnesemia
d. Parkinson disease
e. Volvulus

Ans. e. Acute constipation is secondary to intestinal obstruction, until proven otherwise.

Q3. Which of the following statements is *true* in patients with abdominal pain?

a. Early administration of opioid analgesia should be avoided as it will obscure physical findings, delay diagnosis, or lead to increased morbidity/mortality
b. Elevated serum lipase is highly sensitive and specific for the diagnosis of acute pancreatitis
c. Normal serum lactate rules out mesenteric ischemia
d. Normal white blood cell (WBC) reliably excludes surgical disease
e. The therapeutic value of placing a nasogastric tube in patients who are actively vomiting is well established

Ans. b. An elevated serum lipase has a sensitivity of 90% and a specificity of 93% for the diagnosis of acute pancreatitis.

Q4. Which of the following statements is *true* in elderly patients with abdominal pain?

a. Symptoms tend to manifest sooner

b. Cholecystitis is the most common surgical disease in these patients
c. Fever is a reliable marker for serious abdominal infection
d. It is not crucial to determine the etiology in the emergency department (ED) prior to admission
e. The presence of diarrhea reliably excludes mesenteric ischemia

Ans. b. Cholecystitis is the most common surgical disease in elderly patients with abdominal pain, followed by small bowel obstruction, perforated viscus, appendicitis, and large-bowel obstruction. Fever is not a reliable marker for surgical disease. Instead, the elderly patient with a serious abdominal infection may be hypothermic.

Q5. When evaluating a patient for suspected acute bowel perforation, what is the *most* appropriate initial imaging modality?

a. Cholescintigraphy
b. Computed tomography (CT) of the abdomen with contrast
c. Magnetic resonance imaging (MRI) of the abdomen
d. Plain abdominal films
e. Ultrasonography of the abdomen

Ans. d. If imaging is obtained in cases of suspected acute bowel perforation, then the most appropriate initial imaging modality is plain abdominal films, as they are relatively easy to obtain, and free air visible on a plain abdominal film mandates immediate surgical evaluation without the need for additional imaging. However, abdominal plain films cannot rule out perforation. Up to 20% of patients with perforation will not demonstrate free air. It is important to understand that surgical consultation should not be delayed awaiting the results of imaging in the acute abdomen.

Q6. What is the *most* common cause of traveler's diarrhea in patients returning from developing countries?

a. *Clostridium difficile*
b. *Escherichia coli*
c. Invasive bacteria (*Campylobacter jejuni, Shigella, Salmonella*)
d. Norovirus
e. Protozoa

Ans. b. Diarrhea is a common occurrence in travelers returning from developing countries. Toxin and nontoxin-producing strains of *E. coli* account for most identifiable cases.

Q7. What is the *most* common cause of *lower* gastrointestinal (GI) bleeding?

a. Adenomatous polyps
b. Diverticular disease
c. Infectious colitis
d. Inflammatory colitis
e. Malignancy

Ans. b. Most common source for GI bleeding is from a site proximal to the ligament of Treitz [upper GI (UGI) bleed]. Most UGI bleeds are secondary to peptic ulcer disease. However, in patients with an established lower GI source of bleeding, the most common etiology is diverticular disease, followed by colitis, adenomatous polyps, and malignancy.

Q8. Regarding esophageal perforation, which of the following is *true*?

a. Boerhaave syndrome is responsible for >30% of esophageal perforations
b. Iatrogenic perforation is the most frequent etiology
c. Most iatrogenic perforations occur through the left posterolateral wall of the distal esophagus
d. The absence of mediastinal emphysema rules out esophageal perforation

Ans. b. Iatrogenic perforation from esophageal instrumentation accounts for the majority of cases.

Q9. *True* statement regarding peptic ulcer disease is:

a. All patients with dyspepsia require endoscopy
b. Diet and alcohol use are predisposing factors to the development of peptic ulcer disease, but emotional stress is not
c. GI barium studies are the test of choice for diagnosing peptic ulcers
d. The peptic ulcers mostly caused by infection with *Helicobacter pylori* or by the use of NSAIDs

Ans. d. The majority of peptic ulcers are caused by infection with *H. pylori* or by the use of NSAIDs.

Q10. *True* statement regarding *H. pylori* infection is:

a. Eradication of infection dramatically reduces 1-year recurrence rates for duodenal and peptic ulcers
b. Infection is not a risk factor for adenocarcinoma of the stomach
c. Infection is present in <50% of patients with duodenal and gastric ulcers
d. Most infected people will develop peptic ulcer disease
e. Serologic studies are superior over stool antigens for diagnosing infection

Ans. a. Eradication is typically done with "triple therapy" that includes a proton-pump inhibitor, clarithromycin, and either amoxicillin or metronidazole. Eradication of infection reduces 1-year recurrence rates from 35 to 2% for duodenal ulcers and from 39 to 3% for gastric ulcers.

Q11. Mark the statement True or False regarding drug used to treat peptic ulcer disease and its associated mechanism of action.

a. Antacids—block secretion of acid at the proton pump
b. H2 receptor antagonists—inhibit histamine receptor of parietal cells
c. Misoprostol—protects ulcer from acid exposure by forming a sticky gel
d. Proton-pump inhibitor—buffer gastric acid
e. Sucralfate—prostaglandin analog that increases bicarbonate production

Ans. a. False, b. True, c. False, d. False, and e. False

Histamine receptor antagonists inhibit the H2 receptors of the gastric parietal cells, thereby suppressing acid secretion.

Q12. Most frequent cause of acute pancreatitis is:

a. Alcohol
b. Drug-induced
c. Gallstones
d. Hypercalcemia
e. Hypertriglyceridemia

Ans. c. Gallstones are the leading cause of acute pancreatitis, accounting for at least 35–40% of cases. Alcohol is the second most frequent cause. Hypertriglyceridemia accounts for 1–4% of cases. Drugs account for <2% of cases.

Q13. What is the imaging modality of choice in the ED for diagnosing acute cholecystitis?

a. CT of the abdomen
b. Endoscopic retrograde cholangiopancreatography (ERCP)
c. Magnetic resonance cholangiopancreatography (MRCP)
d. Plain radiographs
e. Ultrasound

Ans. e. Right upper quadrant ultrasound is the imaging modality of choice for diagnosing acute cholecystitis in the ED. It has a sensitivity of 94% and a specificity of 78% for detecting acute cholecystitis. A sonographic Murphy sign has a high positive predictive value (PPV) for acute cholecystitis.

Q14. What is the most common cause of large-bowel obstruction in a 65-year-old patient?

a. Adhesions
b. Hernia
c. Mesenteric ischemia
d. Neoplasm
e. Volvulus

Ans. d. Neoplasms are by far the most common cause of large-bowel obstruction.

Q15. If you suspect that a patient has a small- or large-bowel obstruction, the diagnostic study of choice is:

a. Abdominal series (plain films)
b. Barium enema
c. Barium swallow
d. CT scan
e. MRI

Ans. d. In the ED, flat and upright abdominal radiographs and upright chest X-ray or a lateral decubitus view can be used to screen for bowel obstruction, severe constipation, or free air. Plain X-rays can also localize the site to large or small bowel. However, CT scan is the diagnostic method of choice in the ED if clinical suspicion for obstruction is strong.

Q16. The most common type of hernia in women is:

a. Epigastric
b. Femoral
c. Inguinal
d. Spigelian
e. Umbilical

Ans. c. Seventy-five percent of all hernias occur in the inguinal region making it the most common form of hernia, with two-thirds of these being of the indirect type.

Q17. What is the most common cause of rectal bleeding?

a. Anal fissures
b. Colon cancer
c. Diverticulosis
d. Hemorrhoids
e. Ulcerative colitis

Ans. d. Although the most common cause of rectal bleeding is hemorrhoids, other, more serious causes should be investigated.

Q18. Which anorectal abscess can be appropriately treated in the ED?

a. Intersphincteric
b. Ischiorectal
c. Perianal
d. Submucosal
e. Supralevator

Ans. c. Treatment of perianal abscesses is incision and drainage. An isolated perianal abscess not deep is generally the only type of anorectal abscess that can be adequately treated in the ED. All perirectal abscesses (supralevator, intersphincteric, complicated ischiorectal, and submucosal) should be drained in the operating room.

Q19. Which of the following confirms appropriate placement of a nasogastric tube?

a. Air bubbles when proximal end of tube is placed in water
b. Epigastric auscultation of air insufflated through the tube
c. Patient choking or coughing
d. Patient's inability to speak
e. pH testing of aspirates (indicates gastric placement)

Ans. b. Nasogastric tube placement is confirmed by epigastric auscultation of air insufflated through the tube, aspiration of visually recognizable GI secretions, or pH testing of aspirates (indicates gastric placement).

Q20. What is the most common complication after colonoscopy?

a. Hemorrhage
b. Infection
c. Perforation
d. Splenic rupture
e. Volvulus

Ans. a. Hemorrhage is the most common complication and can be secondary to polypectomy, biopsies, laceration of the mucosa by the instrument, or tearing of the mesentery or spleen.
Potential complications of colonoscopy include hemorrhage, perforation, retroperitoneal abscess, pneumoscrotum, pneumothorax, volvulus, postcolonoscopy distention, splenic rupture, appendicitis, bacteremia, and infection.

Q21. Spontaneous bacterial peritonitis *most* accurately predicts by which of the following tests?

a. Low serum glucose
b. High protein in peritoneal fluid
c. High protein in serum
d. Neutrophil count greater than 250/μL in the peritoneal fluid
e. Total white count greater than 500/μL

Ans. d. Ascitic fluid is tested for cell count, glucose and protein, and Gram stain and culture to identify bacterial peritonitis. A total white blood cell count greater than 1,000/μL or a neutrophil count greater than 250/μL is diagnostic for spontaneous bacterial peritonitis.

Q22. A 22-year-old nonpregnant female presents with acute nausea, vomiting, abdominal pain, and jaundice. Her diagnostic tests reveal an aspartate aminotransferase (AST) of 1,500 and alanine aminotransferase (ALT) of 2,000. Which factor will determine if the patient should be admitted?

a. ALT >1,000
b. AST >2,000
c. Bilirubin >20
d. Glucose >200
e. International normalized ratio (INR) >25% normal

Ans. c. Admit those who have a bilirubin ≥20 mg/dL, prothrombin time 50% above normal, hypoglycemia, low albumin, or any signs of GI bleeding. Patients with acute hepatitis require supportive treatment with pain management and fluid resuscitation. Consider admission for high-risk patients including the elderly and pregnant women.

Q23. Absolute contraindications for liver transplant are following, *except*:

a. Severe cardiopulmonary disease
b. Extrahepatic malignancy
c. Uncontrolled systemic sepsis originating from source other than liver
d. Active substance abuse
e. Advanced age (>70 years)

Ans. e. Relative contraindications for liver transplant are advanced age (>70 years), uncontrolled human immunodeficiency virus (HIV) disease, and diffuse thrombosis of vein.

Q24. An intern sustained a needle stick injury while establishing an intravenous line on a patient in the casualty. The patient was subsequently found to be hepatitis B surface antigen (HBsAg) positive. The presence of which of the following markers in the intern would reliably indicate an early infection?

a. IgM anti-HBsAg
b. IgM anti-HBcAg
c. HBsAg
d. HBeAg

Ans. b. The most reliable indicator of recent hepatitis B virus (HBV) infection is IgM anti HBc in serum. However, the first well logical marker to rise in acute hepatitis B is HBsAg. HBsAg is detectable in serum within 1–12 weeks of infection. Anti-HBc is demonstrable in the serum about 1–2 weeks after this and may sometimes persist in the serum even longer than an anti-HBs antibody. IgM anti-HBcAg is seen early in the infection and persists for about 6 months. It indicates a recent infection.

Note: The risk of transmission of HBV from percutaneous routes that is needle prick is about 6–30% and is about 100 times more infectious than HIV.

Q25. Which of the following is unlikely to be seen as an extrahepatic manifestation in patients with hepatitis C infection?

a. Mixed cryoglobulinemia
b. Lichen planus
c. Porphyria cutanea tarda
d. Polyarteritis nodosa

Ans. d. Polyarteritis nodosa is not characteristically associated with hepatitis C infection. However, it is a common extrahepatic manifestation of hepatitis B infection.

Q26. Which of the following pairs of the viral hepatitis and its management is incorrectly matched?

a. Acute viral hepatitis E—supportive care
b. Acute viral hepatitis B—antiviral therapy
c. Acute viral hepatitis A—supportive care
d. Acute viral hepatitis C—antiviral therapy

Ans. b. Antiviral therapy is not indicated in acute hepatitis B infection. It is only indicated in chronic hepatitis B infection. The majority of acute hepatitis (A, B, E) infections are self-limiting, resulting in viral elimination and complete healing within 6 months. In acute hepatitis C infection, recovery is rare and the risk of progression to chronic hepatitis is high, i.e., 85%. Thus antiviral therapy is started irrespective of the disease stage.

Q27. In which of the following populations should surveillance for hepatocellular carcinoma (HCC)? Mark the statement as True or False.

a. HBV carriers with cirrhosis
b. Asian male HBV carriers between ages of 30 and 40 years
c. Asian female HBV carriers over 50 years
d. HBV carriers with a family history of HCC
e. Patients with high serum levels of HBV DNA and ongoing liver injury

Ans. **a. True, b. False, c. True, d. True, and e. True**

Surveillance for HCC is recommended for Asian male HBV carriers over the age of 40 years the most common etiological factor for HCC in the world is hepatitis B virus infection surveillance programs have been implemented to screen for HCC in the high-risk individuals because it is more cost effective than the treatment of HCC. Surveillance for HCC is recommended in HBV carriers with cirrhosis.

Q28. Which of the following is the most common route of spread of hepatitis E virus?

a. Sexual transmission
b. Blood transfusion
c. Feco-oral route
d. Intravenous (IV) drug use

Ans. c. The most common route of the spread of hepatitis E is feco-oral.

Hepatitis E virus is the most common cause of acute hepatitis in adults specially in endemic countries like India. The most common cause of acute hepatitis in children is hepatitis A virus.

Q29. Patients with alcoholic hepatitis typically have the following features:

a. An elevated serum bilirubin
b. Elevated gamma-glutamyl transferase (GGT)
c. Leukopenia
d. ALT/AST 2:1

Ans. a. True, b. True, c. False, and d. False

Patients with alcoholic hepatitis typically have moderate elevations of AST and ALT typically <300. An AST:ALT ratio >2 elevated serum bilirubin and elevated GGT. A leukocytosis with predominance of neutrophils. An elevated INR

Q30. Marked elevation of serum alkaline phosphatase (that is >4 times of a upper normal limit) is seen in all of the following:

a. Choledocholithiasis
b. AIDS cholangiopathy
c. Infiltrative diseases
d. Third-trimester pregnancy

Ans. a. True, b. True, c. True, and d. False

The major value of serum alkaline phosphatase in the diagnosis of liver disorders is in the recognition of cholestatic diseases. However, an elevation in the alkaline phosphatase concentration is relatively common finding and does not always indicate presence of hepatobiliary disease. The degree of elevation does not distinguish intra- from extrahepatic cholestasis. However, in pregnancy we do get marked rise in serum alkaline phosphatase values and is usually up to two times of upper normal limit.

Q31. In patients with mushroom poisoning *Amanita phalloides* ingestion, which one is True and False?

a. Early administration of activated charcoal is recommended
b. Hallucinations
c. Acute gastroenteritis
d. Toxicity usually happens within minutes after ingestion of potentially lethal mushrooms

Ans. a. True, b. True, c. True, and d. False

Patients who ingest potentially lethal mushrooms like *Amanita virosa* and *A. phalloides* typically develop signs of toxicity >6 hours after ingestion. However, clinical manifestation of poisoning that occurs <6 hours after ingestion does not exclude the potential for life-threatening toxicity especially when more than one type of mushroom has been eaten.

Q32. In acute poisoning of mushroom early administration of activated charcoal is recommended. Write True and False.

a. Hepatitis A is associated with the highest risk of developing fulminant hepatitis
b. Hepatitis B is associated with highest risk of developing fulminant hepatitis
c. Hepatitis E is associated with the highest risk of developing fulminant hepatitis
d. Hepatitis D is associated with the highest risk of developing fulminant hepatitis

Ans. a. False, b. False, c. True, and d. True

Acute viral hepatitis caused by the hepatitis D virus is associated with the highest risk of developing fulminant hepatitis. However, fulminant hepatitis is most commonly caused by hepatitis E specially in endemic countries such as India. This is due to the greater prevalence of hepatitis E infections compared to hepatitis D.

Q33. All are true about caustic injury, *except*:

a. CT scan is right choice to assess severity
b. Endoscopy should be delayed by 48–72 hours
c. Gastric lavage should be avoided
d. Steroid have no roles in management

Ans. b. Upper endoscopy is the modality of choice to diagnose, grade, guide the treatment, and prognosticate the injury. It should be done within 48–72 hours of ingestion.

Genitourinary Emergencies MCQs

Devendra Richhariya

Q1. The imaging modality of choice for urinary tract stone assessment in the present era is which of the following?

a. Excretory urography [intravenous urography (IVU)]
b. Ultrasonography
c. Unenhanced computed tomography (CT)
d. Plain abdomen kidney, ureter, and bladder (KUB) radiograph

Ans. c. Unenhanced CT or stone protocol CT in evaluation of the patients with urinary tract calculi has now emerged as the investigation of choice and has replaced IVU in maximum institutes with reported sensitivity as high as 95% and specificity of 98% compared with 52–69% for IVU. The superior diagnostic performance of CT versus IVU, increased patient acceptability, and equivalent or even lower radiation exposure using low-dose techniques are reasons for the recommendation of CT over IVU. The reported sensitivity and specificity of plain film in the detection of renal and ureteric calculus (>5 mm) are only 45–58% and 60–77%, respectively. The detection rate for stones <5 mm is even low, with a sensitivity of 12% or less. Ultrasonography (USG) usually demonstrates direct signs of obstruction of the urinary tract such as hydronephrosis and hydroureter with a reasonable degree of sensitivity (95%), but at the cost of a low specificity of around 67%. Operator expertise, and poor visualization of midureter due to overlapping bowel gas shadows are the main limiting factors.

Q2. "Whirlpool sign" on sonography suggests the diagnosis of which of the following?

a. Testicular torsion
b. Acute epididymitis
c. Acute ureteric colic
d. Acute pyelonephritis

Ans. a. In the acute phase of testicular torsion, on grayscale sonography, the testis appears enlarged, the spermatic cord immediately cranial to the testis and epididymis is twisted, and an intrascrotal portion of the cord appears as edematous curled echogenic extratesticular mass causing a characteristic "whirlpool pattern." The main objective in case of acute scrotal pain is to diagnose or exclude testicular torsion as this condition requires prompt surgical intervention in order to avoid irreversible testicular damage. However, clinical differentiation between testicular torsion and other causes of acute testicular pain (epididymitis and orchitis) is often difficult. In testicular torsion color, Doppler shows absent or significantly less blood flow in the affected testicle whereas, in acute epididymitis/epididymo-orchitis, there is thickening and enlargement of the epididymis, the echogenicity of the epididymis and testis is usually decreased with significantly increased blood flow on Doppler.

Q3. Primary imaging techniques in the evaluation of the genitourinary tract in a patient who has suffered either blunt or penetrating trauma is which of the following?

a. Ultrasonography
b. IVU
c. Contrast-enhanced computed tomography (CECT)
d. Plain abdomen radiograph

Ans. a. Because up to 10% of traumas have an associated injury to the genitourinary (GU) tract, current guidelines recommend contrast-enhanced abdominal/pelvic CT with delayed imaging in patients with suspected GU injury. The use of delayed imaging, once contrast is in the collecting system is crucial for assessing subtle urothelial abnormalities. The primary role of imaging in suspected trauma to the urinary tract is to accurately assess the severity and extent of injury, evaluate the injured kidney for underlying disorders, evaluate the anatomy and function of the opposite kidney, and assess for other associated injuries. The low sensitivity of IVU for detecting or characterizing injuries limits its usefulness in the routine evaluation of a trauma patient. The role of IVU is currently relegated to situations in which CT may not be available. Point-of-care ultrasound (POCUS) is one of the quickest imaging modalities available and is becoming increasingly prevalent in the emergency department but has low sensitivity and specificity.

Q4. Radiological investigation of choice in acute urinary tract infection (UTI) and acute pyelonephritis (APN) is:

a. Ultrasonography
b. CECT
c. IVU
d. Plain X-ray of KUB

Ans. b. Contrast-enhanced computed tomography is considered the imaging technique of choice for diagnosis or follow-up of patients with acute UTIs. The reported sensitivity and specificity of CT for APNs is 86.8

and 87.5%, compared with 74.3 and 56.7% for the US. Nephrographic-phase imaging is helpful in detecting loss of corticomedullary differentiation with one or more wedge-shaped zones or streaky areas of reduced enhancement extending from the papilla through the medulla to the renal capsule. A striated nephrogram may be observed. Involvement of Gerota's fascia with extrarenal extension may also be noted. The presence of nonenhancing fluid locules within an area of APN suggests fluid liquefaction and abscess formation. APN with diffuse renal involvement causes impaired contrast excretion as per the severity of infection.

Q5. Choose the correction option. The imaging procedure of choice in the evaluation of patients with hematuria is:

a. Computed tomography urography (CTU)
b. Magnetic resonance urography (MRU)
c. IVU
d. Dimercaptosuccinic acid (DMSA) scintigraphy

Ans. a. The American College of Radiology has rated CTU as the imaging procedure of choice as to its appropriateness for evaluating patients with hematuria. CTU has a better diagnostic yield when compared with IVU in patients with hematuria. Detailed anatomy of the major portions of the urinary tract—the kidneys, intrarenal collecting systems, ureters, and bladder can be assessed by CTU. In addition, relative to IVU, CTU can be used to depict structures outside the urinary tract and thus is useful in detecting unsuspected extra urinary disease. MRU may be preferable to CTU for performing imaging examinations of pediatric and younger patients, pregnant women, patients undergoing repeat assessment of the collecting systems (because of the absence of ionizing radiation), patients with a history of allergic to iodinated contrast, and patients with renal dysfunction.

Q6. Which of the following benefits has made USG the first imaging modality in the assessment and follow-up of renal diseases?

a. Portability
b. Cost-effectiveness and availability
c. No radiation exposure to the patient
d. Operator expertise

Ans. a. True, b. True, c. True, and d. False

Ultrasound has the benefits of portability, low cost, availability, and no radiation exposure to the patient. POCUS is one of the quickest imaging modalities available and is becoming increasingly prevalent in the emergency department. Sonography is a real-time modality, interpretation of sonography images, and thus, sensitivity and specificity are dependent on operator experience, expertise, and skills.

Q7. What are the indications of voiding cystourethrogram? Mark each statement as True or False.

a. To image posterior urethra
b. To demonstrate vesicoureteric reflux
c. To assess renal function
d. To image pathologies of the prostate

Ans. a. True, b. True, c. False, and d. False

Voiding cystourethrogram (VCUG) or descending urethrography is used to image posterior urethra and demonstrate vesicoureteric reflux, particularly in pediatric patients. The bladder is initially drained of urine and later filled with water-soluble iodinated contrast medium using a Foley or suprapubic catheter. Anteroposterior and oblique bladder imaging is performed using intermittent fluoroscopy with spot images of abnormal findings. Once the bladder is filled to capacity, the urethra is imaged in profile using an oblique projection after catheter removal and during micturition in supine or while standing.

Q8. Mark each statement as True or False. In patients with trauma presenting with gross hematuria with pelvic fracture evaluation of the urinary bladder can be done by:

a. Conventional cystography
b. CT cystography
c. USG
d. Conventional radiography

Ans. a. True, b. True, c. False, and d. False

Both CT cystography and conventional cystography are similar in their sensitivity and specificity 95% and 100%, respectively for detecting and characterizing bladder injury. On conventional cystography, the identification of contrast material outside the confines of the urinary bladder confirms the diagnosis of bladder rupture. With extraperitoneal leaks, the contrast agent remains confined to the pelvis; with intraperitoneal leaks, contrast material may outline bowel loops and extend into the paracolic gutters, and diffusely into the peritoneal cavity. For CT cystography, active distention of the urinary bladder with contrast material is essential to reliably exclude a bladder leak. Multiplanar reformation may be helpful to better delineate the site of the bladder rupture. USG and CT performed with excreted contrast material (a routine abdominopelvic CT study) only may show intraperitoneal or extraperitoneal fluid but cannot differentiate urine from ascites. Conventional plain radiographs will detect fractures of the pelvis but cannot diagnose bladder injuries.

Q9. Mark each statement as True or False. All radiology departments must be necessarily equipped with emergency drugs and resuscitation equipment because there are:

a. Potential risk of radiation injury
b. Potential risk of anaphylactic reaction with iodinated contrast
c. Potential risk of adverse reaction with barium preparations
d. Potential risk of adverse reactions with ultrasound waves

Ans. a. False, b. True, c. False, and d. False

The frequency of allergic-like and physiologic adverse events related to the intravascular administration of iodinated contrast media (ICM) has decreased considerably with changes in usage from ionic high-osmolality contrast media (HOCM) to nonionic low-osmolality contrast media (LOCM). Statistically acute adverse events occurred in 5–15% of all patients who received HOCM. LOCM is associated with a very low incidence of acute adverse events, and the bulk of these are not life threatening. An overall acute adverse reaction rate (allergic-like + physiologic) for nonionic LOCM reported from various studies is in the range of 0.2–0.6%. Serious acute reactions to IV LOCM are rare, with a historical rate of approximately 0.04%. The majority of adverse side effects of LOCM are mild nonlife-threatening events that usually require only observation, reassurance, and/or supportive measures. Severe and potentially life-threatening adverse events continue to occur rarely and unpredictably. Nearly all life-threatening contrast reactions occur within the first 20 minutes after contrast medium injection. All personnel who inject intravascular contrast media should be prepared to recognize the variety of adverse events that may occur following ICM administration and institute appropriate measures to manage the reaction.

Q10. Mark each statement as True or False. Renal perfusion and excretory functions are best assessed by:

a. IVU
b. CTU
c. Renal scintigraphy
d. MRU

Ans. a. False, b. False, c. True, and d. False

Renal perfusion and excretory functions of the kidney are best assessed by radioactive tracers that are excreted by the kidney, while tracers that are retained in the kidney are helpful in assessing renal anatomy. Currently, the most satisfactory tracer for imaging renal anatomy is 99mTc-DMSA; for investigating renal perfusion and excretion 99mTc-mercaptoacetyltriglycine (MAG3) is now preferred over the earlier tracer 99mTc-diethylenetriaminepentaacetate (DTPA). Analysis of the images and renogram curves obtained during the first pass of the tracer illustrates renal perfusion. The size, shape, and location of the kidneys can be assessed by taking the images obtained 3–5 minutes after injection. During the excretion phase, serial images can be obtained to assess relative renal function, rate of transit of activity through the renal pelvis, drainage from the pelvis, and the residual bladder volume after micturition. Despite improvements in anatomic resolution by various other modalities lessening the role of scintigraphy for anatomic evaluation, scintigraphy maintains a key role in evaluating renal perfusion and function. The sensitivity of IVU and CTU for the assessment of renal function is much less as compared to renal scintigraphy. Evaluation of urinary tract anatomy and pathology are predominantly done by ultrasound, CT scan, and MRI.

Q11. Which is not an indication for dialysis in acute kidney injury (AKI)?

a. Severe acidosis
b. Hyperkalemia
c. Volume overload hypertension
d. Raise of creatinine by three times

Ans. d. As discussed, the indications of dialysis are limited in patients with AKI. The rise of creatinine may define severity but is never an indication of AKI. However, AKI on chronic kidney disease (CKD), with patients on maintenance hemodialysis, might be an exception.

Q12. Which drug does not cause acute interstitial nephritis?

a. Beta lactums
b. Sulfonamides
c. Amphotericin B
d. Acyclovir

Ans. c. Amphotericin B causes direct cell membrane permeability to be increased. Direct cell damage.

Q13. Cystatin C, a novel biomarker for AKI, all are correct, *except*:

a. Indicate glomerular filtration rate (GFR)
b. Good indicator in sepsis patient
c. Indicator of morbidity
d. Not affected by age, muscle mass, and gender

Ans. c. Indicator of morbidity. Cystatin C is an early more accurate predictor of intensity of AKI. It remains unaffected by age, and sex as its production is constant. There is no reference for cystatin C as a morbidity predictor.

Q14. Management of AKI all are recommended, *except*:

a. Adequate volume resuscitation
b. Avoiding colloids
c. Maintain mean arterial pressure (MAP) around 65 mm Hg
d. Low-dose dopamine infusion

Ans. d. There is a strong class IA recommendation by Kidney Disease: Improving Global Outcomes (KDIGO) for using the low-dose dopamine infusion. Hypothetically, low-dose dopamine is believed to cause better blood flow in renal circulation. However, many studies and meta-analyses found, worsening of AKI, increased mortality, and arrhythmias.

Q15. Definition of relapse of UTI is:

a. Recurrent of UTI within 2 weeks with different organisms
b. Recurrent of UTI within 2 weeks with the same organism
c. Recurrent of UTI within 2 months with different organisms
d. Two uncomplicated UTIs in 6 months

Ans. b.

- *Recurrent UTI:* It is defined as two uncomplicated UTIs in 6 months or three or more uncomplicated UTIs in the preceding 12 months
- *Relapse of UTI:* It is defined as the recurrence of UTI within 2 weeks of treatment completion for the same organism
- *Reinfection:* It is a recurrence of UTI with a different organism than the previous one

Q16. Most common organism for complicated and uncomplicated UTI:

a. *Escherichia coli*
b. *Staphylococcus saprophyticus*
c. *Klebsiella*
d. *Proteus mirabilis*

Ans. a. *Escherichia coli* (75–95%) followed by *Staphylococcus saprophyticus* (5–15%) are the most common pathogens responsible for complicated and noncomplicated UTIs.

Q17. Mark each statement as True or False regarding cystitis.

a. Superficial infection of bladder
b. More common in men
c. Patient had no fever usually

d. History of sexually transmitted disease (STD)
e. History of previous instrumentation

Ans. **a. True, b. False, c. True, d. False, and e. True**

Cystitis is a superficial infection of the urinary bladder. A patient who has cystitis presents with localized symptoms such as dysuria, urinary frequency, hesitancy, hematuria, or suprapubic pain. It is more common in women than men. Usually, patients with cystitis have no fever with only the abovementioned localized symptoms. It is necessary to evaluate STD by proper history such as urethral discharge, vaginal discharge, vaginal bleeding, new sexual partner, and sexual partner with STD. All these symptoms are more suggestive of STD than cystitis. Men, with >50 years of age, prostatic abnormality, and a history of previous instrumentation can present with cystitis.

Q18. Emphysematous pyelonephritis is seen in:

a. Prostatomegaly
b. Recurrent UTI
c. Uncontrolled diabetes mellitus (DM)
d. Recurrent renal colic patient

Ans. c. Emphysematous pyelonephritis is a severe necrotizing infection of renal parenchyma and perirenal space caused by *E. coli* mostly in uncontrolled diabetic patients. It is believed that high blood sugar in tissue provides a favorable environment for *E. coli* which ferments sugar and produces carbon dioxide.

Q19. Mark each statement true or false regarding UTI in pregnancy.

a. No need to treat asymptomatic bacteriuria
b. Fluoroquinolones and tetracyclines contraindicated in pregnancy
c. Nitrofurantoin can be given in any trimester
d. Obstetrician opinion is necessary
e. Most common organism is *E. coli*

Ans. **a. False, b. True, c. False, d. True, and e. True**

In pregnancy, asymptomatic bacteriuria also should be treated because there are chances of developing severe sepsis, premature labor, low birth weight, etc. The most common organism is *E. coli*. Fluoroquinolones and tetracyclines are contraindicated in pregnancy. Nitrofurantoin should be avoided in the first trimester and near-term period because of its effect on organogenesis, and potential to cause hemolytic anemia in newborns. Ceftriaxone causes kernicterus by bilirubin displacement. An obstetrician's opinion is necessary.

Q20. Which of the following is *not* a common complication of end-stage renal disease?

a. Bleeding gastric and duodenal ulcers
b. Pericarditis
c. Peripheral neuropathy
d. Subdural hematoma
e. Uremic encephalopathy

Ans. a. The end-stage renal disease causes a number of complications in almost every organ system. Gastrointestinal complications include chronic constipation, gastritis, and increased gastrointestinal bleeding due to the bleeding dyscrasias associated with uremia. However, the incidence of bleeding ulcers is the same as in the general population.

Q21. What is the most common complication of hemodialysis?

a. Air embolism
b. Hyperphosphatemia
c. Hypocalcemia
d. Hypoglycemia
e. Hypotension

Ans. e. Hypotension occurs in up to 30% of hemodialysis treatments, usually caused by excessive ultrafiltration after underestimating the patient's ideal (dry) weight.

Q22. Patients on an alpha-adrenergic receptor blocker for the treatment of urinary retention need to be warned of what possible side effects.

a. Bradycardia
b. Erectile dysfunction
c. Hypotension
d. Tinnitus
e. Urinary incontinence

Ans. c. Postural hypotension, especially with the first dose of an alpha-blocking agent, is the most common side effect of alpha-adrenergic receptor blockade.

Q23. Which of the following conditions requires emergent urologic consultation?

a. Balanitis
b. Balanoposthitis
c. Paraphimosis
d. Phimosis
e. Posthitis

Ans. c. This patient has balanoposthitis which occurs commonly in diabetics. Checking serum glucose is essential because Balanitis, posthitis, and balanoposthitis may be the first presenting signs of diabetes mellitus.

Q24. Which of the following is *not* an indication of emergent dialysis?

a. Blood urea nitrogen (BUN) >100 mg/dL
b. Lithium poisoning
c. Severe metabolic acidosis
d. Uremic encephalopathy with seizures
e. Uremic pericarditis

Ans. a. It is recommended to keep the BUN <100 mg/dL. Each patient should be evaluated by a nephrologist to assess the need for dialysis, there is no absolute BUN value at which to dialyze a patient.

Q25. What is the most critical complication of injection therapy for the treatment of erectile dysfunction?

a. Localized hematoma
b. Penile pain
c. Priapism
d. Prolonged erection
e. Syncope

Ans. c. Priapism is the most critical complication as prolonged engorgement can lead to ischemia. Alprostadil for both intracavernous and intraurethral or papaverine phentolamine for intracavernous injection therapy for erectile dysfunction is used. Emergent urologic consult narcotic analgesia, and injection of terbutaline, 0.25–0.5 mg subcutaneously into the deltoid, repeated in 30 minutes if needed. If this fails, corporal irrigation with phenylephrine or plain saline is required. If this fails as well, surgery may be required. simple or exchange transfusion is required in priapism in Sickle cell.

Neurological Emergencies MCQs

Devendra Richhariya

Q1. A 55-year-old man presented to the emergency department with a headache that started about 12 hours ago. He describes the headache as the worst ever headache that started abruptly. The past medical history is insignificant except for hypertension. A head computed tomography (CT) scan was requested and showed no pathology. What is the recommended diagnostic modality at this point?

a. Brain magnetic resonance imaging (MRI)
b. Repeat CT scan in 24 hours
c. Lumbar puncture
d. Serum D-dimer level

Ans. c.

Q2. A 60-year-old woman was brought to the emergency department with sudden onset of headache, vomiting, and right-sided hemiparesis. A head CT scan was done and revealed a left-sided basal ganglia intracranial hemorrhage without any intraventricular hemorrhage or midline shift. The following managements are recommended for this patient: Mark the statement as True/False.

a. Target systolic blood pressure is <140 mm Hg
b. Target blood sugar is <126 mg/dL
c. The patient should receive an antiepileptic drug
d. Neurosurgical intervention is indicated rarely

Ans. a. True, b. False, c. False, and d. True

Q3. A 64-year-old woman presented to the emergency department with sudden onset of a thunderclap headache. A head CT scan revealed subarachnoid hemorrhage (SAH). She has a previous history of hypertension, diabetes mellitus, and ischemic heart disease. The patient is alert and oriented, but her blood pressure is 210/120 mm Hg, while her heart rate is 75 beats/min. Which recommendation regarding blood pressure control is correct?

a. IV nitroglycerine to a target systolic blood pressure of 140 mm Hg
b. IV labetalol to a target systolic blood pressure of 140 mm Hg

c. IV nitroglycerine to a target systolic blood pressure of 160 mm Hg
d. IV labetalol to a target systolic blood pressure of 160 mm Hg

Ans. d.

Q4. What cerebrospinal fluid (CSF) finding is most diagnostic of SAH?

a. Elevated opening pressure
b. Greater than 50 red blood cells (RBCs)/mL
c. High white blood cell (WBC) count
d. Low glucose
e. Xanthochromia

Ans. e. Xanthochromia is yellow discoloration of the CSF due to bilirubin accumulation from the enzymatic breakdown of hemoglobin in RBCs. It is diagnostic of SAH. Xanthochromia develops within 12 hours of SAH and lasts for up to 3 weeks.

Q5. Which of the following would be atypical for a migraine headache?

a. Duration >12 hours
b. Severe pain
c. Sudden onset
d. Unilateral
e. Vomiting

Ans. c. Migraines, rarely start suddenly.

Q6. Which of the following is associated with a higher risk of stroke after a transient ischemic attack (TIA)?

a. Age <60
b. Anemia
c. Duration of TIA symptoms >10 minutes
d. Family history of coronary artery disease
e. Visual symptoms during TIA

Ans. c. *The following features increase the risk of stroke:* Age >60, hypertension at the time of the TIA, diabetes, duration of symptoms >10 minutes, and weakness or speech disturbance.

Q7. A young woman with a history of autoimmune diseases complains of new onset weakness. You are considering myasthenia gravis. Examination of which of the following is most likely to help confirm this diagnosis?

a. Distal lower extremities
b. Eyes
c. Gait
d. Reflexes
e. Vibratory sense

Ans. b. Both ptosis and ophthalmoplegia are seen; a common examination finding is progressive ptosis during sustained upward gaze.

Q8. Grading of coma can be estimated by the following score. Mark the statement True or False.

a. Glasgow Coma Scale (GCS) score
b. THREE score
c. FOUR score
d. FIVE score

Ans. a. True, b. False, c. True, and d. False

Grading of coma can be done by Glasgow Coma Scale (GCS) and full outline of unresponsiveness score (FOUR)

Q9. Cause of acute flaccid paralysis are all, except:

a. Hyperkalemia
b. Lathyrism
c. Botulism
d. Hypernatremia

Ans. d.

Endocrinal Emergencies MCQs

Devendra Richhariya

Q1. What is the most common cause of primary adrenal insufficiency (AI)?

a. Autoimmune disorders
b. Adrenal hemorrhage
c. Drugs
d. Idiopathic
e. Infectious

Ans. a. Approximately 70% of primary AI is caused by autoimmune disorders.

Q2. A 39-year-old alcoholic presents with ataxia, confusion, and confabulations. What vitamin deficiency is causing these symptoms?

a. Vitamin A
b. Vitamin B_1
c. Vitamin B_6
d. Vitamin B_{12}
e. Vitamin C

Ans. b. Wernicke-Korsakoff syndrome is a complication seen most often in malnourished chronic alcoholics who are suffering from a vitamin B_1 deficiency.

Q3. A 67-year-old female presents with bilateral hand and feet paresthesia, decreased proprioception, anemia, and an elevated lactate dehydrogenase level. What vitamin deficiency is causing her symptoms?

a. Vitamin A
b. Vitamin B_1
c. Vitamin B_2
d. Vitamin B_{12}
e. Vitamin K

Ans. d. Vitamin B_{12} deficiency causes pernicious anemia. Vitamin B_{12} takes several forms: Cyanocobalamin, hydroxocobalamin, aquocobalamin, nitritocobalamin, coenzyme B_{12}, and methylcobalamin.

Q4. A 16-year-old female with acne complains of blurry vision, anorexia, myalgias, and hair loss. What vitamin is causing these symptoms?

a. Vitamin A
b. Vitamin B
c. Vitamin D
d. Vitamin E
e. Vitamin K

Ans. a. *Vitamin A comes in two primary forms:* Retinol, which is commonly used to treat acne, and 3-dehydroretinol. Symptoms of overdose include blurred vision, appetite loss, abnormal skin pigmentation, loss of hair, and occasionally pseudotumor cerebri. Treatment is withdrawal of vitamin A.

Q5. Criteria for diagnosing the diabetes as per the American Diabetic Association include all, *except:*

a. Glycated hemoglobin (HbA1c) ≥6.5%
b. Fasting blood glucose ≥126 mg/dL (fasting—no calorie intake for at least 8 hours)
c. Postprandial blood glucose ≥250 mg/dL
d. Random blood sugars ≥200 mg/dL with symptoms of hyperglycemia or hyperglycemic crisis
e. Oral glucose tolerance test (OGTT) 2-hour plasma glucose ≥200 mg/dL

Ans. c. Diagnosing the diabetes on the basis of following criteria as per the American Diabetic Association: HbA1c ≥6.5%, fasting blood glucose ≥126 mg/dL (fasting—no calorie intake for at least 8 hours), random blood sugars ≥200 mg/dL with symptoms of hyperglycemia or hyperglycemic crisis, and OGTT 2-hour plasma glucose ≥200 mg/dL

Q6. Which of the following is not the rapid-acting insulin?

a. Insulin lispro
b. Insulin aspart
c. Insulin detemir
d. Insulin glulisine

Ans. c. Insulin glargine, biosimilar insulin glargine, and detemir are long-acting insulin.

Q7. Regarding diabetic ketosis, mark the below statement as True or False.

a. Blood glucose >200 mg/dL
b. Metabolic acidosis pH <7.3 and bicarbonate <15 mEq/L
c. Presence of ketones in the blood and the urine
d. An initial bolus dose of insulin is not necessary for initiation of treatment

Ans. **a. True, b. True c. True, and d. True**

The International Society for Pediatric and Adolescent Diabetes (ISPAD) defines diabetic ketoacidosis (DKA) as blood glucose >200 mg/dL with metabolic acidosis (pH <7.3 and bicarbonate <15 mEq/L with presence of ketones in the blood and the urine). An initial bolus dose of insulin is not necessary. The insulin is started as intravenous infusion and this rapidly archives the steady state levels in the serum. The rate of insulin infusion is usually 0.1 unit/kg/hour; however, no difference in rate of fall of blood glucose is seen in some studies with lower doses of 0.05 units/kg/hour.

Q8. Regarding hypoglycemia following statements are true, *except:*

a. Whipple's triad has been used to describe hypoglycemia, which includes recognition of symptoms of hypoglycemia, low blood sugar detection, and relief of symptoms by correction of the low blood sugar levels
b. Tests, such as insulin, proinsulin, and C-peptide levels are of limited value in evaluation of hypoglycemia
c. Elevated insulin levels with elevated C-peptide levels are seen with secretagogue agents such as sulfonylurea administration
d. Neurological recovery to the restoration of a normal glucose is sufficient evidence to confirm hypoglycemic events

Ans. c. Other tests, such as insulin, proinsulin, and C-peptide levels are to be measured, if insulin levels are high in the presence of low C-peptide levels shows that the patient has received the exogenous insulin. Elevated insulin levels with elevated C-peptide levels are seen with secretagogue agents such as sulfonylurea administration.

Q9. Regarding the hyperosmolar hyperglycemic syndrome (HHS), true statements are all, *except:*

a. HHS is the most serious acute hyperglycemic emergency in patients with type 2 diabetes
b. Current diagnostic HHS criteria include a plasma glucose level >600 mg/dL and increased effective plasma osmolality >320 mOsm/kg in the absence of ketoacidosis
c. The reported mortality is lower than with DKA
d. Treatment of HHS is includes replacing volume deficit and correcting hyperosmolality, hyperglycemia, and electrolyte disturbances, as well as management of the underlying illness that precipitated the metabolic decompensation

Ans. c. The reported mortality is about 10 times higher than the mortality rate in patient with DKA.

35 CHAPTER Eye, ENT, Oral, and Dental Emergencies MCQs

Devendra Richhariya

Q1. Which of the following is the one ophthalmologic emergency in which visual acuity and eye examination are not required before starting the treatment?

a. Acute monocular visual loss
b. Acute red eye with photophobia
c. Blunt trauma to the eye
d. Chemical burn to the eye
e. Foreign body to the eye using high-powered tool

Ans. d. Full vital signs, including visual acuity, the vital sign of the eye, and a full eye examination should be done before initiating treatment except for chemical exposure to eye.

Q2. Which of the following diagnoses is likely the cause of this patient's presented to emergency department (ED) with "acute blindness for 1 hour with pain"?

a. Acute optic neuritis if you notice that there is a Marcus Gunn pupil and the posterior chamber is clear
b. Acute retinal artery occlusion secondary to carotid cholesteatoma if visual loss is bilateral
c. Hysterical blindness if the patient exhibits no lateral nystagmus when vertical lines are passed before the eyes
d. Occipital stroke
e. Uveitis

Ans. a. A normal examination with a Marcus Gunn pupil suggests optic neuritis or other causes of afferent papillary defect.

Q3. Which of the following statements about acute hearing loss and tinnitus is most accurate?

a. Antidepressants are the most commonly implicated drugs in tinnitus
b. Metoprolol is the most commonly implicated drug causing tinnitus
c. The majority of tinnitus is drug-induced
d. Tinnitus may be heard by the examiner

Ans. d. Objective tinnitus can be heard by the examiner [i.e., secondary to arteriovenous (AV) malformations, arterial bruits, mechanical abnormalities] and subjective tinnitus can be heard by the patient (i.e., secondary to cochlear/neurosensory insult from toxins or vascular insufficiency).

Q4. Which of the following statements is most accurate about outer ear infections?

a. *Candida* and *Aspergillus* are the most common cause of otomycosis and best treated with topical antifungals
b. Corticosteroid solution eardrops are safe with perforated tympanic membranes (TMs)
c. Otitis externa (OE) is best treated with gently irrigation with hydrogen peroxide and suctioning, alkalinizing agents, topical antimicrobials, and steroids
d. Patients with a history of diabetes and human immunodeficiency virus (HIV), or elderly presented with OE and trismus, cranial nerve palsies, or any systemic signs should get computed tomography (CT) of the brain
e. Topical ofloxacin is contraindicated in OE with perforated TM in a 6-year-old child

Ans. d. Any patients with a history of being immunocompromised present with OE.

Q5. A 54-year-old woman, with a history of alcohol abuse, presents with a well-demarcated 4-cm raised, puffy, warm, erythematous patch without fluctuance on her right cheek that started as a bug bite 6 hours ago. What is the most likely diagnosis?

a. Cellulitis
b. Erysipelas
c. Facial abscess
d. Impetigo
e. Panniculitis

Ans. b. This patient presents with the classic appearance of erysipelas, rapidly spreading, raised, red, puffy appearance with sharply defined borders. Cellulitis, chemical or infectious, is more diffuse in appearance.

Q6. Regarding facial cellulitis the true statement is:

a. Facial cellulitis must be treated more aggressively than cellulitis in other body areas
b. Complications of facial cellulitis include cavernous sinus thrombosis and possible extension of the cellulitis to the brain if not treated

c. Most facial cellulitis is caused by extension of infection from the oral cavity, whereas acute sinusitis accounts for most of the remainder of causes
d. The organisms responsible for facial cellulitis in adults are usually mixed flora

Ans. a. Facial cellulitis must be treated more aggressively than cellulitis in other body areas because of the morbidity and mortality of complications, which include cavernous sinus thrombosis and possible extension of the cellulitis to the brain.

Q7. With regard to temporomandibular joint (TMJ), which of the statements is false?

a. TMJ is formed by articular surface between the mandibular condyles and the temporal bone
b. TMJ is lined by synovial membrane and acts by hinge as well as sliding mechanism
c. Dislocation of mandible can happen in four positions: Anterior, posterior, superior, and lateral
d. Shallow mandibular fossa is not the risk factor for mandibular dislocations

Ans. d. Risk factors for mandibular dislocations are as follows: Shallow mandibular fossa dystonia, convulsions, hypermotility syndrome, and previous history of TMJ dislocation.

Q8. Techniques used for reduction of TMJ are all, *except:*

a. Classic technique
b. Supine technique
c. Recumbent technique
d. Wrist pivot method

Ans. b. Close reduction can be done in emergency under proper analgesia and muscle relaxants. The techniques used are classic technique, recumbent technique, and wrist pivot method.

Q9. A healthy 48-year-old man without any significant past medical history comes in complaining of 12 hours of diplopia. On examination, she has a dilated right pupil and can only abduct and look up with her right eye when range of motion is tested. What is her likely diagnosis?

a. Aneurysm
b. Diabetes mellitus
c. Carotid dissection
d. Wernicke encephalopathy
e. Vertebral artery dissection

Ans. a. This patient is presenting with a third-nerve palsy and pupil dilation. Posterior circulation aneurysm should be considered until proven otherwise [acute cranial nerve (CN) III palsy with ipsilateral pupillary dilatation].

Q10. Which of the following statements is most accurate about peritonsillar abscesses?

a. A physical examination suggestive of peritonsillar abscess with negative needle aspiration requires imaging to rule out abscess
b. Acute tonsillectomy is contraindicated especially in children
c. Adjuvant steroids have not been found to be helpful
d. Needle aspiration effectively treats 65% of patients and often incision and drainage will be required
e. The proper technique of needle aspiration is application of topical anesthesia followed by introduction of an 18-gauge needle halfway between the base of the uvula and the maxillary alveolar ridge penetrating no more than 2 cm

Ans. a. A physical examination suggestive of peritonsillar abscess with negative needle aspiration requires CT or to rule out abscess, also most common mimic is peritonsillar cellulitis. Needle aspiration will effectively treat 90%.

Q11. A 14-year-old male presents with a sore throat. On examination, he is noted to have bilaterally enlarged tonsils and has tender cervical lymphadenopathy. From reviewing his past history, you can see that this is his fifth episode of tonsillitis in the past year. He reports having missed days at school due to his sore throats over the past 12 months. His Centor score is 3/4 and you therefore elect to prescribe a course of antibiotic for him. What other management option should be considered?

a. Screen for infectious mononucleosis
b. Continue antibiotics
c. Advise her to take vitamin C and zinc supplements
d. Check her serum immunoglobulin levels
e. Refer to ear-nose-throat (ENT) for consideration of a tonsillectomy

Ans. e. Refer to ENT for consideration of a tonsillectomy.

Q12. A 64-year-old lady presents with a 7-day history of painful, left-sided neck swelling below the angle of the jaw. She also complains of foulish taste in her oral cavity. On examination, she has a temperature of 103°F and a 2.5 × 4.0 cm submandibular mass which is tender to palpation. There is associated tender lymphadenopathy. What is the most likely diagnosis?

a. Lymphadenitis
b. Viral parotitis
c. Sialadenitis
d. Sjögren's syndrome
e. Malignancy

Ans. c.

Q13. A 5-year-old boy is brought by his mother with complaints of sore throat, fever, and was acting confused. He is leaning forward on hands, in the "tripod" position, with mouth open, tongue out, and head forward and tilted up in a sniffing position. He has a loud inspiratory stridor. Looking at clinical features what should be your treatment plan?

a. Give oral antibiotics and discharge
b. Secure airway at the earliest and involve ENT team
c. Give oxygen inhalation and observe
d. Refer to ENT team as outpatient
e. Secure intravenous (IV) line, give IV antibiotics and admit

Ans. b.

Q14. A 23-year-old female presents to you in ED and complaints of being unwell, having high-grade fever, throat pain, and not being able to swallow and eat for past 3 days. She has muffled, "hot potato voice" with halitosis as well. She is hypotensive, tachycardic, dehydrated, and looks unwell. Upon direct visualization, you see erythematous swollen soft palate, displacement, and inflammation of tonsillar pillar. You have diagnosed this patient as having quinsy. What should be the next steps in management of this patient?

a. Oral antibiotics and outpatient follow-up
b. Surgical intervention at the earliest as outpatient
c. Admission, IV fluids, IV antibiotics, and surgical intervention
d. Saline gargles and analgesia
e. Refer to ENT outpatient

Ans. c.

Q15. A 57-year-old man with history of oropharyngeal cancer presents to ED with pain over floor of mouth, progressive tongue swelling, restricted neck movement, and fever. There is marked tenderness of floor of mouth, neck, and surrounding tissue with crepitus on palpation. Patient also states that his voice has also changed in the past days and you hear a muffled voice. What is the most probable underlying condition?

a. Peritonsillar abscess
b. Retropharyngeal abscess
c. Ludwig's angina
d. Progression of cancer
e. Pharyngitis

Ans. c.

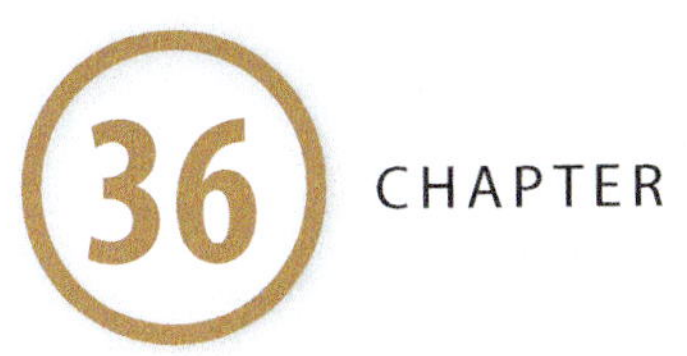

Hematology and Oncology MCQs

Devendra Richhariya

Q1. What are the characteristic features of acute leukemia?

a. Rapid deceleration of abnormal white cells due to bone marrow dysfunction
b. The presence of lymphocyte—predominant cells, sometimes termed "popcorn cells"
c. Rapid deceleration of plasma cells
d. Rapid proliferation of abnormal white cells due to bone marrow dysfunction
e. The presence of mature B cell neoplasms

Ans. d.

Q2. What are the risk factors of acute leukemia?

a. Genetic predisposition, exposure to radiation, exposure to benzene, exposure to household pesticide, obesity, history of hematological malignancy, familial history and smoking
b. Genetic predisposition, exposure to Epstein-Barr virus, exposure to benzene, exposure to household pesticide, obesity, history of hematological malignancy, familial history and smoking
c. Genetic predisposition, exposure to radiation, age, exposure to household pesticide, obesity, history of hematological malignancy, familial history and smoking
d. Genetic predisposition, exposure to Epstein-Barr virus, age, exposure to household pesticide, obesity, history of hematological malignancy, familial history and smoking
e. Exposure to radiation, exposure to benzene, exposure to household pesticide, age, gender, familial history and smoking

Ans. a.

Q3. What are the most common clinical presentations of acute leukemia?

a. Fatigue, amnesia, thrombosis, weight loss, gastrointestinal (GI) symptoms, persistent fever/recurrent infections, generally unwell, night sweats, poor wound healing, and sepsis

b. Fatigue, amnesia, loss of appetite, weight loss, easy bruising/bleeding, persistent fever/recurrent infections, generally unwell, night sweats, poor wound healing, and sepsis
c. Fatigue, GI symptoms, loss of appetite, weight loss, easy bruising/bleeding, persistent fever/recurrent infections, generally unwell, night sweats, poor wound healing, and sepsis
d. Fatigue, shortness of breath, loss of appetite, weight loss, easy bruising/bleeding, chest pain, generally unwell, night sweats, poor wound healing, and sepsis
e. Shortness of breath, amnesia, loss of appetite, weight loss, easy bruising/bleeding, persistent fever/recurrent infections, generally unwell, night sweats, poor wound healing, and sepsis

Ans. b.

Q4. What are the top four indicators for high-risk leukemia?

a. Symptoms for <7 days, absolute neutrophil count (ANC) <100 cells/mm^3, creatinine clearance <30 mL/min, liver function aminotransferase levels >5 times normal value
b. Symptoms for >7 days, ANC >100 cells/mm^3, creatinine clearance <30 mL/min, liver function aminotransferase levels >5 times normal value
c. Symptoms for >7 days, ANC <100 cells/mm^3, creatinine clearance <30 mL/min, liver function aminotransferase levels >5 times normal value
d. Symptoms for >7 days, absolute white cell count <100 cells/mm^3, creatinine clearance <30 mL/min, liver function aminotransferase levels >5 times normal value
e. Symptoms for >7 days, absolute white cell count >100 cells/mm^3, creatinine clearance <30 mL/min, liver function aminotransferase levels >5 times normal value

Ans. c.

Q5. What are the top four indicators for low-risk leukemia?

a. Duration of symptoms for <7 days, normal renal function, normal liver function, few associated symptoms
b. Duration of symptoms for >7 days, normal renal function, normal liver function, few associated symptoms
c. Duration of symptoms for <7 days, normal renal function, gender, few associated symptoms
d. Duration of symptoms >7 days, normal renal function, normal liver function, no comorbidities

e. Duration of symptoms >7 days, MASCC (Multinational Association for Supportive Care in Cancer) >21, normal renal function, few associated symptoms

Ans. a.

Q6. Which *one* of the following findings indicates hyperleukocytosis?

a. Total leukemia blood cell count is >500 × 10/L or 1,000 × 10/L
b. Total red cell count is >50 × 10/L or 100 × 10/L
c. White cell count proliferation occurs to the level of >50 × 10/L or 100 × 10L
d. Total leukemia blood cell count is >50 × 10/L or 100 × 10/L
e. Total white cell count is >500 × 10/L or 1,000 × 10/L

Ans. d.

Q7. The recommended treatment steps for hyperleukocytosis consist of:

a. Administration of oxygen, intravenous (IV) hydration, consider allopurinol, and/or rasburicase, monitor for disseminated intravascular coagulation (DIC), keep platelet count above 200 × 10^9/L
b. Administration of blood transfusion, IV hydration, consider allopurinol and/or rasburicase, monitor for DIC, keep platelet count above 20 × 10^9/L
c. Administration of oxygen, blood transfusion, consider allopurinol and/or rasburicase, monitor for DIC, keep platelet count above 20 × 10^9/L
d. Administration of oxygen, IV antibiotics, consider allopurinol and/or rasburicase, monitor for DIC, keep platelet count above 200 × 10^9/L
e. Administration of oxygen, IV hydration, consider allopurinol and/or rasburicase, monitor for DIC, keep platelet count above 20 × 10^9/L

Ans. e.

Q8. Which *one* of the following statements is true in leukemia patients?

a. Vancomycin is routinely used in the empiric treatment of neutropenic fever.
b. By starting fluid hydration promptly in hyperleukocytosis can cause enhancement of renal blood flow and promotes urinary excretion.

c. By commencing transfusion of packed red blood cells (RBCs) reduces leukocyte production.
d. Keeping a platelet count below 20 × 10^9/L minimizes bleeding risk.
e. Menstruating immunocompromised patients are safe to use tampons.

Ans. b.

Q9. Which *one* of the following five organ systems are affected by leukemia?

a. Lymph nodes, liver, spleen, central nervous system (CNS), and skin
b. Lymph nodes, lungs, spleen, CNS, and skin
c. Lymph nodes, liver, lungs, CNS, and skin
d. Lymph nodes, liver, spleen, heart, and skin
e. Lymph nodes, liver, spleen, CNS, and kidneys

Ans. a.

Q10. Which *one* of the following statements is true?

a. Allopurinol and/or rasburicase reduce the risk of neutropenic sepsis.
b. Patients with hematopoietic stem cell transplantation (HSCT) require isolation.
c. It is safe to administer suppositories to neutropenic patients.
d. Arterial blood gas (ABG) is always indicated for patients with neutropenic sepsis.
e. One set of blood cultures is sufficient for neutropenic patients.

Ans. b.

Q11. Pancytopenia is the laboratory manifestation of underlying bone marrow dysfunction or failure in the production or reduction in the levels of which of the following types of blood cells? Mark as True/False.

a. Erythrocytes
b. Leukocytes
c. Platelets
d. Macrophages
e. CD4 helper cells

Ans. a. True, b. True, c. True, d. False, and e. False

Q12. A rare form of inherited pancytopenia with features of short stature, limb abnormalities, café-au-lait lesions on the skin, microcephaly, vertebral defects, anal atresia, cardiac defects,

tracheoesophageal fistula, renal anomalies, structural malformations of the urogenital tract, or developmental delay may be seen in:

a. Drug-induced conditions
b. Fanconi anemia
c. Paroxysmal nocturnal hemoglobinuria
d. Radiation-induced conditions
e. Acquired aplastic anemia

Ans. b.

Q13. Exocrine pancreatic dysfunction with malabsorption, malnutrition, pancytopenias, and susceptibility to myelodysplasia syndrome is characteristic of:

a. Shwachman-Diamond syndrome
b. Cystic fibrosis
c. Fanconi anemia
d. Wilson's syndrome
e. Johanson-Blizzard syndrome

Ans. a.

Q14. Pancytopenia due to copper deficiency can occur in which of the following situations? Mark as True/False.

a. Total parenteral nutrition (TPN)
b. GI surgery
c. Excessive zinc intake
d. Exercise
e. Cardiac surgery

Ans. **a. True, b. True, c. True, d. False, and e. False**

Q15. Tumor cells released into the bloodstream, either spontaneously or in response to therapy, causing characteristic findings of hyperuricemia, hyperkalemia, hyperphosphatemia, and hypocalcemia are known as:

a. Tumor lysis syndrome (TLS)
b. Rhabdomyolysis
c. Vitamin D intoxication
d. Diabetic ketoacidosis
e. Gout

Ans. a.

Q16. A 60-year-old, chronic smoker presented to the emergency department with complaints of progressive shortness of breath for 1 week. He also gives history of nonproductive cough for

1 month, progressive in nature and increases on lying down. On examination, tachycardia, tachypnea, and facial edema+. Urgent contrast-enhanced CT (CECT) chest was done, which showed a large mass in right lung upper lobe with no evidence of pulmonary embolism. While returning to emergency from radiology department, he developed stridor and altered level of consciousness. Next step in management is:

a. Start heparin (suspected pulmonary embolism)
b. Urgent vascular surgeon referral for endovenous recanalization and superior vena cava (SVC) stenting
c. Urgent cardiothoracic or intervention radiologist referral for tissue biopsy
d. Start steroids

Ans. b. Next step in management is urgent vascular surgeon referral for endovenous recanalization and SVC stenting. This patient has presented to emergency with clinical features suggestive of SVC syndrome. In SVC syndrome, in a patient with suspicion of malignant etiology, pathological diagnosis should always be established prior to initiation of therapy, except in patients presenting with life-threatening signs and/or symptoms of central airway obstruction, laryngeal edema, and/or cerebral edema. In these patients after securing airway and supporting breathing and circulation, immediate vascular intervention of endovenous recanalization with/without SVC stenting should be done. Previously radiation was initial treatment of choice in such patients, but with vascular intervention relieving signs and symptoms faster than radiation, and as radiation may obscure pathological diagnosis, it is now not the initial treatment of choice in patients with life-threatening clinical features.

Q17. Febrile neutropenia is defined as:

a. Fever >100.0°F with ANC <500 cells/mm^3
b. Fever >100.0°F with ANC >500 cells/mm^3
c. Fever >101.0°F with ANC <500 cells/mm^3
d. Fever >100.1°F with ANC >500 cells/mm^3

Ans. c. *Fever:* Single oral temperature measurement of ≥101.0°F (38.3°C) or a temperature of ≥100.4°F (38.0°C) sustained over a 1-hour period; neutropenia: ANC of <500 cells/mm^3 or an ANC that is expected to decrease to <500 cells/mm^3 during the next 48 hours; profound neutropenia: ANC of <100 cells/mm^3.

Q18. All of the following are high-risk febrile neutropenia. Mark as True/False.

a. MASCC score >21
b. Profound neutropenia anticipated to extend >7 days
c. Hemodynamic instability
d. Oral or GI mucositis

Ans. a. False, b. True, c. True, and d. True

Patients of febrile neutropenia are divided into low and high risk based on associated comorbidities or a formal risk classification may be formed using MASCC scoring system. High-risk patient: Patient with any of the following criteria—MASCC score <21, profound neutropenia anticipated to extend >7 days, hemodynamic instability, oral or GI mucositis, abnormal neurologic or mental status, new pulmonary infiltrate or hypoxemia or underlying chronic lung disease, evidence of hepatic insufficiency, or renal insufficiency. Low-risk patient: Patient with any of the following criteria—neutropenia expected to resolve within 7 days, no active medical comorbidity, and MASCC score >21.

Q19. Laboratory abnormalities in TLS. Mark as True/False.

a. Hypokalemia
b. Hypophosphatemia
c. Hypocalcemia
d. Hyperuricemia

Ans. a. False, b. False, c. True, and d. True

Tumor lysis syndrome results from sudden release of intracellular metabolites, nucleic acids and proteins from tumor cells undergoing death spontaneously or post-treatment. Common laboratory abnormalities in it include hyperuricemia, hyperkalemia, hyperphosphatemia, and secondary hypocalcemia.

Q20. Regarding SIADH (syndrome of inappropriate antidiuretic hormone secretion), mark as True/False.

a. Decreased serum osmolality (<275 mOsm/kg)
b. Increased urine osmolality (>100 mOsm/kg)
c. Hypovolemia
d. Urine sodium <20 mmol/L

Ans. a. True, b. True, c. False, and d. False

SIADH is the most common cause of hyponatremia in malignancy and is due to increased production of arginine vasopressin (AVP). In SIADH, increased levels of AVP, result in water resorption/ retention and sodium loss. Causes of SIADH are cancer: Lung cancer, head and neck cancer, etc.; drugs: Cyclophosphamide, vincristine, etc.; infection: CNS and pulmonary; hypothyroidism: Head and neck cancers (paraneoplastic). Diagnosis of SIADH requires serum osmolality <275 mOsm/kg, urine osmolality >100 mOsm/kg, euvolemia, urine sodium >20 mmol/L, and no other cause for hyponatremia (diuretic, hypothyroidism, cortisol deficiency, hyperglycemia, hyperproteinemia, or hyperlipidemia).

Q21. In the evaluation of a patient with anemia, which of the following is *true*?

a. Altered mental status is never attributable to anemia.
b. Folate deficiency causes microcytic anemia.
c. Mean corpuscular hemoglobin concentration (MCHC) is a direct measure of bone marrow activity.
d. Patients with slowly developing anemia may have no complaints even with a hemoglobin concentration as low as 5 g/dL.
e. Serum ferritin is the most useful test in the diagnosis of thalassemia.

Ans. d. Anemia that develops over a long period of time may present with almost no symptoms. Rapidly developing, severe anemia can present with altered sensorium. Folate and vitamin B_{12} deficiencies cause macrocytic anemia. The MCHC is a measure of hemoglobin concentration in the average RBC. Serum ferritin is the most useful test for the diagnosis of iron-deficiency anemia.

Q22. At what platelet count level does the risk for spontaneous bleeding become significant?

a. <10,000–20,000/mm^3
b. 20,000–30,000/mm^3
c. 30,000–40,000/mm^3
d. 40,000–50,000/mm^3
e. 50,000–60,000/mm^3

Ans. a. The risk for spontaneous bleeding, particularly within the brain, is much increased as the platelet count falls below the 10,000–20,000/mm^3 range. Clinicians should consider transfusion of platelets, even in the asymptomatic patient, when the platelet level falls below 10,000/mm^3.

Q23. Which of the following is the most common sign of idiopathic thrombocytopenic purpura?

a. Epistaxis
b. Gingival bleeding
c. Hematochezia
d. Petechiae
e. Subconjunctival hemorrhage

Ans. d. Epistaxis, gingival bleeding, hematochezia, and subconjunctival hemorrhage may be seen in a patient with idiopathic thrombocytopenic purpura. Petechiae, however, are the most common physical finding.

Q24. A 29-year-old man with sickle cell disease presents to the emergency department complaining of bilateral elbow and lower leg pain. These symptoms are typical of his pain crises. Which of the following complications is the leading cause of death in patients with sickle cell disease?

a. Acute chest syndrome
b. Aplastic crisis
c. Bacteremia
d. Hypersplenism
e. Stroke

Ans. a. Acute chest syndrome is the leading cause of death in patients with sickle cell disease. It is also the second most common cause for admission, after vaso-occlusive pain crisis, in patients with sickle cell disease.

Q25. Erythropoiesis needs following:

a. Trophic hormones
b. Bone marrow precursor cells
c. Nutrients
d. All

Ans. d. All stimuli are needed. Trophic hormones: Erythropoietin (secreted from kidney peritubular cells), e.g., reduced in kidney failure, thyroid hormone, e.g., reduced in hypothyroidism; bone marrow precursor cells response to that stimulus, e.g., reduced in aplasia and bone marrow infiltration; nutrients (vitamin B_{12}, iron), e.g., less in dietary lack, celiac sprue; and RBC lifespan (lifespan ~4 months), e.g., less in hemolytic anemia (<100 days).

Q26. Indicators of intravascular hemolysis are all, *except:*

a. Reduced haptoglobin
b. High lactate dehydrogenase (LDH)
c. Urine hemosiderin
d. High indirect bilirubin

Ans. d. High indirect bilirubin is an indicator of extravascular hemolysis.

Q27. Maternal complications of HELLP (hemolysis, elevated liver enzymes, low platelet count) syndrome are all, *except:*

a. Placental abruption
b. Disseminated intravascular coagulation (DIC)
c. Liver hematoma
d. Pulmonary fibrosis

Ans. d. Placental abruption, DIC, renal failure, pulmonary edema, liver hematoma, liver failure, severe ascites, cerebral edema, and cerebral hemorrhage are the complications.

Q28. Choice of IV formulation available is:

a. Ferric carboxymaltose
b. Ferric gluconate
c. Iron sucrose
d. Iron dextran
e. All

Ans. e. A number of IV formulations are available including ferric carboxymaltose, ferric gluconate, oxetol, iron sucrose, iron isomaltoside, and iron dextran, and all of these combinations are equally effective in treating iron deficiency and have a similar safety profile. Major differences include cost formulary agreements and number of visits and time required to administer the full dose. We generally prefer low-molecular-weight iron formulation because of its low cost and ability to administer in a single dose. Others which can be administered as a single dose include ferric carboxymaltose, ferumoxytol, and iron isomaltoside. One exception is high-molecular-weight iron dextran, which has a greater frequency of allergic reactions, so it is no longer available.

Q29. When evaluating anemia, low mean corpuscular volume (MCV) <80 fL is suggestive of:

a. Iron-deficiency anemia
b. Thalassemia
c. Sideroblastic anemia
d. Lead intoxication
e. All of the above

Ans. d. Microcytosis usually reflects a decreased hemoglobin content within the RBCs and is often associated with a parallel production in mean corpuscular hemoglobin producing a hypochromic appearance on blood smear. The three most common causes of microcytosis are iron-deficiency anemia, anemia of chronic disease, and thalassemia.

Q30. A patient with hemolytic anemia develops features of pancytopenia and venous thrombosis. What is the likely diagnosis?

a. Shwachman–Diamond syndrome
b. Pyruvate kinase deficiency
c. Glucose-6-phosphate dehydrogenase (G6PD) anemia
d. Paroxysmal nocturnal hemoglobinemia (PNH)

Ans. d. Paroxysmal nocturnal hemoglobinemia is a type of hemolytic anemia associated with pancytopenia and venous thrombosis. In PNH, there is complement-mediated intravascular hemolysis. Bone marrow dysfunction also occurs resulting in pancytopenia. Transformation to aplastic anemia for acute myeloid leukemia may rarely occur. PNH is also associated with venous thrombosis; this is the most common cause of death in PNH.

Q31. Which of the following would not be seen in a patient with cyanocobalamin deficiency?

a. Glossitis
b. Conjugated hyperbilirubinemia
c. Skin hyperpigmentation
d. Mild fever

Ans. b. Unconjugated hyperbilirubinemia is seen in cyanocobalamin deficiency and not conjugated hyperbilirubinemia. Vitamin B_{12} deficiency causes megaloblastic anemia due to ineffective erythropoiesis. This leads to the formation of nucleated RBCs in the marrow which undergo early lysis. This further leads to increased unconjugated bilirubin in the plasma. The clinical features of cyanocobalamin deficiency include glossitis, angular cheilosis, anorexia and weight loss, diarrhea, leukopenia, thrombocytopenia, ineffective erythropoiesis, unconjugated jaundice, and peripheral neuropathy.

Q32. Microangiopathic anemia is seen in all of the following, *except:*

a. Antiphospholipid antibody syndrome
b. Vasculitis
c. Prosthetic heart valves
d. Eclampsia

Ans. c. Microangiopathic hemolytic anemia (MAHA) is not seen in prosthetic heart valves. It is associated with macroangiopathic hemolytic anemia. MAHA refers to cell fragmentation that occurs in microcirculation. Microvascular lesions lead to lipid narrowing due to deposition of fibrin and platelets.

Q33. Dietary folates are absorbed from which of the following? Mark as True or False.

a. Duodenum
b. Proximal ileum
c. Terminal ileum
d. Jejunum

Ans. **a. True, b. False, c. False, and d. True**

Dietary folate are absorbed from the duodenum and jejunum in the form of monoglutamates. However, vitamin B_{12} is absorbed from terminal ileum.

Q34. Regarding the treatment of hereditary spherocytosis, mark the statement True or False.

a. Cholecystectomy is only indicated for patients with clinical cholelithiasis at the time of splenectomy.

b. Cholecystectomy cannot be performed by laparoscopic root for patients with hereditary spherocytosis and pigment gallstones.
c. Splenectomy is not indicated with mild and asymptomatic disease only after puberty.
d. Lifelong penicillin prophylaxis after splenectomy is mandatory for all adult patients.

Ans. **a. True, b. False, c. True, and d. False**

Cholecystectomy is indicated in patient with hereditary spherocytosis only if they have symptomatic cholelithiasis at the time of surgery. It is usually carried out through laparoscopic approach.

Routine penicillin prophylaxis is not mandatory for adults. It is recommended up to the age of 5 years and at for at least 1 year following splenectomy.

Q35. All of the following drugs are associated with megaloblastic anemia. Mark True or False.

a. Nitrofurantoin
b. Phenytoin
c. Tetracycline
d. Temafloxacin

Ans. **a. True, b. True, c. True, and d. False**

Temafloxacin is not associated with megaloblastic anemia. Megaloblastic anemia is associated with the following drugs:

- Anticonvulsants like phenytoin, primidone, and barbiturates
- Sulfasalazine
- Antibiotics like nitrofurantoin and tetracycline
- Folate antagonists like trimethoprim, methotrexate, pyrimethamine, pentamidine, and cotrimoxazole

Q36. Which of the following is the most common cause of folate deficiency? Mark True or False.

a. Malabsorption
b. Nutritional
c. Use of antifolate
d. Deficiency of enzyme dihydrofolate (DHF) reductase

Ans. **a. False, b. True, c. False, and d. False**

Reduced nutritional intake is the most common cause of folate deficiency.

Q37. A 28-year-old woman presents with fatigue and a red, painful tongue. On examination, there is reduced vibration sense and proprioception in the feet. She is under treatment for Hashimoto's thyroiditis. Peripheral smear reveals macrocytosis

and hypersegmented neutrophils. Which of the following is true in this patient?

a. Intrinsic factor blocking antibodies
b. Antibodies against gastric parietal cells
c. Antibodies against gastrin
d. Intrinsic factor binding antibodies

Ans. a. False, b. False, c. True, and d. False

This clinical scenario in a patient with history of autoimmune thyroiditis is suspected of pernicious anemia. It is an autoimmune cause of vitamin B_{12} deficiency. Antibodies against gastrin are not present in these patients.

The following autoantibodies are seen: Type 1 or blocking antibodies prevent the combination of intrinsic factor and cobalamin; type 2 or binding antibodies prevent attachment of intrinsic factor to ileal mucosa.

Antiparietal cell antibodies target the gastric proton pump located in these cells.

This leads to the deficiency of the intrinsic factor of castle and hydrochloric acid produced by the parietal cells. The resulting atrophic gastritis causes high gastrin and low pepsinogen levels. Lack of intrinsic factor further causes vitamin B_{12} deficiency and megaloblastic anemia.

Dermatology Rheumatology Psychiatry MCQs

Devendra Richhariya

Q1. In patients with acute psychosis which feature is *most* suggestive of organic etiology?

a. Auditory hallucinations
b. Family history of psychosis
c. Normal mental status
d. Onset before 40 years of age
e. Visual hallucinations

Ans. e. While visual hallucinations can occur in functional psychotic illness (schizophrenia or affective disorder), they are much more common and indicative of organic disease.

Q2. The "Mini-Mental State Examination" is *most* useful in determining which of the following?

a. Cognitive impairment
b. Disorientation due to drugs or alcohol
c. Occult depression
d. Prognosis post head injury
e. Psychosis

Ans. a. The Mini Mental Status Examination consists of a series of tasks that assess orientation, memory, attention, calculation, language, and visual construction.

Q3. Which of the following describes a patient group at comparatively high risk of death by suicide?

a. Chronically ill
b. Females
c. Married with children in the home
d. Non-Caucasians
e. Teenagers

Ans. a. The risk of suicide is increasing across all demographic groups. The rate of fatal suicide continues to be highest among older, living alone, with chronic medical illnesses.

Q4. Match the following:

1. Macule	a. A small solid, elevation of the skin <1 cm in diameter
2. Papule	b. A circumscribed elevated area of skin <1 cm in diameter, containing fluid other than pus
3. Vesicle	c. A circumscribed elevated lesion of >1 cm diameter containing free fluid other than pus
4. Bulla	d. A circumscribed area of skin or mucous membrane different in color or texture from its neighboring tissue, measuring <1 cm in diameter

Ans. **1. (d), 2. (a), 3. (b), and 4. (c)**

Q5. Match the following:

1. Lichenification	a. Loss of substance of skin produced by scratching. (linear erosions)
2. Sclerosis	b. Permanent dilatation of capillaries
3. Telangiectasias	c. Thickening of the skin with exaggeration of its normal marking often as a result of chronic scratching or rubbing
4. Excoriation	d. Circumscribed or diffuse hardening of skin usually due to fibrosis

Ans. **1. (c), 2. (d), 3. (b), and 4. (a)**

Q6. Acute complications of Stevens-Johnson syndrome are all, *except:*

a. Fluid and electrolyte dysfunction (if >50% BSA involvement)
b. Anemia and leukopenia
c. Hypalbuminemia
d. Hyperglycemia
e. Bronchiolitis obliterans

Ans. e. Bronchiolitis obliterans is a long-term complication.

Q7. Which of the following is the principal difference between urticaria and urticarial vasculitis?

a. Both are present with pruritus
b. Both have an association with angioedema
c. Both will last for 24 hours
d. None of the above

Ans. c. Urticarial vasculitis is a form of cutaneous vasculitis that lasts for >24 hours. Clinically, patients present with pruritus, wheals, and erythema.

Q8. Which of the following is false regarding pemphigus vulgaris (PV)?

a. PV involves mucosa and skin
b. Rituximab is a United States Food and Drug Administration (US FDA)-approved biologic in the treatment of PV
c. PV is an autoimmune blistering disorder
d. Targeting antigen is desmoglein 1

Ans. d. Pemphigus vulgaris is an autoimmune blistering disorder that targets desmoglein 1 and 3 forming the antibody against it.

Q9. Which of the following is the ideal management in the case of pustular psoriasis?

a. Initially treat with antibiotic then add methotrexate
b. Initially stabilize with fluid resuscitation along with steroids and antibiotics
c. Initially stabilize with fluid resuscitation, sterile dressing, cyclosporine, and add acitretin
d. First, treat with broad-spectrum antibiotics and then add steroid

Ans. c. Pustular psoriasis is a disorder where pustules are sterile so no need for antibiotics in initial management unless the physician notices active signs of infection.

Q10. Staphylococcal scalded skin syndrome (SSSS) is due to:

a. Endotoxin
b. Exotoxin
c. Epidermolysin
d. None of the above

Ans. (b) and (c)

It is commonly seen in infants and children due to exotoxin released by *Staphylococcus aureus* group 2 phage 71. Exotoxin is an epidermolytic toxin also called exfoliating toxin or epidermolysin.

Q11. In which type of herpes zoster steroid is contraindicated?

a. Herpes zoster oticus (Ramsay Hunt syndrome)
b. Herpes zoster ophthalmicus (HZO)
c. Disseminated herpes zoster
d. Glossopharyngeal and vegal herpes zoster

Ans. b. Steroid is contraindicated in HZO because it can precipitate keratitis and corneal ulcers.

Obstetrics and Gynecology Emergencies MCQs

Devendra Richhariya

Q1. In the emergency department (ED), if a pregnant patient is brought in and little can be done to prevent the birth what should be the plan of action?

a. Start intravenous (IV) line and oxygen inhalation even if the patient is conscious and well oriented

b. Take the patient in a lithotomy position to check the presenting parts

c. Bladder should be emptied by catheter if the patient is unable to pass urine herself

d. Give small mediolateral episiotomy while in the second stage of labor to prevent a perineal tear or anal tear

Ans. d. Episiotomy should not be performed routinely in all labor as the benefits of surgical procedures are doubtful, rather it should be performed in specific indications like shoulder dystocia, breech presentation, or very tight perineum.

Q2. In an emergency, if a laboring patient is brought in distress with a fully dilated cervix, the fetal head is delivered spontaneously but no further progress of labor with the head stuck at the perineum. Which statement is False regarding the diagnosis and further management?

a. Shoulder dystocia is a possibility

b. Call the extra help, episiotomy should be performed to make the passage wider to facilitate the delivery

c. From the lithotomy position make the patient to extend the legs outward to make the pelvis roomy

d. Ask the assistant to give suprapubic pressure to dislodge the impacted shoulder

Ans. c. It is a false statement.

If the head is delivered vaginally and the shoulders are stuck inside the pelvis, to facilitate the delivery patient's folded legs are pulled toward the stomach to make the hip joint hyperflexed this is also called McRoberts maneuver it makes the pelvis roomier and 90% of the problem resolves here.

Q3. A laboring patient was brought to ED, on examination she is in distress, per vaginal examination soft parts felt diagnosed as breech presentation. She is not in a condition to shift in the obstetric unit and labor is impending. Which statement is incorrect?

a. Patient is resuscitated IV line started, asked to take deep breathing and not to bear down
b. On examination thick meconium passing through the anal canal is seen, which is not a sign of fetal distress
c. After spontaneous delivery of the lower portion and legs, wrap the warm towel around the fetal abdomen and give steady traction to facilitate delivery of the head
d. Do not hold the fetal trunk >45° above horizontal level while delivering the shoulders and fetal head

Ans. c. As a cardinal rule in successful breach extraction is to employ steady, gentle, downward traction until the lower half of scapulas are delivered outside the vulva, making no attempt at delivery of the shoulders and arms until one axilla becomes visible, as traction to body in an attempt to deliver fetal head may lead to an extension of head and complications.

Q4. A near-term antenatal lady was admitted to ED with bleeding per vagina and shock. Which of the following statements are relevant to this situation?

a. If the degree of shock is more than the bleeding possibility of abruptio placentae should be kept in mind and consumptive coagulopathy, coagulation failure, and disseminated intravascular coagulation (DIC) should be kept in mind and blood sample for prothrombin time, fibrinogen-fibrin degradation products, D-dimer should be sent and act accordingly
b. A gentle PV examination to decide the mode of delivery hemorrhage
c. Fetus is at more risk in concealed hemorrhage than in placenta previa
d. Acute renal failure in pregnancy is more commonly seen in hemorrhage associated with placenta previa, vasa previa than with concealed hemorrhage

Ans. a. True, b. False, c. True, and d. False

Digital palpation to try to ascertain the edge of the placenta and internal os can incite severe hemorrhage. Acute renal failure is more commonly associated with placental abruption, as proteinuria and coagulation complications are more common in abruptio placenta.

Q5. A successful vaginal delivery had happened just at the admission in the emergency ward, followed by profuse bleeding per vagina just after delivery or after births, which of these statements are correct for the given situation?

a. The most common cause of postpartum hemorrhage (PPH) is atonicity of the uterus so uterotonics should be given routinely after each delivery as a prophylaxis
b. Postpartum hemorrhage is an event not a diagnosis; it is a diagnosis when excessive bleeding is encountered, a specific etiology should be sought, and action should be taken without delay
c. As a preventive measure the placenta after births should be removed immediately after delivery of the fetus
d. Sheehan syndrome, acute anterior necrosis followed by impaired endocrinal secretions followed by superinvolution of the uterus, failed lactation, and loss of secondary sexual characters commonly occur after severe postpartum hemorrhage

Ans. a. True, b. True, c. False, and d. False

Delivery of after births and placental separation may take time from 5 to 10 minutes, overzealous attempts to remove the placenta may lead to uterine inversion and retained bits of the placenta, and unnecessary blood loss. Sheehan syndrome is a rare disorder following severe postpartum hemorrhage, exact pathogenesis is unknown.

Q6. Regarding medicolegal issues which of the following statements are relevant?

a. Written consent of maternal condition at the time of admission and thereafter is a must
b. In emergency delivery written consent for fetal condition is not mandatory
c. All hospital delivery records should be kept for a minimum between 3 and 5 years and in medicolegal sensitive cases it must be ideally for lifelong
d. According to Section 29 of the Pre-Natal Diagnostic Techniques (PNDT) Act 1994, requires all the documents to be maintained for a period of 2 years or until the disposal of proceedings

Ans. a. True, b. False, c. True, and d. True

All hospital admissions require proper written consent and documentation. This is the only safeguard and explanation in the court of law if any medicolegal question arises.

Q7. Which of the following is a physiologic change associated with pregnancy?

a. Decrease in cardiac output
b. Decrease in respiratory tidal volume
c. Increase in functional residual capacity
d. Increase in maternal hematocrit
e. Increase in maternal heart rate

Ans. e. There are many physiologic changes associated with pregnancy, an increase in overall blood volume; an increase in maternal cardiac output, increase in the maternal heart rate.

Q8. Which of the following is the most correct statement regarding supine hypotension syndrome?

a. A supine pregnant patient should be placed in a right side-down position
b. It can be relieved with a left lateral decubitus position
c. It most commonly occurs in postpartum patients
d. It is most commonly found in the first trimester
e. It results from the compression of the superior vena cava

Ans. b. Supine hypotension syndrome occurs in the second and third trimester of pregnancy, due to compression of the inferior vena cava by the enlarged uterus.

Q9. Which of the following factors is a major risk factor for ectopic pregnancy?

a. Depression
b. History of ovarian cysts
c. Low socioeconomic class
d. Use of assisted reproduction techniques
e. Young maternal age

Ans. d. The following are major risk factors for ectopic pregnancy: assisted reproduction techniques, pelvic inflammatory disease (PID), history of tubal surgery, use of an intrauterine device, and previous ectopic pregnancy.

Q10. Which of the following is true regarding airway management in pregnancy?

a. Aspiration risk is decreased in pregnancy
b. Respiratory acidosis is normal in pregnancy
c. Because of difficult airway anatomy, intubation should be avoided if possible

d. Functional residual volume remains unchanged
e. Rapid sequence medications, including paralytics, cross the placenta

Ans. e. Because pregnant women are at increased risk for aspiration and more prone to hypoxia due to decreased oxygen reserves, rapid sequence intubation, is recommended as the first-line method for early intubation in critically ill or seriously injured pregnant women used. These medications do cross the placenta but are generally well tolerated by the fetus.

Q11. Which of the following statements regarding preeclampsia and eclampsia is correct?

a. A 34-year-old female gravida 2, para 1 (G2P1) at 16 weeks, seen in the obstetric office on two consecutive visits with a blood pressure of 150/80, should be classified as mild preeclampsia
b. After magnesium, IV angiotensin-converting enzyme inhibitors (ACEIs) are the next line of therapy for hypertension in eclampsia
c. Magnesium should be started in the ED on any patient in the third trimester with a blood pressure >140/90
d. Multiparity is a risk factor for preeclampsia
e. Subcapsular liver hematoma is a potential complication of hemolysis, elevated liver enzymes, low platelet count (HELLP) syndrome

Ans. e. Subcapsular liver hematoma is a potentially life-threatening complication of HELLP.

Q12. Mark the following statement as true or false regarding therapeutic and their adverse effect in pregnancy:

a. *Aminoglycosides:* Dysmorphic syndrome
b. *Lithium:* Ototoxicity
c. *Sulfonamides:* Neonatal kernicterus
d. *Tetracycline:* Congenital heart disease
e. *Valproate:* Fetal teeth and bone abnormalities

Ans. a. False, b. False, c. True, d. False, and e. False

Sulfonamides may cause neonatal kernicterus in the near term.

Q13. Regarding ovarian torsion, which of the following statements is correct?

a. Drugs that stimulate ovulation are a risk factor for ovarian torsion
b. If a patient has vague, bilateral lower abdominal pain, ovarian torsion is extremely unlikely

c. Ovarian torsion most commonly occurs on the left side
d. Pelvic ultrasound is highly reliable for the evaluation of ovarian torsion
e. Pregnancy is not a risk factor for ovarian torsion

Ans. a. Risk factors for developing ovarian torsion include pregnancy, the presence of a large ovarian cyst or mass, and chemical induction of ovulation. Ultrasound is often the first imaging modality to evaluate torsion but should not be relied upon to rule out the diagnosis when clinical suspicion is high.

Q14. Regarding the management of chronic medical illness during pregnancy, which of the following statements is true?

a. ACEI are first-line therapy for chronic hypertension in diabetic pregnant women
b. Labetalol and nifedipine are safe in pregnancy for chronic hypertension
c. Pregnant women are at less risk for diabetic ketoacidosis than nonpregnant women because of a higher basal metabolic rate
d. Methimazole is the drug of choice for hyperthyroidism in pregnancy
e. Trimethoprim-sulfonamide is the best choice for the treatment of urinary tract infections in pregnant women in their third trimester

Ans. b. During pregnancy, labetalol, and nifedipine are safe to use in the management of chronic hypertension because of teratogenic effects and intrauterine growth retardation ACE-I should be avoided in pregnancy.

Q15. When managing a shoulder dystocia which is the first maneuver that should be performed?

a. Clockwise rotation of the baby's torso (Wood corkscrew)
b. Delivery of the posterior shoulder
c. Flexion of the hips (McRoberts maneuver)
d. Fundal pressure
e. Suprapubic pressure

Ans. c. When shoulder dystocia is recognized, the patient's legs should be immediately flexed up to the abdomen with the legs held by the patient or assistant known as the McRoberts maneuver.

Q16. Which of the following is false regarding the anatomical and physiological changes in pregnancy?

a. Aortocaval compression starts at 20 weeks gestation

b. The diaphragm is elevated by 4 cm
c. Plasma volume is reduced by 30%
d. Pharynx and larynx become edematous
e. Relaxation of the lower esophageal sphincter

Ans. c. Plasma volume has increased by 30%.

Q17. During the resuscitation of the pregnant lady:

a. Thoracostomies are done at a higher level than the nonpregnant patients as the diaphragm is elevated by 4 cm
b. Lie the patient flat and manual uterine displacement to the left to achieve the left lateral tilt to relieve aortocaval compression after 20 weeks
c. IV access is preferred in lower limbs
d. Resuscitative hysterotomy may be needed if a return of spontaneous circulation (ROSC) is not obtained in 10 minutes
e. Standard resuscitative guidelines should be followed as there is no modification

Ans. **a. True, b. True, c. False, d. False, and e. True**

Since the diaphragm is raised by 4 cm in pregnancy, high-level thoracostomies are needed to prevent internal organ injuries during the procedure. Aortocaval compression occurs in pregnancy >20 weeks and leads to hypotension in the supine position. The compression can be relieved during resuscitation by tilting the patient to the left lateral position 15–30 using a Cardiff wedge. Still, pillows and sandbags can be used when a Cardiff wedge is unavailable. Because of aortocaval compression by the gravid uterus, IV access is preferred in the upper extremities or above the diaphragm. A resuscitative hysterotomy is a resuscitative procedure if ROSC is not achieved within 4 minutes of resuscitation to deliver the baby and relieve aortocaval compression. There are no modifications in defibrillation and drug dosages while resuscitating pregnant women.

Q18. Regarding airway management in maternal cardiac arrest:

a. Bag-mask ventilation (BMV) can be continued till ROSC is obtained.
b. Large endotracheal (ET) tube sizes are required for intubation
c. The airway is more friable and edematous
d. Hyperventilation is required
e. After two failed attempts of supraglottic airways, ET intubation has to be attempted

Ans. c. During pregnancy, the upper airway becomes edematous and friable. It is necessary that ET intubation has to be done as soon as possible with small-size ET tubes (6–7). BMV is difficult, and if needed, a two-person technique is usually preferred. Intubation is the preferred choice of airway management, but when if two attempts fail, supraglottic airways are to be inserted even if it fails, BMV and prepare for a surgical airway.

Q19. In maternal cardiac arrest:

a. Amiodarone 150 mg has to be given after three shocks
b. Adrenaline 1 mg in 1:1,000 given every 3–5 minutes
c. The maternal cardiac arrest team should include an adult resuscitation team, obstetric team, anesthetist, and neonatal team
d. The fetus should be delivered in 5 minutes if ROSC is not obtained by 4 minutes of resuscitation
e. Consider team briefing irrespective of the outcome

Ans. a. False, b. False, c. True, d. True, and e. True

Medical therapy during cardiac arrest is no different in the pregnant patient than in the nonpregnant patient. It was recommended that perimortem cesarean delivery (PMCD) should begin at 4 minutes to effect delivery at 5 minutes after failed resuscitative efforts. This time interval was chosen to minimize the risks of neurological damage, which begins to develop after 4–6 minutes of anoxic cardiac arrest if there is no ROSC. A comprehensive and sensitive debriefing should be undertaken, with formal counseling and support to follow when required. Units may wish to consider a joint debriefing/review, including the staff involved in the patient's care and their family members.

Q20. In amniotic fluid embolism, which of the following is true?

a. It can occur anytime from the time of delivery till 24 hours postpartum
b. Left ventricular (LV) failure occurs first, followed by right ventricular (RV) failure
c. Diagnosis is by excluding puerperal sepsis, pulmonary embolism (PE), myocardial infarction (MI), and other causes
d. Massive crystalloid resuscitation is required, followed by a massive transfusion protocol
e. The previous history of PE is a risk factor for amniotic fluid embolism (AFE)

Ans. c. Amniotic fluid embolism is a rare obstetric condition that can occur during labor but anytime till 48 hours postpartum. The traditional understanding of AFE describes amniotic fluid embolization into the pulmonary vasculature, resulting in mechanical obstruction of pulmonary capillaries. RV failure occurs initially, and LV failure might happen later. DIC occurs in AFE. Massive crystalloid resuscitation leads to dilutional coagulopathy, which will worsen the bleeding. No clear diagnostic laboratory markers are available. It is essential to rule out PE, puerperal sepsis, aspiration pneumonia, and MI before diagnosing AFE.

Pediatric Emergencies MCQs

Devendra Richhariya

Q1. A child that was injured in a motor vehicle accident requires transfer to a facility that can provide evaluation and treatment of pediatric trauma patients. When arranging for transfer of the patient between the facilities, what is the best way to determine the mode of transport?

a. The referring facility physician should decide
b. The receiving facility physician should decide
c. The referring facility physician and receiving facility physician should discuss and decide together
d. The referring hospital administration should decide
e. The patient's family should decide

Ans. c. When determining the mode of transport for a child between facilities, it is best to decide this based on the communications between the referring and receiving facilities. The patient's family should be included in the discussion regarding the transfer but should not have to decide. The hospital should have established policies regarding transfers of patients, but hospital administration should not be involved in the decision on the mode of transport.

Q2. A 3-year-old male requires transfer to a pediatric facility about 50 miles away, after being diagnosed with likely myocarditis at a small, rural community hospital. When his parents brought him to the hospital, the child was noted to be tachycardic, tachypneic, hypotensive, and somewhat obtunded. Intravenous access was established. Laboratory tests were obtained and the child was given a normal saline bolus. On reassessment, the child's examination is unchanged. Of the following available transportation modes, which would be most appropriate for this child's clinical presentation?

a. Transport via ground ambulance
b. Transport via rotor-wing ambulance
c. Transport via fixed-wing ambulance
d. Parents may transport child in their own vehicle

Ans. b. The most appropriate mode of transportation for the patient in the question is via rotor-wing ambulance. The mode of transport should take into account the condition of the patient, their risk of deterioration during the transfer, the distance between facilities, the weather conditions, and also the cost of the transport. The most important of these are the current condition of the patient and the risk of deterioration. This patient in the question with likely myocarditis is clinically unstable, and their condition will likely worsen over the course of the transport. Thus, the most expeditious transport mode, rotor-wing ambulance in this case, would be most appropriate.

Q3. A team is transporting a child with pneumonia from a small community hospital to a pediatric facility for admission. The child has stable vital signs and is currently on 2 L NC O_2. Which of the following would not be considered standard monitoring for this patient during transport to the higher level of care?

a. Heart rate monitoring
b. Respiratory rate monitoring
c. Pulse oximetry monitoring
d. Cardiac output monitoring
e. End-tidal CO_2 monitoring

Ans. d. Standard monitoring during patient transport includes continuous monitoring of heart rate, respiratory rate, pulse oximetry, and blood pressure. Currently, most transport teams also provide continuous monitoring of end-tidal CO_2. Cardiac output monitoring would not be standard monitoring during transport and would more likely be found in the intensive care unit. Continuous and accurate monitoring is important during transport as a patient's clinical status can change rapidly.

Q4. Of the things listed below, which would a transport team not be expected to provide or perform?

a. Provide pain medications
b. Provide sedation medications
c. Provide resuscitation efforts
d. Perform intubation and manage an airway
e. Perform fracture reduction

Ans. e. A transport team would not be expected to perform a fracture reduction. Transport teams should be able to provide appropriate specialized critical care treatment and interventions. This includes providing medications for pain and sedation needs. The team must also have the essential equipment and skills to provide resuscitation measures as well as manage an airway, which would include performing intubation.

Q5. Which of the following situations would not need administration of prophylactic antibiotics?

a. 4 × 4 cm skin abrasion in a healthy 15-year-old girl
b. Dog bite on hand in healthy a 20-year-old man
c. Nail puncture on sole of foot in a 50-year-old diabetic man
d. Crush injury to index finger in a 30-year-old woman
e. Retained glass piece in big toe in a 10-year-old boy

Ans. a. Answer "a" is a low-risk wound while all others are high-risk traumatic wounds.

Q6. For a type 3 open fracture, following antibiotic is recommended for prophylaxis:

a. Cefazolin
b. Clindamycin
c. Gentamicin
d. a + b
e. a + b + c

Ans. e. The Eastern Association for the Surgery of Trauma guidelines recommend that a first-generation cephalosporin, e.g., cefazolin + methicillin-resistant *Staphylococcus aureus* (MRSA) coverage (clindamycin/vancomycin/linezolid) + gram-negative coverage should be given for 72 hours or till 24 hours after wound closure.

Q7. In a high-risk traumatic wound, tetanus booster is required if ...... years have lapsed since last booster.

a. 2
b. 3
c. 4
d. 5
e. 10

Ans. d. If >5 years have lapsed since the last tetanus booster in case of high-risk wounds or >10 years lapse in case of low-risk wounds, tetanus prophylaxis is needed.

Q8. Bite wounds should be irrigated well with:

a. Povidone-iodine
b. Hydrogen peroxide
c. Chlorhexidine
d. Pressurized saline
e. Any of the above

Ans. d. All bite wounds should be irrigated with large amounts of pressurized saline to reduce bacterial load. Concentrated povidone-iodine, hydrogen peroxide, and alcohol should not be used as these may cause further damage to tissues.

Q9. Endocarditis prophylaxis is needed in the following situations, *except:*

a. Tooth extraction
b. Flexible bronchoscopy
c. Wound debridement
d. Endoscopic sclerotherapy
e. None of the above

Ans. b. As per American Heart Association (AHA), flexible bronchoscopy (with/without biopsy) does not require endocarditis prophylaxis; however rigid bronchoscopy does.

Q10. What comprises the bulk of a tooth?

a. Enamel
b. Dentin
c. Pulp
d. Cementum
e. Composite resin

Ans. b. White enamel forms the external surface of a tooth. The second layer of a tooth is composed of yellow/tan dentin, which makes up the bulk of the tooth. The enamel and dentin layers comprise the crown portion of a tooth. The root of the tooth is covered by the cementum layer and the pulp is in the center and contains the neurovascular supply of the tooth. Composite resin is commonly used by dentists to replace the decayed portion of a tooth.

Q11. A 12-year-old male is brought to the emergency department (ED) after being hit in the mouth with a baseball. On examination of the mouth, you can see that he has sustained an injury to his primary incisor. The injury appears to involve only the enamel and dentin layers. How should this fracture be classified?

a. Uncomplicated crown fracture
b. Complicated crown fracture
c. Crown root fracture
d. Root fracture
e. Alveolar fracture

Ans. a. An uncomplicated crown fracture involves only the enamel and dentin layers of the tooth. A complicated crown fracture involves the enamel and dentin layers but also has exposure of the central pulp. When the enamel, dentin, and cementum layers all involved, the fracture is classified as a crown root fracture. Crown root fracture may also include involvement of the pulp. A root fracture involves the cementum and may sometime be located below the gingival sulcus. An alveolar fracture involves the jawbone in which the teeth are located and are usually combined with luxation of the tooth.

Q12. A 2-year-old child presents after falling on the sidewalk and sustaining an injury to her mouth. The family reports a lot of bleeding was associated with the injury that stopped with direct

pressure to the teeth and mouth. On examination, there is no obvious injury to her teeth, but you do note a frenulum laceration. What is the best management for this child's injury?

a. No intervention needed; provide reassurance only to the family
b. Repair the frenulum laceration
c. Repair the frenulum laceration; refer to dentist to evaluate the dental injury
d. Do repair the frenulum laceration but immediately refer to a dentist to evaluate the dental injury
e. Immediate consultation with orofacial surgeon for repair of laceration and evaluation of the dental injury

Ans. a. On examination, the child in the questions appears to have sustained a dental concussion and a frenulum laceration. Neither of these injuries requires any intervention. Frenulum lacerations may bleed profusely, but once hemostasis is obtained no repair in needed. Dental concussions also require no immediate intervention and do not need dental referral. Thus, providing the parents with reassurance is the most appropriate management in this situation.

Q13. A 5-year-old child falls and hits their mouth on a table and sustains an injury to his upper tooth. On examination, the tooth is slightly tender to touch and is loose in its socket but still in appropriate place and alignment. How would this injury be classified?

a. Concussion
b. Subluxation
c. Intrusive luxation
d. Lateral luxation
e. Avulsion

Ans. b. Subluxation refers to a tooth that is loose in its socket but still in its proper place and alignment. Concussion refers to minor trauma to the tooth with no visible injury. Intrusive luxation refers to a tooth in its socket that has been forced up vertically into its socket. Lateral luxation refers to loosening of a tooth with lateral displacement. Avulsion involves complete displacement of the tooth from its alveolar socket.

Q14. A 16-year-old male presents to the ED after being involved in an altercation with another boy at school. The patient reports that he was punched in the right side of his face and now has pain to his right cheek and jaw area. Which of the following findings on your examination would be suggestive of an alveolar fracture?

a. Swelling to the right cheek
b. Bruising to the right cheek
c. Tenderness to palpation to the right cheek

d. Malocclusion on closure of the mouth
e. Uncomplicated crown fracture of the lower right lateral incisor

Ans. d. Alveolar fractures involve the portion of the jawbone that carries the teeth. This type of fracture is usually associated with pain and malocclusion of the teeth. This is usually noted when the patient attempts to close their mouth. Swelling, bruising, and tenderness on palpation can be associated with many injuries but are not clinical signs indicative of an underlying alveolar bone fracture. An uncomplicated crown fracture can be found in conjunction with an alveolar fracture, but it is not a clinical sign of an alveolar bone fracture.

Q15. Which of the following is *not* a risk factor for severity of illness in a dehydrated diabetic child?

a. Acidosis in a type I diabetic
b. Acidosis in a type II diabetic
c. Age <5 years
d. Hypernatremia
e. Hyperosmolality

Ans. d. Sodium is depleted in the diabetic ketoacidosis (DKA) state and hypernatremia is not a risk factor in determining potential severity of illness. In children presenting with DKA, about 1% will develop significant cerebral edema.

Q16. What is the most reliable indicator for severity of dehydration in an infant?

a. Capillary refill time
b. Mucous membrane appearance
c. Sunken fontanel
d. Urine output
e. Weight loss

Ans. e. Preillness weight is the best way to determine degree of dehydration.

Q17. What is the most common cause of congenital stridor in children?

a. Hemangioma
b. Laryngomalacia
c. Subglottic stenosis
d. Vascular ring
e. Vocal cord paralysis

Ans. b. Laryngomalacia. The condition usually self-resolves as the child grows

Q18. Which of the following would be the most common presentation for a urologic emergency in a 6-month-old boy?

a. High-flow priapism
b. Hydrocele
c. Testicular torsion
d. Tourniquet syndrome
e. Varicocele

Ans. d. Tourniquet syndrome of the penis usually is caused by hair and will lead to diminished tissue perfusion secondary to venous congestion.

Q19. Which is the least likely finding in a child with intussusception?

a. Abdominal pain
b. Abdominal mass
c. Altered mental status
d. Currant jelly stool
e. Vomiting

Ans. d. Currant jelly stool is due to bowel ischemia and is a late finding with intussusception. Altered mental status can be the only presenting finding in up to 10% of cases.

Q20. A 2-year-old child is brought to the emergency room (ER) for fever and difficulty in breathing for 1 day. Child is not vaccinated. There is audible stridor at rest. You also notice that the child is leaning forward and drooling. His vital signs are temperature: 39.8°C, heart rate (HR): 174 beats/min, respiratory rate (RR): 60 breaths/min; blood pressure (BP): 110/68 mm Hg, and room air saturation is 92%. What will be the most appropriate next step in the management for this child?

a. Administer nebulized racemic epinephrine and IM dexamethasone
b. Place an IV line and give a dose of ceftriaxone
c. Prepare for rapid sequence intubation in ER
d. Give oxygen via nasal cannula and observe in ER
e. Give blow-by oxygen and coordinate with otorhinolaryngology or anesthesia to transfer to the operating room for airway management

Ans. e. This child has acute infections airway emergency with features of airway compromise. Epiglottitis and bacterial tracheitis are likely possibilities here. Immediate goal is to minimize any kind of agitation, administer oxygen as tolerated, and contact otorhinolaryngologist or anesthesiologist immediately because the child needs an emergent airway that will be best provided in the controlled setting of the operating room. If intubation is not possible due to the epiglottic swelling, needle cricothyrotomy or tracheostomy will be required. Any invasive procedure that will agitate the child may lead to further airway compromise and should be avoided. IV antibiotic can be administered after the airway has been secured.

Q21. A 5-year-old boy with short gut syndrome on total parenteral nutrition is brought to the ED for fever, chills, redness, and swelling around the central venous catheter site. His vital signs

are temperature: 39.1°C, HR: 168 beats/min, RR: 38 breaths/min, and BP: 96/58 mm Hg. After the blood cultures are obtained from the catheter and a peripheral site, which of the following will be the best next step in the management of this patient after administration of broad-spectrum antibiotic?

a. Obtain a chest X-ray (CXR)
b. Admit for observation
c. Echocardiography
d. Removal of the central venous catheter
e. Normal saline bolus 20 mL/kg

Ans. d. Patient has fever, erythema, and swelling at the catheter site, suggestive of a diagnosis of central line-associated bloodstream infection (CLABSI) associated with catheter site infection. After administration of broad-spectrum antibiotic, removal of the central venous catheter would be the next step as the catheter is likely the source of this infection. Common pathogens associated with IV catheter-related infections are gram-positive bacteria (coagulase-negative *Staphylococcus* and *S. aureus* including MRSA); enterococci; gram-negative bacilli (*Enterobacter, Pseudomonas aeruginosa, Klebsiella pneumoniae,* and *Escherichia coli*); and *Candida* spp.

Q22. You are seeing a 4-year-old girl brought in by the parents with the complaint of fever for 1 week. There is no history of cough, runny nose, vomiting, or diarrhea. Her vital signs are temperature: 39°C, HR: 148 beats/min, BP: 90/60 mm Hg, RR: 40 breaths/min, and room air oxygen saturation of 94%. Chest is clear to auscultation. She has a grade 2/4 diastolic murmur (parents are not aware of any heart murmur). You also notice petechiae over distal extremities. After sending for the laboratory tests you request an echocardiogram that shows a vegetation over the mitral valve. Which of the following is *most* likely to be the cause of this child's infection?

a. *Streptococcus pneumoniae*
b. *Kingella kingae*
c. *Staphylococcus aureus*
d. *Eikenella corrodens*
e. *Candida albicans*

Ans. c. This child's findings are consistent with infective endocarditis (IE). Out of the given choices, most likely pathogen would be *S. aureus*. The other listed pathogens are not common cause of IE. Most common pathogens associated with IE are *Streptococcus viridans* group (*Streptococcus sanguis, Streptococcus mitis, Streptococcus oralis,* and *Streptococcus anginosus*) and *S. aureus*. The *Streptococcus viridans* endocarditis is usually associated with abnormal valves (congenital heart disease and rheumatic fever). *Staphylococcus* spp. endocarditis is seen with both structurally normal and abnormal valves.

Q23. Parents bring a 2-week-old infant for fever. Rectal temperature at home was 38.9°C. Parents report that the infant is little fussy for last 24 hours. The infant was born at term via vaginal delivery to a 30-year-old G1P1 female without any perinatal complications. In ED, temperature: 38.6°C, HR: 190 beats/min, RR: 60 breaths/min, BP: 82/45 mm Hg, and room air saturation is 98%. On examination, infant is irritable and his anterior fontanel is bulging. You collect the blood, urine, and the cerebrospinal fluid shows gram-positive rods. The *best* choice of antibiotic for this infection would be:

a. Ampicillin
b. Ceftriaxone
c. Ceftazidime
d. Vancomycin
e. Cefotaxime

Ans. a. Most likely pathogen is *Listeria monocytogenes* and the treatment of choice for *L. monocytogenes* infections is ampicillin. *Listeria* infection could be acquired through the placenta or during the delivery if the mother is colonized with the bacteria. *Listeria* infections may present with gastroenteritis, bacteremia, pneumonia, and meningitis. *Listeria* organisms are resistant to cephalosporins. Vancomycin has activity against *Listeria* but treatment failures are seen, therefore, vancomycin is not a preferred drug for treatment of *Listeria*.

Q24. A 5-year-old boy is brought to the ED for limping and fever for 2 days. There is no history of fall or any other injury. Parents report mild cough and rhinorrhea about a week ago. In ED, child's vital signs are temperature: 39°C, HR: 130 beats/min, RR: 28 breaths/min, BP: 110/68 mm Hg. On examination, you notice that the child's left lower extremity is abducted and externally rotated and internal and external rotation of the left hip is very painful. There are no rashes and rest of the examination is normal. You send the initial laboratory tests and white blood cell (WBC) count is 20,000/μL (20×10^9/L) with 80% neutrophils and high C-reactive protein (CRP) level. X-ray of the hip in unremarkable. Which of the following will be the next *best* step in management of this child?

a. Give ibuprofen and reassess
b. Start intravenous clindamycin
c. Pain control and follow-up with orthopedics the following day
d. Order ultrasonography of the left hip
e. Aspirate the joint and send fluid for analysis

Ans. d. The child presenting with fever, limp, and limited range of motion of the left hip along with leukocytosis and high CRP puts septic arthritis of the hip on the top of differential diagnosis in this case. Ultrasound of the hip to detect any hip effusion will be the best next step in management to exclude the diagnosis of septic arthritis. Synovial fluid aspiration in septic arthritis is usually turbid or grossly purulent; WBC count of >50,000 cells/mm^3 with a polymorphonuclear leukocytes dominance is highly suggestive of septic arthritis. If the diagnosis of septic arthritis is suspected or confirmed, emergent surgical drainage and irrigation of the joint space is recommended to prevent serious complications (e.g., aseptic necrosis of the femoral head). Bacterial etiology of septic arthritis: neonates—*S. aureus*, group B *Streptococcus*, and gram-negative enteric bacilli. *S. aureus* is the most common cause of septic arthritis in all age groups. *Salmonella* is often the etiology of osteomyelitis and septic arthritis in patients with sickle cell anemia.

Q25. Regarding UTI in children, mark the statement True/False.

a. Girls are at higher risk for urinary tract infections (UTIs) than boys in all age groups except for young uncircumcised boys
b. Rapid urine screening test detects almost all of UTIs, therefore, urine culture is not necessary if the rapid test is negative
c. Urine test is not indicated for a 17-month-old female with a temperature of 39.2°C and no apparent source of infection
d. Risk factors for UTI include young age, circumcised male, and female child
e. Urine dipstick (positive for either leukocyte esterase or nitrites) has a sensitivity of 88%

Ans. **a. True, b. False, c. False, d. False, and e. True**

Risk factors for UTI include uncircumcised status, young age, female sex (girls are at higher risk for UTIs than boys in all age categories except for young uncircumcised boys), and nonblack race. Urine testing is generally indicated in girls younger than 2 years with at least one risk factor for UTI (history of UTI, temperature >39°C, fever without other apparent source, ill appearance, suprapubic tenderness, fever >24 hours, or nonblack race). Circumcised boys between 3 months and 2 years of age without suprapubic tenderness or with no >1 risk factor for UTI (temperature 39°C, fever without other apparent source, fever >24 hours, or nonblack race) have a probability of UTI of ≤2%. Increased risk of UTI in uncircumcised males persists until at least 12 months of age. Urine dipstick (positive for either leukocyte esterase or nitrites) has a sensitivity of 88%. It is important to remember that no rapid screening test detects all UTIs, therefore, urine cultures should be ordered for all of these patients.

Q26. Criteria for diagnosis of multisystem inflammatory syndrome in children (MIS-C) are: mark the statement True/False.

a. Persistent fever >38°C and epidemiological linkage with severe acute respiratory syndrome coronavirus 2 (SARS-CoV-2)
b. Presence of rash or bilateral purulent conjunctivitis or mucocutaneous inflammation
c. Presence of hypotension or shock
d. Presence of pericarditis, myocarditis, endocarditis, or coronary abnormalities
e. Absence of coagulopathy [prothrombin time (PT), partial thromboplastin time (PTT), and elevated D-dimers]

Ans. a. True, b. False, c. True, d. True, and e. False

World Health Organization (WHO) diagnostic criteria of MIS-C: Children and adolescents 0–18 years of age unrelenting temperature 38°C ≥3 days and any two of the following features:

- Rash or bilateral nonpurulent conjunctivitis or mucocutaneous inflammation signs (oral, hands, or feet)
- Hypotension or shock
- Features of myocardial dysfunction, pericarditis, valvulitis, or coronary abnormalities [including ECHO findings or elevated troponin/NT-proBNP (N-terminal, protein B-type natriuretic peptide)]
- Evidence of coagulopathy (PT, PTT, and elevated D-dimers)
- Acute gastrointestinal problems (diarrhea, vomiting, or abdominal pain)
- And raised inflammatory markers such as erythrocyte sedimentation rate (ESR) (>40 mm), CRP (>5 mg/L), or procalcitonin
- And no other possible microbial cause of inflammation, e.g., bacterial sepsis, staphylococcal or streptococcal shock syndromes.
- And evidence of recent coronavirus disease 2019 (COVID-19) infection (RT-PCR, antigen test, or serology positive), or likely contact with COVID-19-infected patient.

Q27. Regarding the three common criteria (Boston criteria, Rochester criteria, and Philadelphia criteria) used for risk stratification of febrile young patients: mark the statement True/False.

a. They are not helpful in neonates
b. They all have following components in common for a patient to be in low-risk category (patient must appear well; no signs of focal

infection on examination; peripheral WBC count within a specific range; no evidence of UTI on rapid urine testing)

c. By using these criteria, risk of serious bacterial infection (SBI) can be ruled out with certainty
d. Rochester criteria are designed for febrile children >60 days of age
e. Boston criteria are designed for febrile children from 1 to 3 months of age

Ans. a. True, b. True, c. False, d. False, and e. True

There are three common criteria (Boston criteria, Rochester criteria, and Philadelphia criteria) commonly used to determine if the patient is at low risk or high risk for SBI. These risk stratification rules are derived for febrile young infants and are not helpful in neonates. They all have following components in common for a patient to be in low-risk category:

- Patient must appear well
- No signs of focal infection on examination
- Peripheral WBC count within a specific range
- No evidence of UTI on rapid urine testing

Boston criteria are designed for febrile children from 1 to 3 months of age.

Rochester criteria are designed for febrile children <60 days old.

Philadelphia criteria are designed for patients between 29 and 56 days of age.

Q28. Kawasaki syndrome is: mark the statement True/False.

a. Acute self-limiting and multiorgan vasculitis
b. Rarely seen in children younger than 3 months or older than 8 years of age
c. Associated with conjunctival injection with exudates
d. Associated with pericardial effusion in 30% of the patients
e. Managed with aspirin and high-dose IV immunoglobulin

Ans. a. True, b. True, c. False, d. True, and e. True

The peak incidence of Kawasaki syndrome is between 6 and 12 months of age. This is the most common cause of acquired coronary artery disease in childhood. Diagnosis of Kawasaki disease/syndrome: high fever lasting 5 or more days with four out of five findings: (1) Bilateral nonpurulent conjunctival injection; (2) Erythematous, cracked lips, and strawberry tongue; (3) Cervical lymphadenopathy; (4) Erythema of palm and sole; (5) Peeling of skin over hands and feet and polymorphous rash.

Patients with acute Kawasaki disease should be given intravenous immunoglobulin (IVIG), 2 g/kg in a single dose, to prevent coronary artery abnormalities. High-dose aspirin, 80–100 mg/kg/day in four divided doses, is given in the acute stage of Kawasaki disease, until the child has no fever for 48–72 hours.

Q29. Indications for admission of febrile children are: mark the statement True/False.

a. All infants <4 weeks of age with a temperature of >38.1°C
b. Toxic appearing irrespective of age or degree of temperature
c. Patients with positive blood culture who is sick looking or febrile.
d. Any child with a temperature of 40°C
e. Well-appearing child with sickle cell anemia with low-grade fever and normal white count

Ans. **a. True, b. True, c. True, d. False, and e. False**

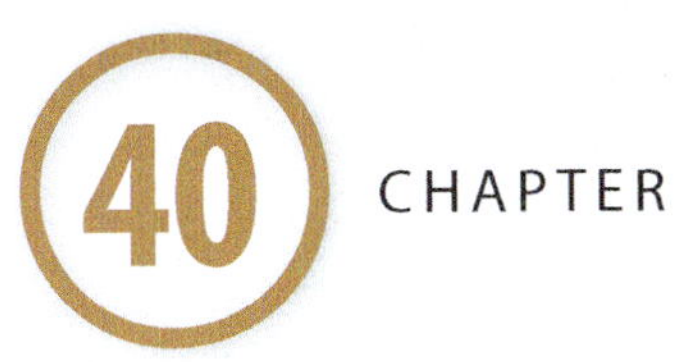

Geriatric Emergencies MCQs

Devendra Richhariya

Q1. Which is not true with physiologic changes in older adults?

a. Decline in hepatic metabolism
b. Decreasing the volume of distribution (*Vd*) of lipid-soluble drugs
c. Decrease clearance of drugs
d. Increased blood-brain barrier permeability
e. Reduced first-pass hepatic extraction

Ans. b. The volume of distribution of lipid-soluble medications, e.g., morphine, benzodiazepines, antipsychotics, and amitriptyline, increases as people age, because they have less lean body weight and muscle mass and a proportionate rise in total body fat, which can lead to longer half-life, prolonged drug effect, and greater potential of adverse effect and toxicity.

Q2. Which medication decreases in pharmacodynamic response in older adults?

a. Benzodiazepines
b. Enalapril
c. Warfarin
d. Propranolol
e. Morphine

Ans. d. Propranolol decreases in pharmacodynamic response in older adults by having less reduction in heart rate with advance age. While benzodiazepines, enalapril, warfarin, and morphine increase in pharmacodynamic response and can initiate higher risk of adverse effects.

Q3. Which one is not recommended when prescribing for older patients?

a. Obtain full list of medications include over-the-counter and complementary/alternative medicines from patient and caretaker
b. Avoid prescribing cascades to treat adverse effects of existing medications
c. Start a new medication with high dose and reduce the dose once the therepeutic goals are acheived.

d. Provide verbal and written instructions on indication, time and route of administration and potential adverse effects of each medication
e. When stopping a medication, check if it can be stopped abruptly or needs to be tapered

Ans. c. For older patients, new medication should be started at the smallest dose and titrate slowly according to response and efficacy (except for drugs in which steady state concentration must be achieved quickly, e.g., antibiotics) to limit potential adverse effects from medication.

Q4. Which drug can cause drug-induced parkinsonism?

a. Donepezil
b. Ibuprofen
c. Atenolol
d. Meperidine
e. Metoclopramide

Ans. e. Metoclopramide can induce parkinsonism and users were three times more likely to begin drug treatment for Parkinson disease as compared to nonusers. This is one of important prescribing cascades that are common in older adults.

Q5. Which one is *not* true about drug–drug interaction from *Beers* criteria?

a. Opioids and benzodiazepines will increase risk of overdose
b. Corticosteroids and nonsteroidal anti-inflammatory drugs (NSAIDs) will increase risk of gastrointestinal bleeding
c. Lithium and angiotensin-converting enzyme inhibitors (ACEIs) will increase risk of lithium toxicity
d. Phenytoin and trimethoprim-sulfamethoxazole will decrease phenytoin efficacy
e. Warfarin and amiodarone will increase risk of bleeding

Ans. d. Phenytoin and trimethoprim-sulfamethoxazole will decrease phenytoin efficacy but will increase risk of phenytoin toxicity.

Q6. Which of the following are true regarding medical presentations of older adults in the emergency department (ED)? Mark the statement as True/False.

a. Compensatory tachycardia is often seen in older adults who are clinically unwell
b. Depression in older adults may not have primarily low mood, but may present as irritability, anxiety, or somatic symptoms
c. Chest pain is the most common presenting symptom for acute myocardial infarction (MI) in patients over the age of 85 years
d. New confusion, or delirium, is an indication for urine investigations in older adults

Ans. **a. False, b. True, c. False, and d. False**

Compensatory tachycardia may not be observed in older adults for several reasons. Maximal heart rate decreases with age, the cardiovascular system is less adrenergically responsive with age, and older adults are often on beta blockers and other medications that prevent tachycardia. Unlike in younger patients, older patients with depression may not present with primarily low mood. They may be more likely to have irritability, anxiety, or somatic physical symptoms. Silent MIs are common with advanced age, and those over the age of 85 years are more likely to present with symptoms other than chest pain such as dyspnea, diaphoresis, nausea and vomiting, and syncope. New confusion, decreased appetite, falls, wandering, or aggression alone are not indications for investigations of a urinary tract infection (UTI). Urine studies should only be sent if there are urinary symptoms such as frequency, urgency, dysuria, suprapubic tenderness, costovertebral tenderness, changed urinary continence, and gross hematuria.

Q7. Which of the following are components of the confusion assessment method (CAM) for delirium? Mark as True/False.

a. Acute-onset and fluctuating progression
b. Inattention
c. Underlying cognitive impairment
d. Disorganized thinking
e. Altered level of consciousness

Ans. **a. True, b. True, c. False, d. True, and e. True**

The CAM, and the numerous variations of CAM, are based on four key components: (1) Acute-onset and fluctuating progression, (2) inattention, (3) altered level of consciousness, and (4) disorganized thinking.

Q8. Regarding comprehensive geriatric assessments (CGA), which of the following is *false*?

a. It includes multiple domains such as medical, functional, psychological, social, and environmental
b. When done in the ED, it has been associated with a decrease in ED visits and reduced functional decline
c. The medical assessment is the most important part of a CGA
d. A CGA is best done with a multidisciplinary approach to cover all domains

Ans. c. The CGA is a multidimensional interdisciplinary approach for the assessment of older adults. While the full CGA is not intended for use in the ED, this framework should be applied to the acute presentations we see in the ED. Domains include medical, functional, psychological, and social and environmental. When CGAs are done in the ED, they have been associated with reduced functional decline and reduced ED visits. While traditionally, the medical domain is what physicians focus on, the other domains are equally important and greatly impact assessment and disposition.

Q9. Which of the following is the most useful assessment tool for screening cognition in the ED?

a. Mini Mental State Examination (MMSE)
b. Montreal Cognitive Assessment (MoCA)
c. Rowland Universal Dementia Assessment Scale (RUDAS)
d. Mini-Cog

Ans. d. The three-step Mini-Cog instrument is a screening tool that can be completed quickly in the ED to aid in identifying cognitive impairment. It consists of a three-item recall component for memory, and a clock drawing test. Although the test cannot be used to rule out mild cognitive impairment, a score of 3 or greater indicates a lower likelihood of dementia. Although the MMSE, MoCA and RUDAS are all validated cognitive assessment tools, they have limited applicability due to time constraints in the ED.

Q10. Which of the following are considered activities of daily living (ADLs)? Mark as True/False.

a. Managing medications
b. Bathing
c. Dressing
d. Preparing meals

Ans. a. False, b. True, c. True, and d. False

The activities of daily living refer to self-care tasks including transferring (i.e., between a bed and chair), toileting, bathing, dressing, feeding, and continence. Instrumental activities of daily living (iADLs) are also important and refer to activities that are needed to live independently including shopping, preparing meals, housekeeping, managing medications, driving, or using public transportation, managing finances, and using a telephone/ technology. Identifying in the ED the patient's baseline function can help clarify the clinical presentation and guide disposition planning.

Q11. Regarding the interpretation of vital signs in older patients in the emergency room (ER), which of the following is *false*?

a. Orthostatic hypotension can be observed in older patients due to the dysregulation of autonomic sensitivity
b. Older adults have a higher core body temperature and present typically with fever when there is an underlying infectious process
c. Compensatory tachycardia may not always be observed in older adults.
d. Hypotension can be a later clinical sign due to stiff peripheral vasculature and loss of responsiveness to sympathetic stimuli

Ans. b. Due to age-associated changes, there can be loss of regulatory and adaptive physiological mechanisms in the older adult. Older adults generally have a lower core body temperature and altered thermoregulatory responses. As such, in the presence of an underlying infectious process, fever response in the elderly may be absent or blunted.

Q12. Following are the components of geriatric syndrome, *except*:

a. Fall
b. Urinary incontinence (UI)
c. Delirium
d. Hard of hearing

Ans. d. Five major geriatric syndromes are: (1) Falls, (2) urinary incontinence, (3) pressure ulcers, (4) delirium, and (5) functional decline.

Q13. What is a common physiological change seen in an elderly patient?

a. Increased chest wall compliance
b. Increased cervical spine mobility
c. Increased myocardial stiffening
d. Increased reflexes
e. Increased lung elasticity

Ans. c. The myocardium is less compliant and progressively stiffens, which decreases the heart's pumping effectiveness. As patients get older, the chest wall becomes more stiff and less compliant, placing them at an increased risk for rib fractures.

Q14. Most common type of elder abuse in society is:

a. Physical abuse
b. Neglect
c. Sexual abuse
d. Emotional abuse

Ans. b. Neglect is a common type of abuse (58%), followed by physical abuse (15%).

Q15. All are the causes of the pelvic organ prolapse (POP) in elderly women, *except*:

a. Multipara
b. Connective tissue abnormalities
c. Obesity
d. Mitral valve prolapse

Ans. d. Causes of POP are:

- *Vaginal childbirth*: Increasing parity increases risk (cesarean section is associated with POP as well)
- *Increases in intra-abdominal pressure:* Obesity, straining with chronic constipation, chronic cough aging/menopause, genetic predisposition, and connective tissue abnormalities.

Infectious Diseases MCQs

Devendra Richhariya

Q1. Which of the following is false regarding the febrile phase of dengue fever?

a. It is a precedent of hemorrhagic fever and dengue shock syndrome
b. Sore throat, anorexia, and nausea are classical symptoms
c. In dengue hemorrhagic fever positive tourniquet test is seen with the presence of 10 or more petechiae
d. Complete blood count shows decreased white blood cell count which is indicative of dengue fever

Ans. c. In dengue hemorrhagic fever, the test is usually positive with the presence of 20 petechiae or more. However, in dengue shock syndrome it may be negative or mildly positive during the heightened period of shock. In the event of a negative result, repeated tests must be taken to ensure confirmation of diagnosis.

Q2. In a patient suffering from dengue hemorrhagic fever (grade III), which of the following will not be seen?

a. Platelet count $<100{,}000/mm^3$
b. Platelet count $>100{,}000/mm^3$
c. High diastolic pressure
d. Altered sensorium

Ans. b. Platelet count in grade III dengue hemorrhagic fever is $<100{,}000/mm^3$.

Q3. The presence of one or more of the following is defined as severe dengue. Mark the sentence as True/False.

a. Signs of respiratory distress secondary to fluid overload
b. Adequate perfusion to all organs thereby preventing end-organ damage
c. Decrease in hematocrit levels
d. Decrease in permeability of vascular blood vessels

Ans. **a. True, b. False, c. False, and d. False**

- Plasma leak from capillaries into extravascular compartment—rise in hematocrit count that may progress to shock
- Signs of respiratory distress secondary to fluid overload

- Fluid overload in the pulmonary or gastrointestinal system: Pleural effusion/ascitis
- Signs of bleeding due to thrombocytopenia
- Decreased adequate perfusion leading to severe organ impairment

The increased permeability of vascular blood vessels increases hypovolemia and progresses to shock. This begins around defervescence, during 3–7th day of illness.

Q4. Regarding hemorrhagic complications, which of the following is not True?

a. Persistent prolonged shock
b. Renal failure patients are not at risk
c. *Refractory shock:* Nonresponsive to fluid therapy
d. Reduced level of hematocrit

Ans. b.

- *Patient with increased risk of bleeding:*
  - Persistent prolonged shock
  - *Associated organ impairment:* Renal failure and liver failure
  - Persistent metabolic acidosis
- *Precursors to bleeding:*
  - Reduced level of hematocrit along with unstable hemodynamic state even after fluid resuscitation
  - Refractory shock—not responding to consecutive fluid resuscitation at 40–50 mL/kg

Q5. Regarding the treatment of dengue fever. Mark the sentence as True/False.

a. Family members should not be counseled regarding the symptoms of the patient
b. Oral hydration with water, juices, or oral rehydration solution (ORS) is encouraged
c. Use of aspirin, ibuprofen, and nonsteroidal anti-inflammatory drugs (NSAIDs) are encouraged
d. Tablet paracetamol 500 mg is advised thrice a day

Ans. a. False, b. True, c. False, and d. True

Oral fluids can be increased with oral rehydration solution (ORS), fruit juices, and electrolyte-rich water with sugar. One must be aware of possible hyperglycemia due to physiological stress in the febrile phase. Tablet Paracetamol 500 mg for high fever is adequate at an interval of 6 hours. In order to reduce body temperature, tepid sponging can be done. Avoid the use of acetylsalicylic acid (aspirin), ibuprofen, and NSAIDs as they may aggravate risks of bleeding with underlying thrombocytopenia. The patient and family need to be counseled regarding signs and symptoms of bleeding, rashes, severe abdominal pain, persistent vomiting, deterioration of mental status, cold clammy extremities, lethargy, irritability, restlessness, black stools, coffee-ground vomiting, and decreased urine output.

Q6. Regarding neurological sequelae of cerebral malaria, which symptom is not seen?

a. Acute confusional state and ataxia
b. Neurosis
c. Tremors and repeated convulsions
d. Cortical blindness

Ans. b. Neurological sequelae of cerebral malaria include hemiplegia, cortical blindness, aphasia, ataxia, tremors, hearing defect, repeated convulsion, behavioral abnormalities, spastic quadriplegia, acute confusional state, and psychosis.

Q7. Mark whether the statement regarding cerebral malaria is True or False.

a. *Plasmodium falciparum* does not invade erythrocytes of all ages
b. High levels of parasitemia and a large number of merozoites are released to infect hepatocytes
c. Presence of coma <6 hours after excluding encephalitis and bacterial meningitis
d. In a patient with severe falciparum malaria, <2% of total erythrocytes are parasitized

Ans. a. False, b. True, c. False, and d. False

Plasmodium falciparum invades erythrocytes of all ages.

Unarousable coma after exclusion of encephalitis and bacterial meningitis with persistence of coma >6 hours after generalized seizure and confirmation of *P. falciparum* parasitemia is a criteria for diagnosing cerebral malaria. In a patient with severe falciparum malaria, more than 2% of total erythrocytes are parasitized.

Q8. Which of the following is not true with respect to laboratory indicators of poor prognosis of cerebral malaria?

a. Total bilirubin >2.5
b. Anemia <7
c. Leukopenia
d. Packed cell volume (PCV) <20%

Ans. c. Laboratory indicators of poor prognosis of cerebral malaria include parasitemia >5%, peripheral schizonts, leukocytosis PCV <20%, anemia <7 g, hypoglycemia <40 mg BUN >60 mg/dL.

Total bilirubin >2.5, aminotransferases more than three times.

Q9. Which of the following is not present in uncomplicated malaria?

a. Mild jaundice
b. Acute respiratory distress syndrome
c. Anemia with elevation of bilirubin
d. Splenomegaly

Ans. b. Physical findings of uncomplicated malaria, include elevated temperatures, perspiration, weakness, enlarged spleen, mild jaundice, enlargement of the liver, and increased respiratory rate. Laboratory findings include demonstrations of parasites in the blood under microscopy along with mild anemia, thrombocytopenia, elevated bilirubin, and aminotransferases. Acute respiratory distress syndrome is seen in severe malaria.

Q10. Regarding chronic complications of malaria, mark which statement as True or False.

a. Abdominal pain and dragging sensation is not one of the clinical symptoms seen
b. Chronic infection of *Plasmodium malariae* gives rise to an immune-mediated injury to the renal glomeruli
c. Immunosuppression induced by malaria infection may give rise to the lymphoma virus
d. Pancytopenia is absent in the clinical picture

Ans. **a. False, b. True, c. True, and d. False**

Tropical splenomegaly or hyperreactive malarial splenomegaly causes sharp abdominal pain suggestive of splenitis, which is one of the chronic complications of malaria. Quartan malaria nephropathy is caused due to *P. malariae* infection that gives rise to an immune-mediated injury to renal glomeruli anemia and pancytopenia is significant in laboratory findings.

Q11. Which of the following is not advisable to be prescribed to pregnant women during malaria?

a. Quinine salt
b. Primaquine
c. Artesunate-based combination therapy
d. Chloroquine

Ans. b. Primaquine is contraindicated in pregnant women.

Q12. **Write True or False for each statement below:**

a. Pleural effusion is a form of extrapulmonary tuberculosis (TB)
b. Cavities are formed in the lungs in the pulmonary TB
c. Night cries are associated with Genital TB
d. Liquefied material in the lungs is responsible for the spread of coughing

Ans. **a. True, b. True, c. False, and d. True**

Q13. **Which of these clinical features is not suggestive of TB as an underlying etiology?**

a. Matted cervical lymph nodes
b. Ascites in young
c. Bilateral pleural effusion
d. Boggy swelling below the inguinal ligament

Ans. c.

Q14. **Write True or False for each statement below:**

a. Ziehl-Neelsen (ZN) staining is the cheapest method for diagnosis of TB
b. Fluorescent staining has negligible false positive rate
c. Cartridge-based nucleic acid amplification test (CBNAAT) comes positive even at a low bacillary load
d. CBNAAT is the gold standard investigation for TB

Ans **a. True, b. False, c. True, and d. False**

Q15. **Which is the best method to diagnose extrapulmonary TB?**

a. ZN staining
b. Culture
c. CBNAAT
d. Histopathology

Ans. c.

Q16. **Which of these is classified as multidrug-resistant (MDR) TB?**

a. Resistance to rifampicin and ethambutol
b. Resistance to isoniazid and pyrazinamide
c. Resistance to rifampicin and isoniazid
d. Resistance to all four first-line drugs

Ans. c.

Q17. **Regarding skin and soft tissue infections, which of the following statements is False?**

a. In necrotizing infections, the etiology may be polymicrobial therefore, broad-spectrum antibiotics should be used

b. If there is purulence, good drainage, and methicillin-resistant *Staphylococcus aureus* (MRSA) antibiotics should be administered
c. If there is no pus, beta-lactam antibiotics can be used which cover β-hemolytic streptococcal infections and MRSA
d. Erysipelas is nonpurulent cellulitis limited to the epidermis
e. Impetigo could be caused by both *S. aureus and Streptococcus pyogenes*

Ans. c. Beta-lactam antibiotics have no effect against MRSA, Oxacillin/methicillin resistance means resistance to all penicillins, monobactams, cephalosporins, carbapenems, and beta-lactam/beta-lactamase inhibitor combinations. While it is true that bet-lactam antibiotics are used to cover β-hemolytic streptococcal infections, MRSA would be resistant, this resistance comes from a penicillin-binding protein called PBP that reduces binding affinity for beta-lactam antibiotics.

Q18. Which of the following statements is the best option regarding the diagnosis and treatment of an abscess?

a. In cases of intravenous (IV) drug use infection *Staphylococcus aureus* is always the only responsible agent, therefore drainage and MRSA-covering antibiotics should be administered
b. The first step in diagnosing an abscess should be to look for a hypoechoic or anechoic cavity with acoustic enhancement deep into the pus collection
c. For deep and intramuscular abscess, ultrasound is most useful to localize the site of the incision
d. Antibiotics should be reserved for large abscess accompanied by fever or systemic inflammatory response signs, >5 cm of surrounding cellulitis, or in an immunocompromised host
e. In all complicated abscess culture and gram staining is required

Ans. d. It is the right answer for those cases where antibiotic therapy is needed, if it is a small uncomplicated superficial abscess, drainage will suffice. An option is incorrect due to the etiology of abscess in IV drug users, normally when an abscess is suspected in an infection site polymicrobial etiology should be ruled out. Option (b) is incorrect, the first step should always be to look for fluctuance if it cannot be found then you can help the diagnosis with an ultrasound. The (c) option is incorrect for deep and intramuscular abscess ultrasound is not useful to determine the incision site for it is not precise and can cause confusion regarding the drainage path. Option (e) is incorrect for empiric treatment is needed in these cases, only in recurrent abscesses staining and culture is required.

Q19. The following question consists of a statement followed by four statements *each* requiring a True or False answer.

The following favors the diagnosis and correct treatment of nonpurulent cellulitis:

a. Ultrasound is useful to differentiate between cellulitis and deep vein thrombosis (DVT)

b. Empiric antibiotic therapy must cover *Streptococcus* species for uncomplicated nonpurulent cellulitis

c. For nonpurulent cellulitis with systemic signs of infection such as a high fever, MRSA should be covered

d. Elevation of the extremity is considered an important component of cellulitis treatment

e. Interdigital fissures, scales, and maceration should be treated with topical antibiotics

Ans. a. True, b. True, c. False, d. True, and e. False

Option (a) is True, the best study for differential diagnosis between DVT and nonpurulent cellulitis is an ultrasound. Option (b) is True most cases of uncomplicated nonpurulent cellulitis are due to *Streptococcus* species, thus requiring therapy that covers this etiological agent. Option (c) is False staphylococcal coverage is not needed if there is no purulence. Option (d) is True, it is important to help circulation and lower edema. Option (e) is False interdigital infection is commonly caused by a fungus, so topical azoles should be administered.

Q20. The following question consists of a statement followed by four statements *each* requiring a True or False answer:

According to clinical, image, and laboratory findings:

a. White blood cell counts of >15.4/mm^3 and sodium of <135 mmol/L in the skin or soft tissue complaint should be considered a necrotizing soft tissue infection (NSTI) at first

b. If an elevated phosphokinase is found one should suspect infection in deep muscle or fascia

c. Plain radiograph is the most useful study in finding subcutaneous gas

d. According to the laboratory risk indicator for necrotizing fasciitis score, a score of >4 should prompt further evaluation (imaging and surgical consultation)

e. Initial imaging of choice in most cases of NSTI is computed tomography scanning.

Ans. a. True, b. True, c. False, d. False, and e. True

Option (a) is True, these clinical and laboratory findings suggest NSTI, and to decrease the chances of complication NSTI should be ruled out first. Option (b) is True, elevated phosphokinase is a sign of muscular injury, in this case, due to the inflammatory progress. Option (c) is False, the best image study to evaluate subcutaneous gas is a computed tomography (CT) scan. Option (d) is False, according to the laboratory risk indicator for necrotizing fasciitis, the score should be >6 to gain further evaluation. Option (e) is True, the initial imaging choice for NSTIs should be a CT scan, as it shows more dimension of the infection as well can evaluate the presence of gas with more accuracy.

Q21. Which of the following is False regarding NSTI?

a. Most NSTIs require prompt surgical exploration and debridement for definitive diagnosis and cure
b. Chances of survival may decrease after a surgical debridement
c. Type 2 NSTIs are associated with streptococcal toxic shock syndrome
d. Gas gangrene typically involves deep muscle tissue and is along the fascial planes
e. NSTIs are not reserved for immunocompromised or elderly patients, any group and healthy individual can be affected by both types of NSTIs

Ans. b. Surgical debridement has shown positive results in early therapy due to the removal of the infectious focus; it is demonstrated that early debridement along with antibiotic therapy increases the survival rate in NSTIs. It is important to remember that also surgical debridement serves as a definitive diagnosis and cure.

Q22. The following are elements of the Multinational Association for Supportive Care in Cancer (MASCC) score. Mark the sentence as True/False.

a. No hypotension [systolic blood pressure (SBP) >90 mm Hg]
b. Age <60 years
c. Dehydration requiring parenteral fluids
d. Chronic obstructive pulmonary disease present

Ans. a. True, b. True, c. False, and d. False

Q23. The following are statements regarding febrile neutropenia. Mark the sentence as True/False.

a. Fever in a neutropenic patient with a single temperature of 101°F
b. The risk of infections in neutropenic patients is directly proportional to the absolute neutrophil count (ANC)

c. Fever in a neutropenic patient with temperature >100.4°F over 1 hour
d. Rectal temperature measurements are recommended

Ans. **a. True, b. False, c. True, and d. False**

Q24. **The only recommended outpatient antimicrobial therapy for febrile neutropenia patients is. Mark the sentence as True/False.**

a. Levofloxacin
b. Clindamycin
c. Azithromycin
d. Amoxicillin/clavulanate

Ans. **a. True, b. True, c. False, and d. True**

Q25. **All of the following statements regarding graft vs host disease are true, *except*.**

a. Combination of calcineurin inhibitors with methotrexate is used for prophylaxis of graft versus host disease
b. Chronic graft versus host disease occurs >100 days after transplantation
c. Skin, gastrointestinal, and liver involvement are characteristic of chronic graft-versus-host disease (GVHD)
d. Steroids are the mainstay of treatment

Ans. c. Skin, gastrointestinal, and liver involvement are characteristics of chronic GVHD.

Q26. **Risk factors for chronic GVHD are:**

a. Older age
b. Cytomegalovirus seropositivity
c. Male patient who received stem cell transplant from a multiparous woman
d. All of the above

Ans. d.

Q27. **Treatment options for postliver transplant biliary complications are all, *except:***

a. Endoscopic retrograde cholangiopancreatography (ERCP)
b. IV steroids
c. IV antibiotics
d. Drainage of biloma

Ans. b.

Q28. **Which travel-related disease can still be commonly acquired despite proper vaccination?**

a. Hepatitis A
b. Hepatitis B

c. Rabies
d. Typhoid fever
e. Yellow fever

Ans. d. Vaccination history is extremely important. The vaccine for typhoid fever is highly recommended, as it is widely prevalent in the developing world and is easily transmitted by contamination of food with feces or urine. However, the vaccine is only 75% effective.

Q29. What is the most common cause of serious opportunistic viral disease in patients with advanced AIDS?

a. Cytomegalovirus
b. Herpes simple virus (HSV)
c. Influenza virus
d. Human papillomavirus
e. Varicella zoster virus

Ans. a. While HSV, human papillomavirus, and varicella-zoster virus all have a higher prevalence and a tendency for disseminated disease in human immunodeficiency virus (HIV)-infected individuals, cytomegalovirus is the most common. It can establish itself in many organ systems and becomes a serious risk with CD4+ T-cell counts below 50.

Q30. A resident experiences a needlestick after attempting to place a central line in a septic patient. The source patient has liver cancer from chronic hepatitis B. The intern received the vaccination series for hepatitis B, but there are no records of antibody titers. What is the proper course of action?

a. If the source is positive for hepatitis B core antigen (HBcAg), test the intern for hepatitis B surface antigen (HBsAg). If inadequate, treat with a vaccine booster
b. No treatment is necessary; the intern has received proper vaccination
c. Test the intern for anti-HBs. If adequate, give only hepatitis B immune globulin (HBIG)
d. Test the intern for anti-HBs. If inadequate, treat with HBIG and vaccine booster
e. Treat the intern with HBIG

Ans. d. Documentation of antibody to hepatitis B surface antigen (anti-HBs) >10 mIU/mL demonstrates a proper response to the vaccine and signifies immunity. No intervention is necessary if exposed. However, if the exposure is unvaccinated or the response to the vaccine is unknown, then testing begins with the source.

Toxicology MCQs

Devendra Richhariya

Q1. Clinical features of β-adrenergic antagonists (BAAs) toxicity include all of the following, *except:*

a. Peripheral vasoconstriction and cool peripheries
b. Hyperglycemia
c. Sodium channel blockade
d. Central nervous system (CNS) depression

Ans. b. Hypoglycemia favors the diagnosis of BBA toxicity.

Calcium channel blocker (CCB) toxicity is likely to result in hyperglycemia as there is blockage of pancreatic L-type of calcium channels in the pancreas resulting in decreased insulin secretion.

Q2. All of the following statements are true regarding the use of glucagon in the treatment of BAAs and calcium channel antagonists (CCAs) toxicity.

a. Glucagon is used late in the course of both BAAs and calcium channel antagonists toxicity because of the minimal adverse effect profile
b. Hemodynamic improvement should occur within 5 minutes of the initial bolus of glucagon
c. There is no established maximum dose of continuous infusion of glucagon
d. Hyperglycemia which may occur by the use of glucagon does not typically require any intervention

Ans. a. Minimal adverse effect profile supports the use of glucagon early in the course of both CCA and BAA. Glucagon acts rapidly. It responses in heart rate (HR) and blood pressure (BP) often occurs within minutes. Transient hyperglycemia is expected based on glucagon's stimulation of glycogenolysis and typically does not require any intervention.

Q3. Calcium chloride and calcium gluconate both can be used in the treatment of BAA and CCA toxicity. All of the following statements are true, *except:*

a. Intravenous calcium is used as a first-line agent in CCA toxicity and BAA toxicity as well
b. Calcium chloride contains less calcium in terms of milliequivalents than calcium gluconate
c. Calcium chloride should be given by central venous access
d. Calcium should not be given inadvertently in a digitalis intoxicated patient

Ans. b. Calcium is available in two forms: (1) chloride and (2) gluconate. Calcium chloride contains more calcium in terms of milliequivalents than calcium gluconate. A 10 mL vial of 10% calcium chloride solution contains 13.5 mEq of calcium, whereas a similar volume and concentration of calcium gluconate provides 4.5 mEq.

Q4. Adverse effect of high-dose insulin euglycemia therapy includes all, *except:*

a. Hypoglycemia
b. Hyperkalemia
c. Hypophosphatemia
d. Hypomagnesemia

Ans. b. The primary complications of high-dose insulin euglycemia therapy include hypoglycemia and electrolyte imbalance, particularly hypokalemia. As insulin shifts potassium intracellularly, its concentration should be monitored closely.

Q5. Digoxin toxicity can result in almost any dysrhythmia, *except:*

a. Sinus bradycardia
b. Atrial fibrillation or flutter with slow ventricular response
c. Ventricular tachycardia
d. Rapidly conducted supraventricular tachycardia

Ans. d. Digoxin is used to treat patients with congestive heart failure and/or rate control of rapid ventricular response caused by atrial fibrillation or flutter. Clinically, there is a combination of increased ventricular automaticity and increased vagal effects resulting in atrioventricular (AV) nodal blocking. This lethal combination can lead to almost any type of dysrhythmias except rapidly conducted supraventricular tachycardia.

Q6. A 6-year-old boy was brought to the emergency department (ED) with the history of ingestion of large amount of drain cleaner. Which of the following is most likely to be associated with this ingestion?

a. Coagulative necrosis
b. Hypocalcemia and hypomagnesemia

c. Liquefaction necrosis of the esophagus
d. No significant injury

Ans. c. Caustic materials are categorized as acids or alkali. Alkali causes liquefaction necrosis, which results in extremely rapid and deep penetration into tissues. Alkali commonly causes severe esophageal injuries due to rapid penetration and partial neutralization of the substance in the stomach. Common alkali includes laundry and dishwasher detergents, drain cleaners, and bleach. In contrast, acid causes coagulative necrosis, thereby creating an eschar and preventing deeper spread into tissues. Common acids include battery fluid, metal cleaner, and rust remover. Hypocalcemia and hypomagnesemia is characteristic of hydrofluoric acid burns. The fluoride ions in hydrofluoric acid form complexes with calcium and magnesium ions leading to systemic hypocalcemia and hypomagnesemia. Alkali being more corrosive than acids, no significant injury is expected in this case. The severity of a caustic ingestion is related to the amount and concentration of the substance, duration of contact, and the corrosiveness of the substance.

Q7. A 24-year-old male patient presents to the hospital with the history of ingestion of drain cleaner 30 minutes back. He appears uncomfortable and reports burning sensation of chest. The active ingredient of the drain cleaner is sodium hydroxide. Which of the following is true regarding this patient's care?

a. Activated charcoal should be given as the patient presented within 1 hour of ingestion.
b. He should be kept nil per os (NPO) in preparation for endoscopy.
c. Gastric lavage should be performed to prevent systemic toxicity.
d. Induction of vomiting may be attempted.

Ans. b. For caustic ingestions, endoscopy should be performed early within 12–24 hours of ingestion. Alkaline ingestions cause severe damage with liquefactive necrosis. Endoscopy will help in determining the extent of injury and also guide in management, disposition, and follow-up decisions. Endoscopy should be avoided after the first 2 days postingestion and for at least 2 weeks thereafter because wound strength is at its weakest during this time, increasing the risk of esophageal perforation during the procedure. Activated charcoal is contraindicated in case of an alkaline ingestion as there is an increased risk of perforation and leakage of charcoal into the mediastinum. Gastric lavage and induction of vomiting is also contraindicated because it can cause further esophageal damage and perforation.

Q8. Which of the following factors determines the extent of injury caused by caustic agent ingestion? Mark the below statement True/False.

a. Duration of tissue contact
b. Ability of substance to penetrate tissue
c. Absence of oropharyngeal burns
d. Volume and concentration

Ans. a. True, b. True, c. False, and d. True

The severity of tissue injury is determined by factors, such as pH, concentration, volume, duration of contact, ability of substance to penetrate the tissue, and the corrosiveness of the substance (i.e., acid versus alkali). Significant injuries occurred with acid at a pH <3 and alkalis at a pH >11. Solid or granular caustics often cause oropharyngeal and proximal esophageal injury, whereas liquid ingestions are characterized by extensive esophageal and gastric injuries. The presence or absence of oropharyngeal burns does not predict or rule out esophageal or gastric injury.

Q9. Which of the following are the major signs of impending airway obstruction caused due to caustic ingestion? Mark the below statement True/False.

a. Hoarseness
b. Cough
c. Tachypnea
d. Bradycardia
e. Dysphonia or aphonia

Ans. a. True, b. True, c. True, d. False, and e. True

Major signs of impending airway obstruction caused by caustic ingestion include stridor, hoarseness, dysphonia or aphonia, respiratory distress, tachypnea, and cough. Other signs of injury includes tachycardia, drooling, hematemesis, subcutaneous air, acute peritonitis, and oropharyngeal burns (these oropharyngeal burns are important when identified; however, significant esophageal involvement may also occur in the absence of oropharyngeal lesions). Indications of severe injury include altered mental status, hypotension, peritoneal signs, evidence of viscous perforation, stridor, and shock. Bradycardia is not a sign of impending airway obstruction.

Q10. What are the late developing complications in caustic ingestion patients who survive the initial phases of injury? Mark the below statement True/False.

a. Strictures
b. Fistula

c. Hypocalcemia
d. Hypomotility disorder
e. Increased risk of gastrointestinal cancer

Ans. **a. True, b. True, c. False, d. True, and e. True**

Initial complications of caustic ingestion are airway obstruction which occurs secondary to edema, bleeding, and the presence of necrotic material. Airway protection is the mainstay of management as airway obstruction can develop rapidly. Delay in securing the airway can results in increased difficulty due to progressive airway edema. Other than airway obstruction, initial complications include esophageal, gastric, bowel, airway, or vascular perforation. Fluid loss from vomiting, bleeding, and third spacing may lead to hypovolemia and shock. Significant acid ingestion may cause metabolic acidosis, hemolysis, and acute renal injury including multiorgan failure. Hypocalcemia develops precipitously after ingestion of significant amounts of hydrogen fluoride. Late developing problems in patients who survive the initial phases include strictures, fistula, hypomotility disorder, and increased risk of gastrointestinal cancers.

Q11. In which of the following condition nails and hairs are commonly preserved?

a. Lead poisoning
b. Arsenic poisoning
c. Copper poisoning
d. All of them

Ans. b.

Q12. Which one of the following is the most common mode for lead poisoning?

a. Inhalation
b. Dermally
c. Ingestion
d. None

Ans. a.

Q13. A patient came to the ED with a history of iron poisoning. He has a history of vomiting, abdominal pain, diarrhea along with hematemesis. On presentation, patient is at shock. Acid-base analysis shows high anion gap metabolic acidosis (HAGMA). He also has hepatorenal failure along with coagulopathy. Most likely he had taken poison how many hours ago?

a. 1–4 hours ago
b. 6–8 hours ago
c. 8–12 hours ago
d. 12–48 hours ago

Ans. d.

Q14. Which one of the following is an antidote for iron poisoning?

a. British anti-Lewisite (BAL)
b. Ethylenediaminetetraacetic acid (EDTA)
c. Atropine
d. Deferoxamine

Ans. d.

Q15. Burton's line is a feature of:

a. Lead poisoning
b. Arsenic poisoning
c. Copper poisoning
d. Iron poisoning

Ans. a.

Q16. When does the seed of rosary pea (*Abrus precatorius*) become poisonous?

a. After heating
b. After mixing with water
c. After crushing
d. After swallowing intact

Ans. c. Oral ingestion of whole seeds often does not produce any serious illness since the shell protects the toxin from digestion. Crushing and chewing of seeds disrupts the hard shell, exposing more abrin to the gastrointestinal tract. Most effects of this toxin are usually to gastrointestinal symptoms.

Q17. Which is the common presentation in acute cannabis inhalational poisoning?

a. Vomiting and abdomen cramps
b. Dyspnea
c. Hyperthermia
d. Neuroexcitatory symptoms

Ans. d. Tetrahydrocannabinol (THC) is detectable in plasma only seconds after inhalation with a peak plasma concentration at 3–10 minutes. Cannabis acts through cannabinoid receptors (CB1 and CB2), CB1 receptors are found mainly on neurons in brain, spinal cord, and peripheral nervous system, which cause various neuroexcitatory and depressive symptoms. CNS excitation after inhalational use may be explained by the rapid absorption of THC (primary psychoactive component).

Q18. What is the primary site of action of nicotine in tobacco poisoning?

a. Preganglionic acetylcholine receptors
b. Postganglionic acetylcholine receptors
c. Adrenergic receptors
d. Dopaminergic receptors

Ans. a. Nicotine diffuses readily into brain tissue, where it binds to preganglionic nicotinic acetylcholine receptors, which are ligand-gated ion channels. This agonistic action causes opening of channel, allowing the entry of ions mainly sodium and calcium.

Q19. Mention True or False for the paired plants with their primary toxin:

a. *Castor plant:* Capsaicin
b. *Rosary pea:* Abrin
c. *Calotropin:* Calotoxin
d. *Cleistanthus:* Atropine

Ans. a. False, b. True, c. True, and d. False

Ricinus communis is castor plant of Euphorbiaceae family. Toxicity is caused by ingestion of seeds containing highly toxic protein ricin (toxalbumin). *Cleistanthus collinus* is toxic shrub of Phyllanthaceae family. The toxic substances are cleistanthin A, cleistanthin B, collinusin, and diphyllin.

Q20. Mention True or False for the plant toxin and mechanism of action.

a. *Thevetin:* Inhibition of 3Na/2K pump
b. *Hyoscine:* Acetylcholine receptor agonist
c. *Myristin:* Sympatholytic
d. *Strychnine:* Stimulate glycine receptors

Ans. a. True, b. False, c. False, and d. False

Tropane alkaloids—atropine, hyoscine, and hyoscyamine are the toxins produced by *Datura metel.* They are competitive antagonist of central and peripheral acetylcholine receptors. Myristicin is the toxic element produced by *Myristica fragrans.* It metabolizes into 3-methoxy, methylenedioxyamphetamine which has sympathomimetic action. Strychnine is the toxin produced by *Strychnos nux-vomica.* It competitively inhibits glycine (inhibitory neurotransmitter) receptors in the spinal cord.

Q21. A 20-year-old lady arrives to the ER after vomiting and collapsing during a dance party. She is arousable yet confused when she first arrives. Her vital signs include temperature of 101°F, HR of 115 beats/min, blood pressure (BP) of 150/88 mm Hg, and respiratory rate (RR) of 18 breaths/min. Her creatinine level was 1.4 mg/dL, her sodium level was 128 mEq/dL, and her creatine phosphokinase level was 12,000 IU/L. Her pupils are equal and responsive, and she exhibits mild clonus in her lower extremities. Which of the drugs listed below is the most likely cause of this patient's symptoms?

a. Cocaine
b. Lysergic acid diethylamide (LSD)
c. 3,4-methylenedioxymethamphetamine (MDMA)
d. Methamphetamine
e. Phencyclidine (PCP)

Ans. c. In this case, the patient is intoxicated on MDMA (ecstasy). MDMA is a popular nightclub drug with sympathomimetic and serotonergic properties. Euphoria, agitation, heat, dehydration, rhabdomyolysis, and increased creatinine are all signs of toxicity. MDMA acts by stimulating the release and inhibiting the reuptake of norepinephrine, dopamine, and serotonin neurotransmitters. Multiple causes contribute to hyperthermia, including vigorous exertion, dehydration, and serotonergic effects. Hepatotoxicity, renal failure, and disseminated intravascular coagulation are all possible causes of serotonin syndrome. Hyponatremia is another associated clinical characteristic, which arises as a result of gastrointestinal losses and changes in antidiuretic hormone release. Seizures, comas, and death have all been recorded on occasion. Rehydration, electrolyte replacement, intravenous crystalloids for rhabdomyolysis, cooling measures for hyperthermia, benzodiazepines for seizures, and creating a safe environment for the patient are all part of the treatment for MDMA intoxication.

Cocaine intoxication (answer A) is comparable to MDMA in that it causes sympathomimetic symptoms such as agitation and tachycardia as well as the following complications: seizures, dysrhythmias, ischemia, and rhabdomyolysis. In contrast to MDMA, cocaine intoxication seldom results in clonus or hyponatremia. LSD (answer B) is a hallucinogen.

Patients often have heightened awareness as well as auditory and visual hallucinations. Gastrointestinal discomfort and sympathomimetic symptoms such as hypertension and tachycardia are other common side effects. Coma, seizures, hyperthermia, and rhabdomyolysis have all been described as side effects of LSD use; however, hyponatremia is rare. In terms of clinical appearance, methamphetamine intoxication (answer D) resembles cocaine and MDMA intoxication, although hyponatremia is infrequent, and central nervous system effects are evident. PCP (answer E) is a dissociative anesthetic that induces agitation and excitation of the central nervous system. Although nystagmus, rhabdomyolysis, renal failure, and severe injuries are all possible, serotonergic effects and hyponatremia are rare.

Q22. After consuming an unknown narcotic, an 18-year-old male arrives at the ED. The patient's vital signs include a blood pressure of 170/85 mm Hg, a HR of 122 beats/min, a temperature of 98°F, a RR of 18 breaths/min, and a pulse of 99% on room air. He is agitated and diaphoretic during the examination. His pupils are reactive and measure 7 mm in diameter. Which of the following drugs was most likely used by this patient?

a. Cocaine
b. Dextromethorphan
c. Fluoxetine
d. Phencyclidine

Ans. a. It is prevalent in those who abuse cocaine, amphetamines, or decongestants. Dopamine, epinephrine, norepinephrine, and serotonin are all released when people take cocaine. Adrenergic activation by norepinephrine and epinephrine has the greatest impact. By stimulating α-adrenergic receptors on vascular smooth muscle, norepinephrine produces vasoconstriction. Epinephrine stimulates $\beta 1$-adrenergic receptors, which raise myocardial contractility and HR. The reuptake of these neurotransmitters is also inhibited, in addition to producing catecholamine release. Patients with mydriatic pupils are hypertensive, tachycardic, and have mydriatic pupils. Cardiovascular collapse can occur in shock and wide-complex dysrhythmias in severe overdoses. Seizures are one among the CNS's side effects. Anticholinergic toxidrome might be difficult to differentiate from sympathomimetic toxidrome. The distinction is that individuals with an anticholinergic excess frequently have dry mucous membranes, whereas sympathomimetics cause diaphoresis. The majority of treatment is supportive.

Agitation, hypertension, and heat should all be treated with benzodiazepines.

Dextromethorphan (answer B), a popular component in cold remedies, has effects that are comparable to those of PCP and other opioids. It disrupts the N-methyl-D-aspartate receptor at the PCP-binding site, inhibiting serotonin absorption. Overdosing results in lethargy, agitation, dysarthria, ataxia, diaphoresis, hypertension, and nystagmus in patients. Intoxication is similar to LSD at large dosages including euphoria and hallucinations. Dystonic responses in children have been recorded following therapeutic administration. When used with a serotonin reuptake inhibitor, dextromethorphan decreases the intake of serotonin, resulting in serotonin syndrome. Fluoxetine (answer C) is a serotonin reuptake inhibitor that is selective [selective serotonin reuptake inhibitor (SSRI)]. The gastrointestinal (nausea, vomiting, and abdominal pain), cardiovascular (tachycardia, bradycardia, and QTc prolongation), and central neurological systems are the most affected by elevated serotonin in overdose (dizziness, hyperreflexia, and agitation). Serotonin syndrome is rare when fluoxetine is used in excess. PCP (answer D) is a dissociative drug that produces a wide range of effects when smoked. Patients may exhibit bizarre behavior, agitation, and violence. A blank or catatonic stare is common. Vertical, horizontal, and rotary nystagmus are often present.

Q23. For the past hour, a 38-year-old guy has been experiencing chest discomfort. He is anxious, diaphoretic, and has dilated pupils. A temperature of 101.1°F, a HR of 135 beats/min, and a BP of 210/130 mm Hg are significant vital indicators. Prior to the commencement of chest trouble, he admits to consuming cocaine. The lateral leads of an ECG exhibit sinus tachycardia with ST-segment depression. Troponin is at a high level of 0.13. Which of the following drugs should not be given?

a. Hydralazine
b. Metoprolol
c. Nitroglycerin
d. Phentolamine

Ans. b. Hyperthermia, hypertension, tachycardia, diaphoresis, and dilated pupils are all signs and symptoms of a sympathomimetic toxidrome in this patient. He also exhibits cocaine-induced myocardial ischemia as demonstrated by ECG abnormalities and increased troponin. Cooling for hyperthermia and benzodiazepines such as lorazepam and diazepam for drowsiness and anxiety symptoms are the mainstays of cocaine toxicity treatment. Infusing saline, packing with ice, and using wet blankets and big fans to generate evaporative cooling are all options for cooling. Cocaine can produce chest discomfort by a variety of processes including pneumothorax, pneumomediastinum, and aortic dissection, which are noncardiac causes. Cocaine produces coronary vasoconstriction while also raising myocardial oxygen demand, which can lead to heart ischemia or infarction. Aspirin and nitrates should be given to this patient since he exhibits signs of heart ischemia. If myocardial infarction is suspected, heparin and antiplatelet medications may be used. If nitrate therapy fails to control hypertension, phentolamine or hydralazine may be administered. Because of the potential of unopposed α-stimulation, which might aggravate coronary vasoconstriction, β-blockers like metoprolol are contraindicated with cocaine usage.

Hydralazine (answer A) is a vasodilator and a direct-acting smooth muscle relaxant that is used to treat hypertension by lowering peripheral resistance. It is most commonly utilized as a second-line treatment for cocaine-induced hypertension. Nitroglycerin (answer C) lowers cardiac preload and, to a lesser extent, afterload. It is used to treat myocardial ischemia and cocaine-induced hypertension. Phentolamine (answer D) is a nonselective α-antagonist that causes vasodilation by blocking α-1 receptors. It is usually reserved for pheochromocytoma-induced hypertension, although it can also be utilized for cocaine-induced hypertension.

Q24. A 35-year-old guy is experiencing nausea and stomach pain. His vital signs are normal, and he has a soft and nontender abdomen. When he passes the packets, he becomes uncomfortable and admits to swallowing 50 plastic packets containing cocaine in exchange for a big quantity of money. Which of the following is the best course of action?

a. Administer polyethylene glycol and admit for observation
b. Endoscopic retrieval of the packets
c. Laparotomy and surgical removal of packets
d. Reassure and discharge home since he will pass the packets on his own.

Ans. a. As part of a drug smuggling scheme, individuals ingest sealed packets carrying cocaine, as seen in this clinical scenario. Telemetry should be used to monitor patients with cocaine body packing, and large-bore intravenous access should be established. To accelerate gastrointestinal passage of the packets, whole-bowel irrigation with polyethylene glycol is utilized. It is also possible to use activated charcoal at a rate of 1 g/kg of body weight. Patients with intact packets may have gastrointestinal discomfort or bloating, but their vital signs are usually normal and they show no evidence of cocaine poisoning. The deadly dosage of cocaine released when packets burst is typically fatal. Sudden mortality or signs and symptoms of cocaine poisoning, such as tachycardia, severe hypertension, heat, diaphoresis, chest discomfort, and cardiac arrhythmias, may occur in patients. In the event of a rupture, a patient may be rushed to the operating room to remove the packets and preserve his or her life.

Endoscopic retrieval of the packets (answer B) is not first-line treatment because of concern for packet rupture during the procedure. Laparotomy and surgical removal of the packets (answer C) is typically reserved for cases of packet rupture. This patient has normal vital signs and does not manifest signs and symptoms of a sympathomimetic toxidrome, so it is unlikely the packets have ruptured. Reassurance and discharge home (answer D) is incorrect because this is a high-risk situation and patients require hospital admission and observation.

Q25. The toxic syndrome for anticholinergic overdose is similar to sympathomimetic toxicity and includes all of the following signs with the exception of:

a. Altered mental status
b. Diaphoresis
c. Hyperthermia
d. Increased HR
e. Urinary retention

Ans. b. Anticholinergic (antimuscarinic) syndrome includes all of the signs above except for diaphoresis. Typically, anticholinergic poisoning presents with dry skin and mouth but otherwise has similar features to sympathomimetic toxicity. Sympathomimetic overdose often presents with diaphoresis. Anticholinergic patients are also less paranoid and violent.

Q26. Intoxication with morning glory seeds will mimic intoxication with which of the following hallucinogens?

a. Ecstasy
b. Ketamine
c. LSD
d. Marijuana
e. PCP

Ans. c. Several plants contain alkaloids similar to LSD including morning glory and Hawaiian baby woodrose.

Q27. Which unique life-threatening electrolyte abnormality is seen with the use of *N*-methyl-3,4-methylenedioxyamphetamine (MDMA)?

a. Hyperkalemia
b. Hypernatremia
c. Hypokalemia
d. Hypomagnesemia
e. Hyponatremia

Ans. e. Hyponatremia can occur with MDMA use and can be severe and life-threatening. MDMA alters the release of vasopressin and will induce a clinical syndrome resembling the syndrome of inappropriate secretion of antidiuretic hormone (SIADH). The patients have concentrated urine with high urine sodium content. Seizures can occur and should be treated with hypertonic saline. In the absence of seizures or other life-threatening conditions, general supportive care with water restriction is adequate treatment.

Q28. What is the preferred primary method for controlling a combative patient suffering from a sympathomimetic overdose?

a. Chlorpromazine
b. Diazepam
c. Droperidol
d. Haloperidol
e. Physical restraints

Ans. b. Diazepam and other benzodiazepines are the most effective medications for sedating and calming an agitated patient. They promote drowsiness and lower muscular tone, both of which can help with hyperthermia. They can also help with the initially elevated blood pressure that comes with sympathomimetic usage. Lorazepam is more predictably absorbed than diazepam in the agitated patient when IV access is difficult to obtain. Chlorpromazine can be administered intramuscularly for fast sedation; however, it has anticholinergic side effects that might worsen hyperthermia. Butyrophenone medications (e.g., haloperidol and droperidol) are used to treat more severe agitation and are considered secondary treatments when benzodiazepine dosages have been met. Additionally, they may have dysrhythmic effects that are additive to cocaine's. Physical constraints may be necessary at first, but they are not desired since they might raise the risk of hyperthermia and agitation, both of which are linked to a higher risk of death.

Q29. How long does a typical urine drug screen result remain positive after use of cocaine?

a. 1 day
b. 3 days
c. 1 week
d. 2 weeks
e. 1 month

Ans. b. Urine drug screens detect the cocaine metabolite benzoylecgonine, which is typically present in the urine for 3 days after the last use.

Q30. Police observed a 24-year-old male using crack cocaine on a street corner. The patient complains of a bad headache on the way to jail, so the police take him to the ED for medical clearance. The patient is conscious and has a normal mental condition, but she still has widespread headache. His vital signs include BP of 195/99 mm Hg, HR of 102 beats/min, RR of 18 breaths/min, and temperature of 37.2°C. His physical check shows that he is in good health. What criteria should be used to assess his headache?

a. Acetaminophen administration, discharge if headache resolves
b. Blood pressure reduction, discharge if headache resolves
c. Head computed tomography (CT) scan, discharge if normal
d. Head CT scan, lumbar puncture if normal, discharge if both are normal.
e. No evaluation needed; cocaine is not associated with headache.

Ans. d. Subarachnoid hemorrhage (SAH) is linked to cocaine use. Patients who have a severe headache after using cocaine should be evaluated thoroughly for SAH, which includes a head CT scan and lumbar puncture. Additionally, while the examination is being done, increased blood pressure should be reduced.

Trauma MCQs

Devendra Richhariya

Q1. A 20-year-old male is brought in by emergency medical service (EMS) with a history of a road traffic accident. He is conscious but drowsy and able to speak to you. He has saturation of 85% on room air, respiratory rate of 28 breaths/min, pulse rate 110 beats/min, and a blood pressure of 98/65 mm Hg. He already has a c-collar in place. Also he has reduced air entry on the left side and focused assessment with sonography for trauma (FAST) is positive. After taking the patient onto the bed, what would your next steps be?

a. Intubate the patient, blood transfusion, chest tube placement, and tranexamic acid
b. Chest tube placement, tranexamic acid, intubate the patient, and blood transfusion
c. Supplemental oxygen, tranexamic acid, blood products, chest decompression, and intubate the patient
d. Tranexamic acid, chest decompression, supplemental oxygen, and blood products

Ans. c. The abovementioned patient requires intubation urgently *but not* immediately, as he is self-ventilating with an oxygen saturation of 85% and is protecting his airway. With a positive FAST and shock index (SI) >1.0, the team leader should choose to achieve hemodynamic optimization before rapid sequence intubation (RSI), specifically a presumed right-sided tension pneumothorax and intra-abdominal injury.

Q2. Which of the following is not a physiologically difficult airway?

a. Uncorrected hypoxia
b. Uncorrected hypotension
c. Uncorrected acidosis
d. Difficult cricothyrotomy
e. Right ventricular failure

Ans. d. Physiologically, difficult airways comprise uncorrected hypoxia, shock, severe unresolved metabolic acidosis, and right ventricular failure. Difficult cricothyrotomy, difficult bag mask, difficult intubation, and difficult extraglottic device placement are anatomically difficult airways.

Q3. **The following may be clinical indicators of occult shock. Mark the below statement True/False.**

a. Vital signs
b. Thromboelastography
c. Base deficit
d. Shock index
e. Point-of-care ultrasound (POCUS)

Ans. **a. True, b. False, c. False, d. True, and e. True**

Clinical indicators of shock comprise vital signs, shock index, and bedside ultrasound. Laboratory indicators comprise base deficit, lactates, international normalized ratio (INR), and viscoelastic assays.

Q4. **Standard tourniquet use may be difficult in injuries of: mark the below statement True/False.**

a. Forearm
b. Axilla
c. Neck
d. Leg
e. Thigh

Ans. **a. False, b. True, c. True, d. False, and e. False**

The groin, neck, and axilla are certain anatomic regions where standard tourniquet use has been proved to be difficult. Junctional tourniquets and hemostatic dressings have been developed for the same.

Q5. **Damage control resuscitation has the following components: mark the below statement True/False.**

a. Damage control surgery
b. Hemostatic resuscitation
c. Permissive hypotension
d. Recognition of shock
e. Management of critical airway

Ans. **a. True, b. True, c. True, d. False, and e. False**

Damage control resuscitation has three key components—(1) hemostatic resuscitation, (2) permissive hypotension, and (3) damage control surgery.

Q6. **Primary brain injury involves:**

a. Skull fractures
b. Brain parenchymal injury
c. Blood vessel injury
d. All of the above

Ans. d. The initial insult associated with moderate and severe traumatic brain injury (TBI) imparts mechanical forces that produce high levels of direct damage and strain to the brain parenchyma. The primary injuries include contusions (bruises to brain parenchyma), hematomas (subdural, epidural, intraparenchymal, intraventricular, and subarachnoid), diffuse axonal injury (stress or damage to axons), direct cellular damage (neurons, axons, and other supportive cells), loss of the blood-brain barrier, disruption of the neurochemical homeostasis, and loss of the electrochemical function.

Q7. Goal of treatment in TBI is: mark the below statement True/False.

a. Prevention of primary injury
b. Prevention of secondary injury
c. Recognition and treatment of raised ICP
d. Identify and treat other life-threatening injuries

Ans. a. False, b. True, c. True, and d. True

The primary goals of treatment are to maintain cerebral perfusion and oxygenation by optimizing intravascular volume and ventilation; prevent secondary injury by correcting hypoxia, hypercapnia, hyperglycemia, hyperthermia, anemia, or hypoperfusion; recognize and treat elevated intracranial pressure (ICP); arrange for neurosurgical intervention to evacuate intracranial mass lesions; and treat other life-threatening injuries. Both intracranial and systemic events contribute to increased ICP after TBI. In the first hours after trauma, expansion of hematomas is the main threat, whereas in the following days, other mechanisms including water accumulation, disrupted autoregulation, ischemia, and contusion expansion, lead to further increases in ICP. Herniation is a medical emergency, requiring prompt treatment to prevent irreversible and often fatal damage to the brain stem.

Q8. What is true about basilar skull fracture? Mark the below statement True/False.

a. Raccoon's eye
b. Battle's sign
c. Cerebrospinal fluid (CSF) leak from ear and nose
d. Meningitis

Ans. a. True, b. True, c. True, and d. True

Basilar skull fractures most commonly involve the temporal bones but may involve the occipital, sphenoid, ethmoid, and the orbital plate of the frontal bone as well.

Q9. Secondary brain injury is accentuated by: mark the below statement True/False.

a. Hypoxemia and hypercapnia
b. Hypotension
c. Hyperthermia
d. Hyperglycemia

Ans. **a. True, b. True, c. True, and d. True**

Hypotension, hypoxemia, and hyperglycemia that accelerate neurotoxic damage and worsen long-term outcome. Treat hypotension, hypoxemia, hypercarbia, and hyperglycemia. A single occurrence of hypotension and hypoxia after brain injury is associated with a 150% increase in mortality.

Q10. Cushing's triad includes:

a. Hypotension, tachycardia, and irregular breathing
b. Hypertension, bradycardia, and irregular breathing
c. Hypotension, bradycardia, and unequal pupils
d. Hypertension, tachycardia, and unequal pupils

Ans. b. The Cushing reflex is a physiological nervous system response to acute elevations of ICP, resulting in the Cushing triad of widened pulse pressure (increasing systolic, decreasing diastolic), bradycardia, and irregular respirations.

Q11. Indication of anticonvulsant in TBI: mark the below statement True/False.

a. To prevent late onset post-traumatic seizure (PTS)
b. To prevent early onset PTS
c. Skull fracture and penetrating head injury
d. Post-traumatic amnesia of >30 minutes

Ans. **a. False, b. True, c. True, and d. True**

Prophylactic use of phenytoin or valproate is not recommended for preventing late PTSs. Phenytoin is recommended to decrease the incidence of early PTS (within 7 days of injury). However, early PTS has not been associated with worse outcomes [irritant-induced asthma (IIA)]. Risk factors for early seizures include younger age (especially <5 years), acute intracerebral hematoma, acute subdural hematoma, diffuse cerebral edema, intracranial metal fragment retention, focal neurologic deficits, depressed/linear skull fractures, and loss of consciousness (LOC)/amnesia for >30 minutes.

Q12. A 24-year-old male meets with a motor vehicle crash at a speed of 100 km/hour and is brought to the hospital not moving his lower limbs. He is moving his upper limbs. There is a fracture dislocation at T9 level. Which of the following is he likely to have? Mark the below statement True/False.

a. Spinal shock
b. Neurogenic shock
c. Quadriplegia
d. Paraplegia

Ans. **a. True, b. True, c. False, and d. True**

Injuries in the cervical cord and thoracic level T6 and above cause neurogenic shock which is paralysis of the sympathetics to the heart and blood vessels. Spinal shock is flaccid paralysis and loss of reflexes due to spinal cord injury. Quadriplegia occurs when injury is at the level of the cervical spine while thoracic and lumbar injuries cause paraplegia.

Q13. A 70-year-old male falls and strikes his chin on the car bonnet. He develops weakness more in the upper than the lower limbs. Which one of the statements is True/False?

a. Anterior cord syndrome
b. Central cord syndrome
c. Prognosis is poor
d. Magnetic resonance imaging (MRI) is the primary imaging modality for this and shows increased T2 signal secondary to cord edema

Ans. **a. False, b. True, c. False, and d. True**

Hyperextension injury in the elderly with associated spinal canal stenosis produces central cord syndrome where there is stretch of the fibers located centrally and thereby the upper limbs are affected more than the lower limbs. It has good prognosis and recovery occurs from the lower, then the upper limbs. Anterior cord syndrome is due to thrombosis of the anterior spinal artery and carries poor prognosis.

Q14. A patient falls on his head while diving in a shallow swimming pool. He is conscious but complains of neck pain. A fracture of the atlas is diagnosed on investigation. Mark the below statement True/False.

a. Open mouth view X-ray can confirm the diagnosis
b. The incidence of quadriplegia is high following this injury
c. Computed tomography (CT) scan is necessary for definitive diagnosis
d. Fractures of C2 do not occur with this mechanism of injury

Ans. **a. True, b. False, c. True, and d. False**

Falls on head (axial loading) during shallow dives are the most common cause of atlas (C1) fractures. Jefferson's fracture is when the ring splits and moves apart. They are commonly missed due to absence of neurological deficit. Diagnosis can be made on open mouth view and confirmed on CT scan. Ligamentous instability on X-rays is noted when the lateral mass displacement is 7 mm or greater. MRI may be needed to evaluate the ligamentous structures. Fractures of axis (C2) are commonly associated.

Q15. Regarding the fractures of the vertebrae, mark the below statement True/False.

a. Flexion teardrop fractures are seen in the cervical spine and are unstable
b. Clay-shoveler's fracture is a spinous process avulsion injury
c. Compression fractures of thoracolumbar spine are usually unstable
d. Chance fracture is a horizontal fracture through the body of the thoracic or lumbar vertebra

Ans. **a. True, b. True, c. False, and d. True**

Flexion teardrop fractures in the cervical spine are unstable, while extension teardrop fractures are stable. Compression fractures of the thoracolumbar spine are usually stable as only one column is involved. Chance fracture is commonly seen following seatbelt injury, involves all three columns, and is associated with intra-abdominal injury. Spinous process fractures were initially described in Clay-shoveler's.

Q16. Regarding neurogenic shock which occurs after trauma, mark the below statement True/False.

a. It is due to peripheral vasodilatation and sympathetic paralysis
b. Manifest as bradycardia and hypotension
c. There is loss of anal tone and reflexes
d. Treated initially with IV fluids and vasopressors

Ans. **a. True, b. True, c. False, and d. True**

Neurogenic shock occurs due to spinal cord injury T6 and above involving upper thoracic and cervical cord. It is due to sympathetic paralysis and vasodilatation. Bradycardia and hypotension are diagnostic of the condition. Treatment is initially with IV fluids and followed by vasopressors. Loss of anal tone is noted in spinal shock.

Q17. A 30-year-old male is brought after a polytrauma with cervical collar and long spine board. He is resuscitated as per advanced trauma life support (ATLS) principles. Which one of the statements is true?

a. Spine board can be kept for a maximum of 3 hours
b. Canadian C spine rule for radiological assessment states that alcohol intoxication is an indication
c. NEXUS criteria include X, i.e., extremes of age
d. Absence of pain, tenderness in cervical spine, and negative X-ray indicates cervical collar can be removed
e. Most common site of spine injury is dorsolumbar junction

Ans. d. Spine board should be kept a maximum of 2 hours. Canadian C spine rule is dangerous mechanism of injury, age above 65 years and paresthesia. NEXUS (National Emergency X-Radiography Utilization Study) criteria, X is extreme distracting injury. The most common region to be affected is the cervical spine.

Q18. A 26-year-old male is being evaluated for spine injury and neurological deficit post-trauma. Which one of the statements is true?

a. The minimum power to localize the level of injury is 2/5
b. Vertebral level and neurological level usually correspond to each other
c. Myotome is a muscle supplied by a single nerve root
d. Dermatome is an area of skin supplied by a single nerve root
e. The likelihood of recovery decreases from category A to D in ASIA score

Ans. d. The minimum power to localize a level of injury is 3/5. Usually, the vertebral and neurological levels do not correspond as the spinal cord ends at L1, the nerve roots exit from below and there is ascending edema. Myotome is a group of muscles and not a single muscle supplied by a nerve root. The likelihood of recovery increases from category A to D.

Q19. Patients with injuries to the vertebrae may need surgery. The following statements are true, *except:*

a. Indications for surgery are instability and neurological deficit
b. Best results are obtained by surgery within 48 hours of injury
c. Surgery involves relieving pressure on the cord, removing bony fragments, and stabilizing the spinal column
d. Fixation is done up to 1–2 levels above and below the fracture
e. Improvement continues to occur for 3–6 months after surgery

Ans. b. Best results are obtained when patient is operated within 24 hours of injury or after 6–8 weeks. The three main components of any spinal column injury evaluated are as follows: (1) Displacement—is reduction needed? If left in that position, will functional disability occur? Does it therefore need any reduction? (2) Stability—if left untreated, will the position change? Does it therefore need fixation? (3) Biology—will it heal? Is there any cord and/or root injury-and will that heal?

Q20. After spinal trauma with paraplegia, there is a high incidence of deep vein thrombosis (DVT). Cord edema also occurs which

contributes to the neurological deficit and the immobilization leads to bedsores. Which one of the statements is false?

a. Low molecular weight (LMW) heparin should be started in all case of spine trauma with paraplegia immediately to prevent DVT
b. Vena cava filters are useful if associated bleeding is expected to continue beyond 72 hours
c. Vacuum-assisted closure (VAC) therapy is useful in large pressure sores
d. The role of steroids in the acute phase is controversial
e. LMW heparin may have to be continued for 3 months

Ans. a. Low molecular weight heparins are started only after ruling out intracranial, abdominal, and pelvis bleed. Elastic compression stockings can be applied immediately. Steroids are controversial. Studies state that methylprednisolone infusion can be given within 8 hours of injury.

Q21. Which one of the statements is true regarding spine injuries?

a. Spinal cord injury without radiographic abnormality (SCIWORA) is usually seen in the elderly
b. Chance fracture is common in the cervical vertebrae
c. Fracture with dislocation is usually stable fractures
d. Swimmer's view is used to view the dens
e. For instability, at least two columns should be affected

Ans. e. Spinal cord injury without radiographic abnormality is usually noted in children. Chance fracture is seen in dorsolumbar region. Fracture with dislocations is unstable. Swimmer's view is needed for the C7 vertebra. Denis described the spine as a three column concept where there are anterior, middle, and posterior columns. Anterior or posterior along with central column involvement leads to instability. Single column affected is stable. The three columns are: (1) anterior column—anterior longitudinal ligament (ALL) anterior two-thirds of the vertebral body, (2) middle column—posterior one-third of the vertebral body and posterior one-third of the intervertebral disk (annulus fibrosus), and (3) posterior column—everything posterior to the posterior longitudinal ligament (PLL) and pedicles.

Q22. Which is the most common type of dislocation of the hips?

a. Anterior
b. Posterior
c. Central
d. Dislocation with fracture shaft

Ans. b.

Q23. Von Rosen splint is used in:

a. Congenital talipes equinovarus (CTEV)
b. Congenital dislocation of the hip (CDH)
c. Fracture of shaft of femur
d. Fracture tibia

Ans. b.

Q24. What is the formula of dry plaster of Paris?

a. $CaSO_4 \cdot 1/2\ H_2O$
b. $CaSO_4$ only
c. $CaSO_4 \cdot 5H_2O$
d. $MgSO_4 \cdot 2H_2O$

Ans. a.

Q25. Treatment of choice for fracture shaft femur in children is:

a. Gallows or Russell's traction
b. Internal fixation
c. Kuntscher nail
d. Thomas splint

Ans. a.

Q26. The most important factor in fracture healing is:

a. Good alignment
b. Organization of blood clot
c. Accurate reduction and 100% opposition of fractured fragments
d. Immobilization
e. Adequate calcium intake

Ans. d.

Q27. Stellate ganglion block is mainly used for:

a. Compound palm ganglion
b. De Quervain's synovitis inflammation
c. Sudeck's dystrophy
d. Osteoarthritis of carpometacarpal joint

Ans. c.

Q28. Volkmann's ischemia contracture is commonly due to:

a. Tight plaster
b. Tight splint
c. Both
d. None

Ans. c.

Q29. Ideal treatment with fracture neck of the humerus in a lady will be:

a. Triangular sling
b. Hemiarthroplasty
c. Chest arm bandage
d. Internal fixation

Ans. a.

Q30. In anterior dislocation of the shoulder, the nerve involved is:

a. Radial nerve
b. Circumflex nerve
c. Ulnar nerve
d. Median nerve

Ans. b.

Q31. A 65-year-old female presents with impacted fracture surgical neck of humerus. Treatment of choice is:

a. Arthroplasty
b. Arm chest strapping
c. Triangular sling
d. Wait and watch

Ans. c.

Q32. The bony triangle is maintained in:

a. Supracondylar fracture of humerus
b. Posterior dislocation of elbow
c. Intercondylar fracture of humerus
d. Lateral condylar fracture of humerus

Ans. a.

Q33. Which one of the statements is false?

a. In sprain, the ligament is often torn
b. In dislocation, there is no contact in-between both the components of the joint
c. Sclerosis of the fracture ends indicate absolute nonunion
d. None of the above

Ans. d.

Q34. Which one of the statements pertaining to green stick fracture is correct?

a. Any fracture in child
b. It is generally incomplete
c. Fracture only in rickety children
d. All of the above

Ans. b.

Q35. All of the following statements about dislocation of the shoulder are true, *except:*

a. The injury is produced by a fall with the cup fully abducted
b. The most common position for the head of the humerus to move into the subspinous
c. The axillary (circumflex humeral) nerve is likely to be injured
d. The easiest way to reduce it is by simple pressure with the patient under general anesthetic with muscle relaxation

Ans. d.

Q36. Strike the false statement(s):

a. Reversed Colles is called Smith's fracture
b. If the lower limb is externally rotated, it is most likely due to fracture neck of femur
c. If the thigh consumes flexion, adduction, and internal rotation following a history of severe injury, a posterior dislocation is the likely cause
d. None of these

Ans. d.

Q37. Match the list 1 with list 2 and write the correct answer.

List 1	*List 2*
a. Intracapsular neck of femur fracture	1. Thomson prosthesis
b. Extracapsular subtrochanteric fracture	2. Conservative treatment
c. Shaft fracture in children	3. Internal fixation using screw and plate
d. Supracondylar fracture	4. K-wire fixation

Ans. **a. (1), b. (3), c. (2), d. (4)**

Q38. Gustilo-Anderson grade IIIC involves:

a. Exposed bone
b. Exposed bone with soft tissue loss
c. Exposed bone with soft tissue loss, with contamination
d. Exposed bone with soft tissue loss, contamination with vascular injury

Ans. d. Open injuries are classified using Gustilo-Anderson classification and grade IIIC involves open fracture with soft tissue loss requiring cover and with involvement of the neurovascular bindle which need early recognition and treatment.

Q39. Grossly contaminated wounds should be treated with:

a. Cephalosporins
b. Aminoglycosides
c. Tetanus toxoid
d. All of the above

Ans. d. Contaminated injuries are prone for infection and it is prudent to treat them with broad-spectrum antibiotics and tetanus toxoid.

Q40. Shoulder trauma series X-rays consists of:

a. Shoulder anteroposterior (AP)
b. Shoulder AP and axial and Y view
c. Shoulder axial
d. Shoulder AP and axial

Ans. b. Trauma series X-rays should include optimum views so that full profile of the bone and joint is visible. Taking the necessary X-rays' assessment of the joint congruity and displaced, minimally displaced fractures can be made easily.

Q41. Knee dislocation/subluxation with neurovascular injury should be suspected in:

a. High velocity injuries
b. Low velocity injuries in obese patients
c. Knee injuries with ligamentous instability
d. All of the above

Ans. d. Knee dislocations should be suspected in both high-velocity injuries and low-velocity injuries in obese patients and understanding the mechanism is very important to suspect the neurovascular injury which needs prompt attention and treatment.

Q42. Triage is done for:

a. To assess the trauma patient
b. To categorize the patient's injuries into life threatening, limb threatening
c. To communicate with concerned departments
d. All of the above

Ans. d. Triage forms important part of the emergency. This is the place where decisions are made which patients need immediate care and which can wait.

Q43. According to estimation of burns by Wallace's "rule of nines", which one of the following statements is false?

a. Though being an efficient tool to evaluate the percentage of burns over body surface, it overestimated the area by 15%
b. Burns over each arm and head are 9%
c. Burns over perineum are 1%
d. Burns over chest, back, and legs are 18%

Ans. a. Though being an efficient tool to evaluate the percentage of burns over body surface, it overestimated the area by 3%.

Q44. Determine whether the following statement is True or False regarding the severity of burns on basis of depth.

a. The integrity of an epidermis is intact in second-degree burns and when the extent of the burn is limited to upper layers of the epidermis it is a superficial second-degree burn

b. The skin may present as dark, dry, hard, and painless in second-degree burns
c. Deeper second-degree burns have decreased pain and a blunt pressure feeling in affected areas
d. First-degree burns include all layers of skin and subcutaneous fat as well as deeper tissues

Ans. **a. True, b. False, c. True, and d. False**

The skin may present as dark, dry, hard, and painless in third-degree burns. Fourth-degree burns include all layers of skin and subcutaneous fat as well as deeper tissues.

Q45. Regarding wound care in second-degree burns, which one of the following statements is false?

a. Aseptic dressing with paraffin and woven fabrics ensure the wound does not stick to the dressing
b. Small blisters may be left intact however larger blisters need unroofing to be done along with serial dressings
c. There is no risk of hypertrophic scar formation, keloid, discoloration, and contractures in second-degree burns
d. Application of silver sulfadiazine, mupirocin, and nitrofurazone over the burns directly or underneath the gauze along with paraffin is mandatory

Ans. c. There is increased risk of hypertrophic scar formation, keloid, discoloration, and contractures in second-degree burns.

Q46. Which one of the following statements is True or False regarding clinical signs and symptoms of inhalational injury?

a. Voice hoarseness, mucosal edema, black sputum, and presence of carbon particles are present in mucosa
b. Burns over hair, face, nose, and ear are absent
c. Neck burns are present horizontally in a few cases
d. Nausea, vomiting, fatigue, dizziness, and headache are present

Ans. **a. True, b. False, c. False, and d. True**

Burns over hair, face, nose, and ear are present. Neck burns are present circumferentially along with perioral and facial burns.

Q47. Which one of the following statements is false regarding the transfer of patient to tertiary care burns unit?

a. Maintain a urinary output of 10 mL/hour in adults and children at 1 mL/kg/hour
b. Enteral nutrition should be initiated early in the stabilization of patient

c. Two large bore venous cannulas are established preferably in upper extremities
d. Lactated ringer's solution is the fluid of choice in the initial 24 hours of burns prior to transfer

Ans. a. Maintain a urinary output of 30 mL/hour in adults and children at 1 mL/kg/hour.

Q48. A 20-year-old male patient is brought to the emergency department (ED) after being stabbed in the anterior aspect of the neck just inferior to the cricoid cartilage. Which one of the following choices identifies the zone of injury for this patient and associated anatomic structure of concern for this particular injury?

a. Zone I, pharynx
b. Zone I, vertebral arteries
c. Zone II, jugular vein
d. Zone III, carotid arteries
e. Zone III, vertebral arteries

Ans. b. Zone I includes the vertebral and proximal carotid arteries, major thoracic vessels, superior mediastinum, lungs, esophagus, trachea, thoracic duct, and spinal cord.

Q49. Which of the following is *most* accurate with respect to penetrating neck injury?

a. Angiography is the preferred imaging modality for injuries in the pediatric population
b. CT scans can effectively exclude laryngotracheal injury
c. Penetrating esophageal injuries are often initially asymptomatic
d. The preferred treatment for injuries to zones I and III is operative
e. Ultrasound can be particularly useful in evaluation of zone I and zone III injuries

Ans. c. Penetrating esophageal injuries are frequently initially asymptomatic. Nonoperative management is preferred for injuries to zones I and III.

Q50. A 25-year-old male presents to the ED after blunt trauma to neck. He has no complaints and the examination is unremarkable except for left-sided ptosis and pupillary constriction. These findings are most concerning for injury to which of the following structures?

a. Left carotid artery
b. Left vertebral artery
c. Right carotid artery
d. Right vertebral artery
e. Spinal artery

Ans. a. The patient demonstrates findings consistent with Horner syndrome, which can occur as a result of injury to the ipsilateral carotid artery.

Q51. Which of the following is true regarding vascular injury in trauma?

a. An ankle brachial index (ABI) of 0.5 is concerning for arterial injury
b. An ABI of 1.0 is concerning for arterial injury
c. Duplex ultrasound is a useful modality to diagnose vascular injury in open fractures
d. Multidetector CT angiography is safe to use in patients with iodine allergy
e. Underlying preexisting vascular disease will not affect the ABI

Ans. a. An ABI of 1.0 is normal. An ABI of <0.9 is concerning for arterial injury. Preexisting vascular disease and hypothermia will lower the ABI. Duplex ultrasonography has an accuracy of 96–98% for vascular injury but is operator dependent and is not useful with open fractures, large hematomas, or bulky dressings. Multidetector CT angiography is less invasive and has a similar cost to angiography, but the limitations include the inability to perform the test on patients with iodine allergies and the artifact caused by bullet fragments.

Q52. Which one of the following statements is *true* regarding genitourinary trauma?

a. Infection is the most common complication after circumcision
b. Male straddle injuries are at greatest risk for posterior urethral injuries
c. Testicular rupture should be managed conservatively with ice and analgesics
d. With penile fractures, perform a retrograde urethrogram (RUG) to evaluate for urethral injury
e. Zipper injuries to the penis often have to be managed in the operating room

Ans. d. Obtain a CT retrograde urethrogram for penile fracture or penetrating penile injury because of the high incidence of coexisting urethral injury. Bleeding is the most common complication after circumcision and is often controlled by direct pressure. Infection occurs in up to 10% of patients and requires urologic consultation.

Q53. Which one of the following soft tissue foreign bodies is usually not visible on X-ray?

a. Bone
b. Glass
c. Gravel
d. Metal
e. Wood

Ans. e. Materials, such as glass, metal, gravel, or bone are usually visible on plain films. Organic materials such as wood are more difficult to identify with plain films, but ultrasound can be useful. CT scanning is more accurate for finding both radiolucent and opaque foreign bodies.

Q54. According to the New Orleans Criteria, which of the following is an indication to obtain a head CT after minor head trauma?

a. Absence of intoxication
b. Age <60 years
c. Fall from standing
d. Unwitnessed fall
e. Visible trauma above the clavicle

Ans. e. The New Orleans Criteria for obtaining a head CT after minor head injury are based on the presence of any of the following seven criteria: age >60 years, headache, vomiting, intoxication, persistent anterograde amnesia, evidence of trauma above the clavicles, or seizure. The reported sensitivity of this decision rule is 100%.

Q55. Which one of the following injuries of the cervical spine is considered *stable*?

a. Bilateral interfacetal dislocation
b. Extension teardrop fracture
c. Flexion teardrop fracture
d. Fracture of the posterior arch of the atlas
e. Traumatic spondylolisthesis

Ans. d. A fracture of the posterior arch of the atlas is considered a "stable" fracture. All the remaining fractures are considered "unstable."

Q56. Which one of the statements is *true* of Brown-Séquard syndrome?

a. Most common cause is penetrating injury to the spine
b. Patients have decreased strength in the upper compared with lower extremities
c. Quadriparesis is present
d. Saddle anesthesia is present
e. Vibration, position, and crude touch are preserved

Ans. a. The most common cause of Brown-Séquard syndrome or transverse spinal cord hemisection occurs in the setting of penetrating trauma.

Q57. Which of the following is not part of "the primary survey" in trauma patients?

a. Airway assessment
b. Breathing assessment
c. Circulation assessment
d. Digital rectal examination
e. Exposure

Ans. d. The goal of the primary survey is to identify immediate life threats and to stabilize them. The primary survey includes airway, breathing, circulation, disability (gross neurologic deficit), and exposure of the patient.

Q58. Which of the following may prevent secondary brain injury?

a. Hyperventilation to a PCO_2 of <20
b. Maintaining a PaO_2 of >60
c. Permissive hyperglycemia
d. Permissive hypotension
e. Wearing a motorcycle helmet

Ans. b. Secondary brain injury occurs as a result of metabolic and pressure insults to the brain.

Q59. Regarding risk of developing a wound infection, which one of the following factors is most predictive?

a. Smoking
b. Immunosuppressive medication use
c. Location of the wound
d. Collagen vascular disease
e. Diabetes mellitus

Ans. c. Wound characteristics, such as location, age, depth, and configuration are the most predictive factors for wound infections.

Q60. Which one of the following statements is *true* regarding the use of sterile technique for wound closure?

a. Basic cleanliness, including the use of nonsterile gloves, is appropriate for wound closure
b. Chlorhexidine can be used to clean skin margins, but iodine-containing solutions can prevent wound healing
c. Full sterile technique should be used for dirty wounds
d. Probing of the wound with a sterile, gloved, and finger is recommended for palpation of foreign bodies prior to wound closure
e. Skin disinfectants should be used to cleanse the wound and wound margins prior to closure

Ans. a. Full sterile technique is not necessary for wound closure in the ED. Nonsterile gloves, along with basic cleanliness, are appropriate and adequate.

Q61. Which one of the following statements regarding wound preparation for closure is correct?

a. All wounds should be irrigated with high-pressure irrigation
b. Debridement of wound margins is not recommended secondary to cosmetic concerns
c. Hair should never be removed
d. Wet-to-dry dressings are an appropriate method for debridement of a nonexudative wound
e. Wound soaking is not recommended as an adequate method for wound decontamination

Ans. e. In preparation for wound closure, all wounds should be visualized fully. Hair should be trimmed approximately 2 mm above the roots, if needed, to aid in visualizing the wound. Alternatively, hair can be used to help close the wound.

Q62. Regarding the use a tissue adhesive to close a forehead laceration, which one of the following statements best applies to the use of tissue adhesives?

a. Cyanoacrylate tissue adhesives have a lower rate of wound dehiscence as compared with other forms of primary closure
b. Octyl cyanoacrylate and butyl cyanoacrylate are similar in their water resistance and burst strength
c. The patient should be placed in Trendelenburg to avoid leakage of the adhesive into the eyes
d. Tissue adhesives are appropriate for use in high-tension wounds
e. Tissue adhesives should cover the entire wound and extend to 5–10 mm on either side of the wound edges

Ans. c. Tissue adhesives are a useful method of wound closure in the ED.

Q63. A 44-year-old man presents to the ED after a deep upper thigh laceration after dropping his chain saw. What is the appropriate way to close this wound?

a. Deep absorbable sutures
b. Horizontal mattress suture
c. Multilayered closure
d. Tissue adhesive
e. Running sutures

Ans. b. Deep absorbable sutures are not recommended for wounds with a high rate of contamination (such as chain saw injuries to the thigh). Horizontal mattress sutures or skin staples are ideal for wounds that have a high propensity for infection.

Q64. Which one of the following statements is true regarding the management of puncture wounds?

a. Debridement of a puncture wound should always be performed to better visualize the base
b. High-pressure irrigation will enable better visualization of the entrance site
c. Prophylactic antibiotics should always be prescribed in cases where the puncture wound involves the foot
d. *Pseudomonas* should be considered in puncture wounds involving sneakers or rubber soled shoes
e. *Staphylococcus aureus* is infrequently associated with infected puncture wounds

Ans. d. When treating a patient with a puncture wound, one of the most important questions to ask is what the patient was wearing at the time the puncture occurred.

Q65. Which of the following is the best recommendation provided to a patient with a large facial laceration closed with sutures?

a. A mandatory wound check should be done in 2 days
b. No washing or scrubbing of the face should occur for the first 72 hours
c. Prophylactic antibiotics are necessary
d. Sun exposure will help achieve the best cosmetic repair
e. Suture removal should occur in 3–5 days

Ans. e. Suture removal for facial lacerations should occur within 3–5 days in order to prevent scar formation from the sutures themselves (hatch marks and sinus tracts).

Q66. Which of the following is not a part of primary survey in case of traumatic injury?

a. Airway with cervical spine immobilization
b. CT scan brain
c. Exposure of patient
d. Circulation
e. Breathing and ventilation

Ans. b. According to ATLS guidelines, the primary survey consists of five important steps: (1) airway with restriction of cervical spine movement, (2) breathing and ventilation, (3) circulation and control of hemorrhage, (4) disability, and (5) exposure and control of environment.

Q67. What does disability involve in a primary assessment?

a. Fractures of limbs
b. Amputation of any part of body or limb
c. Wounds, such as abrasion, laceration, and avulsion
d. Glasgow Coma Scale (GCS) and neurological deficits to assess neurology
e. Inability to mobilize any part of body

Ans. d. Disability involves monitoring of the patient's neurological status by assessing GCS and pupil examination is very important to identify rapid deterioration in neurology. If the patient's GCS <8, then airway protection via an endotracheal tube is of utmost importance to prevent hypoxia and aspiration.

Q68. Which is the appropriate location for needle thoracocentesis in pediatric patient?

a. Fifth intercostal space midaxillary line
b. Second intercostal space midaxillary line
c. Second intercostal space midclavicular line
d. Fifth intercostal space midclavicular line
e. Fifth intercostal space anterior axillary line

Ans. c.

Q69. Which of the following is true for lethal triad of trauma?

a. Acidosis, coagulopathy, and hyperthermia
b. Alkalosis, coagulopathy, and hypothermia
c. Acidosis, hypothermia, and coagulopathy
d. Shock, hypothermia, and coagulopathy
e. Acidosis, hypothermia, and shock

Ans. c.

Q70. Which of the following physiological parameters do not require damage control resuscitation?

A. Temperature <35°C
b. Feeble pulse
c. Systolic blood pressure (SBP) <100 mm Hg
d. Pulse <100 beats/min
e. Cold extremities

Ans. d.

Environmental Emergencies MCQs

Devendra Richhariya

Q1. Hypothermia can occur in:

a. Anorexia nervosa

b. Diabetic ketoacidosis

c. Malnutrition

d. All of the above

Ans. d.

Q2. Clinical features of hypothermia are:

a. Amnesia, dysarthria, and impaired judgment

b. Tachycardia progressing to bradycardia, raised blood pressure (BP)

c. Increased muscle tone followed by fatiguing, anoxia

d. All of the above

Ans. d.

Q3. Hypothermia should be considered in a patient:

a. If there is history of exposure to cold

b. Is having burns

c. Having a cold trunk or a core temperature of <35°C

d. All of the above

Ans. d.

Q4. Regarding temperature measurement in a case of hypothermia all of the following are true, *except:*

a. Mercury or alcohol-containing thermometer cannot measure temperature below 35.6°C

b. Core temperature lags behind rectal and bladder temperature by up to 1 hour

c. Esophageal temperature is the most accurate and minimally invasive method of core temperature measurement

d. Epitympanic probes are not accurate in the field settings as they are designed to be used in operating theaters.

Ans. b. It is rectal and bladder temperature which lag behind core temperature changes by up to 1 hour. They can give the false impression that the patient is still cooling during rewarming. Until a patient is in a warm environment rectal or bladder temperature should not be performed as exposing a hypothermic patient causes further heat loss. The rectal probe should be inserted to a depth of 15 cm.

Q5. All of the following are True regarding rewarming in frostbite, *except:*

a. Rewarming is best achieved by warm bath emersion.
b. Dry heat is recommended because it is easy to regulate.
c. In the early stage, rewarming by exercise, rubbing, or friction is contraindicated.
d. Rapid rewarming at temperatures slightly above normal body temperature may significantly decrease tissue necrosis and reverse tissue crystallization.

Ans. c. Dry heat is not recommended because it is more difficult to regulate and increases the chances of accidental burns.

Q6. What are the risk factors for high-altitude illness? Mark the statement as True/False.

a. Coronary heart disease
b. Poor acclimatization
c. Altitude >4,000 m
d. Chronic pulmonary disease
e. Male

Ans. a. True, b. True, c. True, d. False, and e. False

Risk factors for developing high altitude disease are classified into two categories: (1) Individual (i.e., women, people younger than midadulthood, history of migraine, obesity, coronary heart disease, and permanent resident <900 m) and (2) altitude (i.e., poor acclimatization, rate of ascent, absolute change in altitude, and altitude >4,000 m). Early identification of these factors is crucial in identifying patients at risk.

Q7. What advice should be given to a patient to limit the risk of high-altitude illness?

a. Sleep well before the climb
b. Limiting hydration to limit the risk of cerebral edema
c. Avoid alcohol
d. Increase your physical activity before the climb
e. If headaches occur, stop the climb, and remain at the same altitude for acclimatization

Ans. a. True, b. False, c. True, d. False, and e. False

Prevention is one of the most important points: Avoid alcohol and sleeping medications. In case of mild acute mountain sickness (AMS), avoid further ascent until symptoms are resolved. Acclimatization for 1–2 days at the same altitude is recommended. Hydration by water and reducing activity levels could help the patient. In case of moderate or severe AMS, the patient must descend at a lower altitude.

Q8. Mark the statement as True/False.

a. Mild AMS is defined by a Lake Louise score of 6 or more.
b. The Lake Louise score is based on the evaluation of five symptoms.
c. In case of high-altitude pulmonary edema (HAPE), the electrocardiogram could is always pathologic
d. Acetazolamide remains the best choice for the prevention of AMS.
e. HAPE seems to be due to pulmonary vasoconstriction

Ans. a. False, b. True, c. False, d. True, and e. True

The Lake Louse score should be performed for diagnosis of acute high-altitude illnesses but also for monitoring patients. Based on five symptoms (i.e., headache, gastrointestinal symptoms, fatigue and/or weakness, dizziness/lightheadedness, and difficulty of sleeping), this score is simple to use. A score of five or less corresponds to mild AMS. In the case of HAPE, the electrogram could only report sinus tachycardia.

Q9. What is the first-line treatment in high-altitude pulmonary edema?

a. Acetazolamide
b. Oxygen
c. Dexamethasone
d. Budesonide
e. Nifedipine

Ans. b. First-line therapy for HAPE supplemental oxygen; if oxygen is not available descent, is primary therapy. Combined measures, e.g., oxygen and descent are more effective than drug therapy. Thus, oxygen should be part of the equipment when climbing at high altitudes.

Q10. What are common adverse events of acetazolamide?

a. Headache
b. Fatigue
c. Hypotension
d. Gastrointestinal bleeding
e. Nausea

Ans. a. True, b. True, c. False, d. False, and e. True

Acetazolamide remains the best choice for prevention of AMS, so knowing the side effects is important. Especially since acetazolamide can give symptoms close to high-altitude illness.

Q11. Arthropods consist of various morphologies. Which one below is False?

a. Adult insects have six legs and three body regions (head, thorax, and abdomen), and some insects have wings.
b. Adult spiders have eight legs and two body regions (cephalothorax and abdomen).
c. Adult mites and adult ticks have six legs and one body region but no true mouth (with mouthparts only).
d. Adult scorpions have eight legs with a broad, flat body region and a tail with a stinger.
e. Adult centipedes have a pair of legs in each body segment. The number of body segments is numerous, and the shape is usually flat.

Ans. c. Adult mites and adult ticks have eight legs and one body region but no true mouth (with mouthparts only). Recognition of different arthropods' various morphologies may help in making the right diagnosis.

Q12. Which of the following is true? Allergic reaction or hypersensitivity is usually classified as:

a. Type I [immunoglobulin E (IgE)-mediated], usually with delayed onset.
b. Type II (cytotoxic reaction), usually with delayed onset.
c. Type III (antibody-antigen complex), usually with delayed onset.
d. Type IV (T-lymphocytes and macrophages), usually with delayed onset.
e. Type IV (T-lymphocytes and macrophages), usually with acute onset.

Ans. d. Allergic reactions or hypersensitivity are usually classified as type I (IgE-mediated), type II (cytotoxic reaction), type III (antibody-antigen complex), or type IV (T-lymphocytes and macrophages). Types I, II, and III are usually immediate in onset whereas type IV usually has a delayed onset of a few hours to days. The venom, protein substances, and foreign bodies left behind by stings and bites can certainly cause an allergic reaction.

Q13. Which one of the following is True?

a. Sandflies may transmit Leishmaniasis
b. Earwigs may transmit *Trypanosoma cruzi*, which causes Chagas disease
c. Deer flies may transmit African trypanosomiasis (*Trypanosoma brucei*)
d. Beetles may transmit scrub typhus in Asia
e. Horse flies may transmit Lyme disease

Ans. a. Sandflies may transmit Leishmaniasis. Conenose bugs (in the Americas) may transmit *Trypanosoma cruzi*, which causes Chagas disease. Tsetse flies (tropical Africa) may transmit African trypanosomiasis (*Trypanosoma brucei*). Chigger mites may transmit scrub typhus in Asia. Ticks may transmit Lyme disease.

Q14. Mosquito bites may cause the following, *except:*

a. Malaria
b. Yellow fever
c. Dengue fever
d. Chikungunya fever
e. Tularemia

Ans. e. Deer flies and ticks may transmit tularemia. Mosquitoes are involved in the transmission of malaria, yellow fever (flavivirus), dengue fever, Rift Valley fever, Ross River virus disease, chikungunya fever, lymphatic filariasis (*Brugia malayi*), Eastern equine encephalomyelitis, Western equine encephalitis, Venezuelan equine encephalitis, Japanese encephalitis, St Louis encephalitis, West Nile encephalitis (West Nile virus), and La Crosse encephalitis.

Q15. The following are true in terms of treatment after exposure to arthropods, *except:*

a. Local wound care
b. The victim's tetanus status is irrelevant
c. A local or oral antihistamine is usually enough to treat a mild reaction
d. IV antihistamine (e.g., diphenhydramine 1 mg/kg) and IV steroid may be necessary for moderate reaction
e. Adrenaline, subcutaneous (SC), intramuscular (IM), or intravenous (IV) is necessary to treat a severe, life-threatening reaction.

Ans. b. Because bites or stings may carry soil, the patient's tetanus status should be checked.

Q16. Mark True or False regarding: Exposure (whether causing disease or not) to arthropods can be experienced via.

a. Bites
b. Stings
c. Local irritation, causing local infection, systemic hypersensitivity, anemia, etc.
d. Ingestion

Ans. **a. True, b. True, c. True, and d. True**

Exposure to arthropods may occur in many ways other than bites and stings. Some diseases result from crushing a louse.

Q17. After exposure to arthropods, which of the following local effects may occur? Mark the below statement as True/False.

a. *Blockage of orifices and skin attachment:* Small arthropods may enter and block any body orifices. Sometimes, arthropod body parts remain lodged. A tick may stick strongly to the skin.
b. *Local wounds:* Bites, stings, and even scratching by arthropod feet might result in local wounds. The wounds are usually small. Some wounds may carry foreign bodies.
c. Bees leave their stingers behind.
d. Cellulitis, necrosis (and sepsis may follow).

Ans. **a. True, b. True, c. True, and d. True**

After exposure to arthropods, the local effect ranges from nothing to cellulitis and necrosis. If the effect is untreated, sepsis may occur.

Q18. After exposure to an arthropod, which of the following systemic effects may happen? Mark the below statement as True/False.

a. Anaphylaxis
b. Fever
c. Anemia
d. Alternation in consciousness

Ans. **a. True, b. True, c. True, and d. True**

Allergic reactions or hypersensitivity, fever, sepsis, anemia, weight loss, alternation in consciousness, coma, and even death may result from contact alone or the diseases or venom transmitted. Never underestimate exposure to arthropods.

Q19. Which of the following is true in terms of preventing arthropod-related diseases?

a. Malaria (drug) prophylaxes are always 100%.
b. Proper food storage and preparation .
c. Proper use of repellents such as DEET (N,N-diethyl-meta-toluamide) or the use of insecticides in the garden.
d. Do not handle any sick or dead animal, even pets, and unprotected. Always wear gloves, etc.

Ans. **a. False, b. True, c. True, and d. True**

The efficacy of malaria prophylaxes is high but never 100%. You must supplement them with other preventive measures.

Q20. After exposure to an arthropod, which of the following is True?

a. You should immediately crush the arthropod.
b. The usual wound care must be conducted. Check for foreign bodies. Look for unusual swelling, necrosis, or signs of infection.
c. *Blockage of orifice:* If an arthropod block an orifice, you must remove it carefully. You must plan the removal of embedded

arthropods, such as maggots, carefully. Breakage of maggots may lead to hypersensitivity.

d. You must remove the remaining sting carefully so as not to squeeze the remaining toxins and chemicals into the skin.

Ans. **a. False, b. True, c. True, and d. True**

You can transmit epidemic typhus (*Rickettsia prowazekii*), trench fever (*Bartonella quintana*), and louse-born relapsing fever (*Borrelia recurrentis*) by crushing the lice and their feces on the skin. Crushing also prevents the identification of arthropods.

Q21. Which of the following statements is false regarding the pathophysiology of electric burns?

a. According to Ohm's law, electric current is directly proportional to the voltage of the source.

b. Least resistance is seen in fat, tendon, and bone.

c. Electrical energy passes through highly resistant skin and disperses through tissues with lesser resistance.

d. Burns may appear mild on the surface however may have deranged underlying tissues.

Ans. b. The highest resistance is seen in fat, tendon, and bone followed by skin.

Q22. Regarding the mechanism of electrical injuries, a state which of the following is True or False?

a. Indirect mechanism involves severe muscle contraction

b. Primarily affected areas will be those areas away from the source point on the ground.

c. Direct mechanism involves the primary impact on various body tissues.

d. Electric current dissipates as thermal energy causing further burns in other vital tissues.

Ans. **a. True, b. False, c. True, and d. True**

Primarily affected areas will be those in contact with the source point with the ground.

Q23. Which of the following statements is false regarding clinical symptoms of electrical injuries?

a. Ventricular fibrillation and asystole are uncommon.

b. Pneumonitis, pulmonary effusion, hypoxia due to direct central nervous system (CNS) dysfunction, and fluid shift are a few of the major respiratory complications.

c. Necrosis and thermal burns of the myocardium may cause infarction, pericardial injury, and heart failure.
d. Excessive myoglobin release will lead to myoglobinuria.

Ans. a. Ventricular fibrillation and cardiac standstill [pulseless electrical activity (PEA)/asystole] are the most fatal and dreaded complications in early management.

Q24. Which of the following statements is true or false with respect to taser injuries?

a. Taser devices may produce an initial shock of 50,000 V followed by multiple subsequent shocks.
b. Fractures of long bones are rare.
c. Chest pain along with shortness of breath is indicative of an increase in sympathetic tone.
d. Pneumothorax is a clinical finding in taser injuries.

Ans. **a. True, b. False, c. False, and d. True**

Q25. Which statement is True or False regarding lightning injuries?

a. Side flash includes a direct strike of lightning to a person and a resultant discharge to a second person in close proximity.
b. Flashover phenomena include the lightning striking the ground then entering the body from one foot and exiting from the other.
c. Lichtenberg figures are permanent and deep, healing is prolonged.
d. Vasospasm may mimic stroke, myocardial infarction, and bowel ischemia or cause signs of compartment syndrome.

Ans. **a. True, b. False, c. False, and d. True**

Flashover phenomena include lightning current moving along the body and resulting in a blast effect on the clothing. Lichtenberg figures are a fine branching rash that resembles branches of trees and are temporary and superficial and fade within weeks.

Q26. Write True or False.

a. Snakes have excellent visual acuity.
b. Snakes have an excellent auditory system capable of picking low-pitched sounds.
c. All snakes are venomous and capable of causing toxicity in humans.
d. Snakes can have either a rounded or an elliptical pupil.

Ans. **a. False, b. False, c. False, and d. True**

Q27. The "pit" in pit viper species.

a. Is capable of receiving sound waves and creating an image of a prey through ultrasound.
b. Is a heat-sensitive device capable of forming a thermal image of the prey.
c. Is used by pit viper species to store venom.
d. Is highly sensitive to vibration and helps detect prey.

Ans. **a. False, b. True, c. False, and d. False**

Q28. With regards to sea snakes write True or False.

a. All sea snake species are venomous
b. Sea snake bites are very common in India
c. The available polyvalent antisnake venom (ASV) is very effective against all sea snake species.
d. All sea-snakes have a modified paddle-like tail which helps them to swim.

Ans. **a. True, b. False, c. False, and d. True**

Q29. Venom is predominantly

a. Protein rich
b. Glycoprotein rich
c. Carbohydrate rich
d. Lipid rich

Ans. a.

Q30. Write True or False.

a. Cobra venom causes a predominant postsynaptic neuromuscular paralysis
b. Krait venom is predominantly presynaptic in action
c. Symptoms of neuroparalysis in krait bite victims show excellent resolution with an injection of a cocktail of atropine and neostigmine.
d. Krait envenomation results in significant local inflammation at the bite site.

Ans. **a. True, b. True, c. False, and d. False**

Q31. Write True or False. Enzymes present in snake venom include:

a. Hexokinase
b. Phospholipase
c. Hyaluronidase
d. Lectin

Ans. **a. False, b. True, c. True, and d. False**

Q32. All of these could occur in a Russel's viper bite, *except:*

a. Ptosis
b. Respiratory paralysis
c. Gum bleeding
d. Acute kidney injury

Ans. b.

Q33. All of the following could be attributed to cobra bite, *except:*

a. Descending paralysis
b. Significant local inflammation at the bite site
c. Albuminuria
d. Cardiac involvement

Ans. c.

Q34. Sea anemones and soft corals envenomation present as:

a. Painful lesion with central pallor and petechial hemorrhage
b. Halo of erythema with muscular tetani is evident
c. Weakness with urethritis
d. Necrosis with bristles to break off into the skin and urticarial rash

Ans. a.

Q35. Select incorrect with respect to antivenom and anaphylaxis.

a. Most reactions and side-effects occur within 15–30 minutes and nearly last 6 hours.
b. A recipient of antivenom should be pretreated with 50–100 mg of IV diphenhydramine in children.
c. Antivenom should be administered in one vial over 5 minutes.
d. If anaphylaxis develops, after antivenom injection, aliquots of antivenom should be alternated with epinephrine.

Ans. b.

Q36. Amongst the listed contents which is not present in the stingray's venom gland's secretion?

a. Serotonin as vasoconstrictor
b. 5'-nucleotidase
c. Conotoxins targeting receptors and channels
d. Phosphodiesterase

Ans. c.

Q37. Select the most rational option among the following:

a. The "Irukandji syndrome" is local vasoconstriction attributed to the parasympathetic nervous system.
b. A lidocaine-containing product is an effective contaminant along with 5% acetic acid in jellyfish sting pain.
c. Occasional residual hyperpigmentation may be caused due to stinging of the tentacle of a Portuguese man of war (*Physalia physalis*)
d. Erythema multiforme or dyshidrotic eczema develops as an immediate systemic complication due to the manifestation of crinotoxins by sponges

Ans. c.

Q38. Select the erroneous statement.

a. Conotoxins are injected through the parrot-like beak that causes paralysis
b. Edrophonium can be given for paralysis with atropine
c. Severe envenomation-induced paralysis lasts for 12–36 hours and takes weeks for symptom resolution
d. Treatment of blue-ringed octopus bite centers on neural and renal support

Ans. d.

Q39. All of the following are marine animals, *except:*

a. Box jellyfish
b. Cobra
c. Sea snake
d. Stone fish

Ans. b.

Q40. Which immunization is the key for the treatment of all marine animals?

a. Tetanus
b. Bacille Calmette-Guérin (BCG)
c. Vitamin A
d. Diphtheria, tetanus, and pertussis (DPT)

Ans. a.

Q41. Clinical features of Irukandji jellyfish are all, *except:*

a. Muscle pain
b. Hypertension
c. Heart failure
d. Dyspnea

Ans. d.

Q42. Hot water is applied for how much time in the treatment of sea urchins?

a. 10–20 minutes
b. 30–90 minutes
c. 20–30 minutes
d. 90–120 minutes

Ans. b.

Q43. Sponges have spicules of:

a. Sodium bicarbonate
b. $Ca(OH)_2$
c. Sodium carbonate
d. Calcium carbonate

Ans. d.

Q44. Regarding considerations prior to travel, which of the following statements are True or False?

a. Since the stay is for longer periods, travelers are more likely to experience gastrointestinal symptoms in countries with poor sanitation and overpopulation.

b. Pretravel counseling is not essential for every trip one takes and does not prevent diseases.

c. It is ideal to undergo a medical evaluation 6 weeks prior to traveling especially if the traveler is in an immunocompromised state.

d. Individual risk assessment of travel must include the duration of stay, country of destination, medical condition, and any history of travel in the last 6 months.

Ans. **a. True, b. False, c. True, and d. True**

Pretravel counseling is advice for all travelers to countries with poor hygienic conditions. Studies have shown a link between those travelers who avoided pretravel consultation and then contracted diseases, such as malaria and dengue.

Q45. Which of the following is false regarding acute altitude sickness?

a. It is present in individuals ascending above 2,500 m and 25% of travelers that ascend rapidly.

b. In cases of high risk, prophylaxis treatment with tablet acetazolamide 4 days prior to ascending.

c. Acute altitude illness comprises of acute altitude sickness, high-altitude cerebral edema, and high-altitude pulmonary edema.

d. In adults with sulfa allergies, prophylactic treatment with tablet dexamethasone can be started 24 hours prior to ascending.

Ans. b. In cases of high risk, prophylaxis treatment with tablet acetazolamide 2 days prior to ascending.

Q46. With regard to travel to malaria-endemic areas, which statement is true or false?

a. Permethrin-treated clothing should not be worn during dawn, dusk, or daytime.

b. Local application of DEET and picaridin in 20% overexposed areas can help in the prevention of mosquito bites.

c. Wearing long-sleeved shirts, jackets or coats is helpful.

d. Avert areas of water pooling or stagnant water bodies collection and vegetation around accommodation.

Ans. **a. False, b. True, c. True, and d. True**

Permethrin-treated clothing should be worn during dawn, dusk, or daytime.

Q47. Which of the following statements is True or False regarding the prevention and treatment of gastrointestinal infections?

a. Encourage oral fluids or unsweetened juices to replenish the loss of water in mild dehydration.
b. Oral rehydration solution (ORS) is prepared at home by mixing one teaspoon of salt and one teaspoon of sugar in 1 L of bottled juice.
c. In Southeast Asian countries, the use of ciprofloxacin is advised for the treatment of severe diarrhea.
d. Avert eating at restaurants with poor hygiene and sanitation.

Ans. a. True, b. False, c. False, and d. True

The oral rehydration solution is prepared at home by mixing half a teaspoon of salt and half a teaspoon of sugar in 1 L of bottled water for moderate hydration. In Southeast Asian countries, azithromycin is preferred due to fluroquinolone resistant enteropathogens.

Q48. Regarding sea sickness, which of the following statements is False?

a. Always engage in water sports activities under the supervision of a certified and licensed guide or company.
b. Exposure to brackish and salt water is encouraged.
c. For high-risk travelers, prevention of infections of schistosomiasis and leptospirosis through early prophylaxis treatment with tablet doxycycline is advisable once a week.
d. Sound knowledge of marine sea life and venomous stings is essential.

Ans. b. Exposure to brackish water and salt water should be avoided. Proper and timely cleaning of wounds with antiseptic solution and clean dressing is recommended.

Q49. Which of the following conditions is most likely to be observed in an alcoholic man found in an alley in January with a core temperature of 31°C?

a. Delta wave on the electrocardiogram (ECG)
b. Coma
c. Hypercoagulability
d. Respiratory distress
e. Volume overload

Ans. b. Hypothermia causes multiple metabolic changes. As temperature decreases, the victim becomes initially uncoordinated, progressively confused, and finally comatose.

Q50. Which of the following is *not* a complication of high-voltage electric injury?

a. Blunt trauma from being hurled from the source
b. Cardiac or respiratory arrest
c. Compartment syndrome
d. Fern patterns burn
e. Tetanic contractions

Ans. d. High-voltage direct current (DC) electricity can throw the victim from the electrical source causing blunt traumatic injuries. High-voltage alternating current (AC) injury can result in tetanic contractions where the victim cannot let go of the source of injury. High-voltage injury is associated with deep tissue destruction and may cause compartment syndrome. Any type of electrical injury may cause cardiac or respiratory arrest. Fern pattern burns, also known as Lichtenberg figures, are seen with lightning injuries. These are not true burns and resolve quickly.

Index

A

B

C

D

E

F

G

H

I

M

N

O

P

Q

R

T

U

V

W

Y

Z